Internet Resources for Nurses, 2nd Edition

Joyce J. Fitzpatrick, PhD, MBA, RN, FAAN, is a Professor of Nursing, Frances Payne Bolton School of Nursing at Case Western Reserve University in Cleveland, Ohio, where she was Dean from 1982 through 1997. She earned her BSN at Georgetown University, her MS in Psychiatric-Mental Health Nursing at The Ohio State University, her PhD in Nursing at New York University, and an MBA from Case Western Reserve University in 1992. She was elected a Fellow in the American Academy of Nursing in 1981 and received the *American Journal of Nursing* Book-of-the-Year Award 17 times. Dr. Fitzpatrick is widely published in nursing and health care, having over 250 publications. She is coeditor of the *Annual Review of Nursing Research* series, now in its 20th volume, and editor of the journals *Applied Nursing Research* and the National League for Nursing's *Nursing Education Perspectives*. From 1997 to 1999, Dr. Fitzpatrick was the President of the American Academy of Nursing.

Kristen S. Montgomery, PhD, RN, is a Postdoctoral Research Fellow at the University of Michigan School of Nursing. She received her PhD in nursing from the Frances Payne Bolton School of Nursing, Case Western Reserve University, Cleveland, Ohio. She earned her MSN from The University of Pennsylvania, in Philadelphia, Pennsylvania, and her BSN from Oakland University in Rochester, Michigan. She is Co-Editor of the *Maternal Child Health Nursing Research Digest*, which received the *American Journal of Nursing* Book of the Year Award, as did the first edition of this book.

Internet Resources for Nurses, 2nd Edition

Joyce J. Fitzpatrick, PhD, RN, FAAN
Kristen S. Montgomery, PhD, RN
Editors

 Springer Publishing Company

Springer Publishing Company, Inc.
536 Broadway
New York, NY 10012-3955

Acquisitions Editor: Ruth Chasek
Production Editor: Pamela Lankas
Cover design by Joanne Honigman

03 04 05 06 07/5 4 3 2 1

Library of Congress Cataloging-in-Publication Data

Internet resources for nurses / Joyce J. Fitzpatrick, Kristen S. Montgomery, editors.—2nd ed.
    p. ; cm.
   Includes bibliographical references and index.
   ISBN 0-8261-1785-6
    1. Nursing—Computer network resources. 2. Internet.
  3. Nursing informatics. 4. Medical care—Computer
network resources. I. Fitzpatrick, Joyce J., 1944-
II. Montgomery, Kristen S.
   [DNLM: 1. Internet—Resources Guides. 2. Medical
Informatics—Resource Guide. 3. Nursing—Resource Guides.
WY 26.5 I617 2002]
RT50.5 I57 2003
025.6'61073—dc21   2002030922
                                          CIP

Printed in the United States by Capital City.

Contents

Part I.   Professional Topics

Part III. Evaluation Information

Contributors

Mary K. Bailey, APN/CNP, ND(c)
Assistant Professor
Mennonite College of Nursing
Illinois State University
Normal, IL

Jane H. Barnsteiner, PhD, RN, FAAN
Professor of Pediatric Nursing
School of Nursing
University of Pennsylvania and
Director of Nursing Practice and
  Research
The Children's Hospital of
  Philadelphia
Philadelphia, PA

Suzanne Hetzel Campbell, PhD, APRN, WHNP
Assistant Professor
School of Nursing
Fairfield University
Fairfield, CT and Nurse
  Practitioner
Breastfeeding Resources
Stratford, CT

Stephen J. Cavanagh, PhD, RN
Associate Dean for Academic
  and Clinical Affairs
College of Nursing
Wayne State University
Detroit, MI

Joseph P. Colagreco, MS, RN, ANP-C
Clinical Assistant Professor
Division of Nursing
New York University
New York, NY

David A. Conner, BSN, RN
Graduate Student
Division of Nursing
New York University
New York, NY

Christine R. Curran, PhD, RN, CNA
Assistant Professor
Director, Informatics Program
and Director, Research
  Resources
School of Nursing
Columbia University
New York, NY

Emily E. Drake, MSN, RN
Instructor
School of Nursing
University of Virginia
Charlottesville, VA

Paulette Espina-Gabriel, MA, EdD(c), RN, C
Nurse Manager, Telemetry
  Monitoring Center
Columbia Presbyterian Medical
  Center
New York, NY

Lucinda Farina, MSN, CNM
PhD Student
Frances Payne Bolton School of
  Nursing
Case Western Reserve
  University
Cleveland, OH

Sarah Farrell, PhD, RN, CS
Associate Professor
School of Nursing
University of Virginia
Charlottesville, VA

Maria Donovan Fitzpatrick, BA
PhD Student
Department of Economics
University of Virginia
Charlottesville, VA

Joan Fleitas, EdD, RN
Associate Professor
School of Nursing
Fairfield University
Fairfield, CT

Shelia C. Grossman, PhD, APRN
Professor
School of Nursing
Fairfield University
Fairfield, CT

Kristen A. Guadalupe, MSN, RN, CS
Nurse Manager
Louis Stokes Cleveland VA
  Medical Center
Cleveland, OH

Patricia G. Hinegardner, MLS, AHIP
Coordinator of Special Services
Health Sciences and Human
  Services Library
University of Maryland
Baltimore, MD

Bette K. Idemoto, MSN, RN, CCRN, CS
Clinical Nurse Specialist
University Hospitals of Cleveland
Cleveland, OH

Gail L. Ingersoll, EdD, RN, FAAN, FNAP
Director of Clinical Nursing
  Research
Strong Memorial Hospital and
Professor of Nursing
School of Nursing
University of Rochester
Rochester, NY

Deborah M. Joers, MPA, BSN, RN, CNA
Nursing Informatics Coordinator
The Children's Hospital of
  Philadelphia
Philadelphia, PA

Trudy Johnson, MA, RN, CNAA
Director, Performance
  Improvement Services
New York Presbyterian Hospital
New York, NY

Françoise Juste, MA, BSN, RNC
Logician Clinical Implementation
  Specialist
Mount Sinai-NYU Health
New York, NY

Carl A. Kirton, MA, RN, ACRN, ANP-C
Nurse Practitioner and Nurse
  Manager
AIDS Center
Mount Sinai Hospital Medical
  Center
New York, NY

Jean W. Lange, PhD, RN
Assistant Professor
School of Nursing
Fairfield University
Fairfield, CT

Felissa R. Lashley, PhD, RN, ACRN, FACMG, FAAN
Dean and Professor
College of Nursing
Rutgers, The State University of
  New Jersey
Newark, NJ

Jenifer Lasman, MSN, RN, FNP
Doctoral Student
Frances Payne Bolton School of
  Nursing
Case Western Reserve
  University
Cleveland, OH

Doris Troth Lippman, EdD, APRN, CS
Associate Professor
School of Nursing
Fairfield University
Fairfield, CT

Erin V. Messett, MSN, C-FNP/ GNP, CCM
Director, Nurse Practitioner Case
  Management
Memorial HealthCare IPA
Signal Hill, CA

Georgia L. Narsavage, PhD, RN
Associate Professor
Frances Payne Bolton School of
  Nursing
Case Western Reserve
  University
Cleveland, OH

Jeanne M. Novotny, PhD, RN, FAAN
Dean and Professor
School of Nursing
Fairfield University
Fairfield, CT

Jennifer Okonsky, MA, APRN, BC
Clinical Instructor
Frances Payne Bolton School of Nursing
Case Western Reserve University
Cleveland, OH

Eileen R. O'Shea, MSN, RN
Adjunct Faculty
School of Nursing
Fairfield University
Fairfield, CT

Joan T. Panke, MA, RN, APRN
Executive Director
DC Partnership to Improve End-of-Life Care
A Robert Wood Johnson Community–State Partnership
Washington, DC

Kathleen Perfetto, BSN, RN
RN Care Coordinator
Saint Mary's Hospital
Waterbury, CT

Cynthia R. Phyillaier, MSLS
Information Specialist and Liaison to School of Nursing
Health Sciences and Human Services Library
University of Maryland
Baltimore, MD

Barbara K. Redman, PhD, RN, FAAN
Dean and Professor
College of Nursing
Wayne State University
Detroit, MI

Carol A. Romano, PhD, RN, C, CNAA, FAAN
Chief, Clinical Informatics Services for Nursing, NIH Clinical Center
National Institutes of Health
Bethesda, MD

Laree J. Schoolmeesters, MSN, RN
Nurse Educator
School of Nursing
Mercy Hospital
Pittsburgh, PA

Patricia W. Stone, PhD, RN, C
Assistant Professor
Director of Advanced Clinical Management
School of Nursing
Columbia University
New York, NY

Hussein Tahan, DNS(c), RN, CNA
Director of Cardiovascular Nursing
New York Presbyterian Hospital
New York, NY

Tener Goodwin Veenema, PhD, MPH, CPNP
Assistant Professor
Center for High Risk Children and Youth
School of Nursing
University of Rochester and Department of Emergency Medicine
School of Medicine and Dentistry
University of Rochester
Rochester, NY

Antonia M. Villarruel, PhD, RN, FAAN
Associate Professor and
Director, Center for Health
Promotion
School of Nursing
University of Michigan
Ann Arbor, MI

Patricia Hinton Walker, PhD, RN, FAAN
Dean and Professor
Graduate School of Nursing
Uniformed Services University of
the Health Sciences
Bethesda, MD

Meredith Wallace, PhD, RN, CS-ANP
Assistant Professor
School of Nursing
Fairfield University
Fairfield, CT

Dara B. Walls, MSN, RN
Nurse Practitioner
New York, NY

Patricia A. Wilke, MSN, RN
Clinical Instructor
College of Nursing
Kent State University
Kent, OH

Introduction

Joyce J. Fitzpatrick, PhD, RN, FAAN

This second edition of *Internet Resources for Nurses* is expanded in scope and depth; it includes more content headings and additional features. Since the publication of the first edition in 2000, there has been a substantial increase in the information available to nurses through the Internet. We can expect that this trend will continue and that the number, depth, and scope of health care Web sites will increase dramatically as health care organizations more fully embrace the information resources available. This book is designed as a quick resource and reference guide for professional nurses who are developing familiarity with the Internet and the many Internet resources that are available to them to improve their practice.

The specific content areas chosen for inclusion were those judged most useful for professional nurses. Authors familiar with the Internet were selected to write brief descriptions and evaluations of key Web sites in areas of their expertise. Each author was asked to select the top six to ten Web sites in the particular area, to list these alphabetically within the category, and to provide a brief description and evaluation of each site. The guidelines for site review were consistent across the chapters.

This book is not meant to be exhaustive of all of the sites available to nurses and other health professionals. Rather, the sites selected for inclusion are representative of the best resources available today. It is recognized that several hundred new health care and nursing sites appear daily, and that this number will continue to increase. In today's changing and chaotic health care environment nurses often do not have enough time to locate the Internet resources that would be most helpful to them. This book is a handy guide for the busy professional. Each site is introduced by the use of the Uniform Resource Locator (URL), or Web address, which makes it possible for the reader to easily locate the site on the Internet.

Content is organized according to the general categories of clinical web sites and professional web sites. An initial chapter provides brief guidelines for browsing the Internet. For those wanting more detail, the last chapter describes Web sites that give evaluation guidelines. A chapter is included which provides helpful information to the nurse who wishes to evaluate health care information on the Internet. Additional new features for the second edition include Web site reviews focused on career development and other professional functions such as outcomes management and evaluation, nursing administration, and evidence-based practice. Since many professional organizations now provide information for consumers as well as professionals, we have marked those Web sites that are also suitable for patient's use with an asterisk.

Access to the Internet will increase for clinicians everywhere. While today the Internet is often viewed as a supplement to usual health care practice, we envision a time when the Internet will be at the clinician's fingertips, to be accessed whenever a question, concern, problem, or curiosity arises. For many, this book will serve as the introduction to the journey. For others it will serve as a resource guide. For all, it is meant to enhance professional nursing practice by providing more information in a usable, friendly manner.

Guidelines for Browsing the Internet

*Carol A. Romano, Patricia G. Hinegardner, and
Cynthia R. Phyillaier*

The Internet offers a vast amount of information via the World Wide Web and is an exciting and attractive communication medium for health care providers and consumers alike. The Internet benefits health professionals because it is a source of clinical research findings and guidelines, an information exchange medium among colleagues, and a communication forum with patients and families. The Internet benefits consumers because it contributes to their sense of control about health care conditions. They can take an active role in locating information about prevention, diagnosis, and treatment of illness. The Internet also increases consumers' abilities to participate in health care decisions, to improve self-help skills, and to reduce the financial burden of care (Jadad & Gagliardi, 1998; Widman & Tong, 1997).

NEED FOR EVALUATION CRITERIA

Several recent journal articles on the accuracy of Web sites have indicated a need for evaluation criteria (Beredjiklian, Bozentka, Steinberg, & Bernstein, 2001; Pandolfini, Impicciatore, & Bonati, 2000; Li, Irvin, Guzman, & Bombardier, 2001). A 1999 study that systematically examined the content of 400 Web sites for a specific type of cancer (Biermann, Golladay, Greenfield, & Baker, 1999) previously reached the same conclusion. Results noted erroneous information in 6% of the sites and misleading information in many others when compared with information presented in a preeminent oncology textbook. Schloman (1999) also noted that studies of Web sites for management of childhood fevers and diarrhea identified sites with significant misinformation, potentially harmful instruction, and contradictions with established treatment guidelines. Health care consumers and providers need a healthy skepticism and criteria to evaluate Internet sites to protect against fraudulent claims, inaccurate information and potential harm. To identify quality consumer health resources on the Internet requires establishment of evaluation criteria to judge the quality of the site.

EVALUATING WEB SITES

In order to identify evaluation criteria, we searched the professional literature and reviewed key nursing and medical library science Web sites. Literature searches were performed in two of the authoritative databases used by nurses, MEDLINE and CINAHL. An article from ONLINE (Hawkins, 1999) was also consulted. In addition to the literature searches, two major Web sites for nursing and medical library science were searched—the American Nurses Association (ANA) Web site, and the National Library of Medicine (NLM) Web site. These organizations represent two of the major disciplines, nursing and medical library science, involved with the critical review of consumer health information.

A comparison of selection criteria yielded five common criteria: authority/source, purpose/objectivity, content, currency, and design (derived from Hawkins, 1999; Kim, Eng, Deering, & Maxfield, 1999; Schloman, 1999; U.S. National Library of Medicine, 1999). These are described in the text that follows.

- Authority/Source: The author or organization should be identified. If it is a person, then what are his/her credentials or experience with the subject? If it is an organization, is it reputable? Is there a way to contact the authors or sponsors of the site?
- Purpose/Objectivity: Is the purpose of the site clearly stated (educational, commercial, etc.)? Who is the intended audience? If there is sponsorship, is it fully disclosed?
- Content: Is the information accurate, useful, and relevant to the needs of the audience? Is the scope appropriate? Are selection

criteria included? Are there relevant and authoritative links? Is factual information verifiable? Are spelling and grammar accurate?

- Currency: Is the production date of posted information clearly indicated? Are revision dates included? Are links up to date?
- Design: Is it well organized and easy to navigate? Are graphics meaningfully used or do they clutter the screen? Is the site stable?

We hope you will find these evaluation criteria useful as you begin your search on the Internet. More detail on evaluation is given in the final chapter of this book.

REFERENCES

Beredjiklian, P. K., Bozentka, D. J., Steinberg, D. R., & Bernstein, J. (2001). Evaluating the source and content of orthopaedic information on the Internet. The case of carpal tunnel syndrome. *Journal of Bone & Joint Surgery, 83A,* 951–952.

Biermann, J., Golladay, G., Greenfield, M. L., & Baker, L. (1999). Evaluation of cancer information on the Internet. *Cancer, 86,* 381–390.

Hawkins, D. T. (1999). What is credible information? *ONLINE, 23*(5), 86–89.

Jadad, A., & Gagliardi, A. (1998). Rating health information on the Internet: Navigating to knowledge or to Babel? *Journal of the American Medical Association, 279,* 611–614.

Kim, P., Eng, T. R., Deering, M. J., & Maxfield, A. (1999). Published criteria for evaluating health related Web sites. *British Medical Journal, 318,* 647–649.

Li, L., Irvin, E., Guzman, J., & Bombardier, C. (2001). Surfing for back pain patients: The nature and quality of back pain information on the Internet. *Spine, 26,* 547–557.

Pandolfini, C., Impicciatore, P., & Bonati, M. (2000). Parents on the web: Risks for quality management of cough in children. *Pediatrics, 105*(1), e1.

Schloman, B. F. (1999). Whom do you trust? Evaluating Internet health resources. *Online Journal of Issues in Nursing.* Accessed October 13, 1999. Available: *http://www.nursingworld.org/ojin/infocol/info_1.htm.*

U.S. National Library of Medicine. *MEDLINEplus Selection Guidelines.* Accessed October 11, 1999. Available: *http://www.nlm.nih.gov/medlineplus/criteria.html.*

Widman, L., & Tong, D. (1997). Requests for medical advice from patients and families to health care providers who publish on the World Wide Web. *Archives of Internal Medicine, 157,* 209–212.

_____ Part **I**

Professional Topics

Chapter 1

Professional Nursing Organizations

Bette K. Idemoto

P rofessional nursing organizations serve as a framework for professional relationships, networking, and organization of members with similar goals and interests. Professional organizations generally provide their members with various services, information resources, and opportunities. Many also have an annual conference or meeting. Professional organizations vary in scope and function. For example, many professional nursing organizations exist which cater to all nurses. Other professional nursing organizations are specific to a certain type of specialty practice, such as AIDS care or geriatric nursing. Still other professional nursing organizations are organized according to nursing role or job function, for example, nurse practitioner organizations. Other professional organizations may include all health care providers, such as the American Red Cross, or a variety of disciplines, like The Society for Research on Adolescence. The Web sites listed below are some of the best professional nursing organization resources.

GENERAL PROFESSIONAL NURSING ORGANIZATIONS (ALL NURSES)

1. American Nurses Association

http://www.nursingworld.org

The official Web site of the American Nurses Association, a full-service professional organization representing the nation's 2.6 million Registered Nurses through the federation of 54 Constituent Member Associations (CMAs), this organization provides an influential and effective network of registered nurses who support nursing with over 180,000 memberships. The purpose of the site is to provide statements of the mission, vision, and values of the organization; national, state, and local nursing and health information exchange through government affairs; The Nursing code of ethics; access to affiliate organizations; a bookstore; liability insurance; and access to issues of significance to nurses including: ethics and human rights, workplace advocacy, and certification. The Web site is designed to be useful to all nurses. Information is current and updated daily. The most important features of this site include membership information, certification information, conferences and meetings, online CE, standards of nursing practice, and government affairs/lobbying the Congress and regulatory agencies on health care issues. Information is presented in English at an average level. The site is attractive and easy to use.

2. Sigma Theta Tau International

http://www.nursingsociety.org

This is the official Web site of Sigma Theta Tau International, The Honor Society of Nursing. The society was founded in 1922 and is dedicated to support and connect the global community of nursing scholars who enhance health care worldwide. The membership of STTI is more than 300,000 with more than 90 countries represented. The purpose of the site is to provide information on the organization and its services. The site is intended for all nurses. Information is current and updated on a weekly basis. The most important features of the site are the directory of nurse experts, *The Online Journal of Knowledge Synthesis for Nursing,* The STTI International Virginia Henderson Library, research data sets, *The Journal of Nursing Scholarship,* and online continuing education. Information is presented in English at an average level. The site is attractive and easy to use.

SPECIALTY ORGANIZATIONS FOR PROFESSIONAL NURSES

3. American Academy of Nurse Practitioners

http://www.aanp.org/

This is the official Web site of the American Academy of Nurse Practitioners (AANP), an organization formed in 1985 to promote the high standards of health care delivered by nurse practitioners and to act as a forum to enhance the identity and continuity of all nurse practitioner specialties. The AANP currently has over 60,000 nurse practitioner members. Highlights of the site include practice and legislative information, resources for nurse practitioners, and care standards. The site is intended for all nurse practitioners. Information is current and updated weekly to bi-weekly. Information is also provided on certification, scholarship, legislative activities, conferences, and position statements. The text is available in English at an average level. The site is attractive and easy to use.

4. American Association of Critical Care Nurses

http://www.aacn.org/

This is the official Web site of the AACN which was founded in 1969. The association is designed to help educate nurses working in newly developed intensive care units. AACN is the world's largest specialty nursing organization with more than 65,000 members representing the United States and 45 countries. The purpose of the site is to provide members with the knowledge and resources necessary to provide optimal care to critically ill patients through career development, education, publications, research, scholarships and grants, and local chapters. Critical care nurses are the intended audience. Information is current and up-to-date. The most important features include information on the National Teaching Institute (NTI), certification, clinical practice, careers, and online journal abstracts for the *American Journal of Critical Care,* and *Critical Care Nurse* with selected online CE. Information is available in English at an average level. The site is attractive and easy to use.

5. American Association of Occupational Health Nurses (AAOHN)

http://www.aaohn.org/forum.htm/

This is the official Web site of the AAOHN, which focuses on workplace health and safety. The association was founded in 1942 to promote excellence in occupational health nursing. More than 12,500 nurses belong to AAOHN. Information is current and updated often. The most important features of this Web site include continuing education, certification, conferences, practice resources, the AAOHN Journal, and legislative links. Information is available in English at an average level. The site is easy to use.

6. American Nephrology Nurses Association (ANNA)

http://www.annanurse.org

The ANNA was founded in 1969 and now has a membership of over 12,000 nephrology professionals with varying experience and expertise in such areas as conservative management, peritoneal dialysis, hemodialysis, continuous renal replacement therapies, and renal and extrarenal transplantation. The purpose of the site is to promote research, practice, and certification; set forth and update high standards of patient care; educate practitioners; stimulate research; disseminate new ideas through the field; promote interdisciplinary communication and cooperation; and address issues encompassing the practice of nephrology nursing. The intended audience is all nurses, primarily nephrology.

Information is current and updated monthly. The most important features of this site are career opportunities, conferences, online ordering, and the *Nephrology Nursing Journal*. Certification is also available through the Nephrology Nursing Certification Commission: *http://www.nncc-exam.org/*. Information is provided in English at an average level. The site is attractive and easy to use.

7. AORN Online: The Association of Perioperative Registered Nurses

http://www.aorn.org/

The AORN was founded in 1954 to encourage cooperative action by registered nurses to improve the quality of patient care before, during, and after surgery. The association has 41,000 members. The purpose of the Web site is to disseminate information on standards of practice, legislation, research, and career and promote education. Information is current and up-to-date. Information is available in English at an average level. The site is attractive and easy to use.

8. Oncology Nursing Society (ONS)

http://www.ons.org/

ONS is a national organization of more than 30,000 nurses dedicated to excellence in patient care, teaching, research, administration, and education in the field of oncology. Information is current and updated daily/weekly. The most important features of the site include online CE, conferences, certification, scholarships, chapter information, research and career opportunities, education, leadership development, clinical practice, publications, and what's new. Information is available in English at an average level.

_____ Chapter **2**

Nursing Administration

Patricia Hinton Walker

_____

The role and scope of accountability for nurse administrators has expanded significantly as many health care delivery systems now provide care across the continuum (from acute care, to ambulatory care, home health, and even long-term care settings). Issues related to health care regulation and accreditation are more complex, particularly with patient safety as highlighted by the recent reports from the Institute of Medicine. In addition, the current (and future) nursing shortage requires that nurse administrators have up-to-date information about regional workforce supply and demand. Administrators can benchmark their strategies, services, and products by keeping informed about what the competition is doing in recruitment and retention, programs, and services by visiting Web pages. Web sites selected address the broader, changing role of the administrator who is a nurse. Also, "supersites" are included; these sites emerged in the Internet search for "healthcare managers and healthcare administrators" and have been developed in order to facilitate access to and address varied needs of health care professionals through one site.

1. Agency for Healthcare Research and Quality

http://www.ahrq.gov

The Agency for Healthcare Research and Quality (AHRQ) is a Public Health Service agency in the Department of Health and Human Services (DHHS). AHRQ sponsors and conducts research that provides evidence-based information on health care outcomes; quality; and cost, use, and access. *AHRQ* was formerly known as *the Agency for Health Care Policy and Research.* This Web site is relatively easy to use. For nurse administrators, topics related to patient safety, error reduction, evidence-based practice, workforce issues, patient safety, and quality of care would be of interest. A new section on the Web site—"nursing research"—provides information about nursing research at AHRQ and about nurses who work at AHRQ who can serve as contacts or resources to nurses seeking information related to nursing interests. This Web site is very responsive and one can easily get research reports and information about the availability of grants and workshops through use of the site. The AHRQ User Liaison Program also disseminates health services research findings for state and local health policymakers through interactive on-site workshops, teleconferences, distance learning programs, and research syntheses. Web links are available for sister agencies including the National Institutes of Health, the Centers for Disease Control and Prevention, the Food and Drug Administration, the Health Care Financing Administration, and the Health Resources and Services Administration.

2. American Organization of Nurse Executives

http://www.aone.org

This site was designed by the American Organization of Nurse Executives (AONE), a subsidiary of the American Hospital Association, to provide information and resources to its members. This organization provides leadership, professional development, advocacy, and research to advance nursing practice and patient care. In addition, the AONE promotes excellence in nursing leadership and develops strategies to impact health care public policy. The major purpose of the Web site is to serve the members of the AONE. The site is easy to access and links allow the user to locate services and resources easily. Pages provide information in a format that is easy to read with a sidebar table of contents of interest to nursing administrators. Sections are marked "members only" and these parts of the Web page can only be accessed by the members of the AONE.

3. Council on Graduate Education for Administration in Nursing (CGEAN)

http://www.unc.edu/~sengleba/CGEAN/

CGEAN's purpose is to further the development and improvements of graduate education for administration in nursing. This Web site is simple and straightforward, providing a limited amount of information. Schools of Nursing offering nursing administration programs are available along with their Web pages and the site offers links to the member home pages (however there are only a very few members who have provided home pages). There is a link to the AACN-ANOE position statement on nursing education and the essentials for baccalaureate and masters education in leadership and management. One of the most informative sections is the learning resources section which includes but is not limited to links to ANA's Nurse Sensitive Quality Indicators, selected standardized nursing languages such as the Nursing Intervention Classification and Nursing Outcomes Classification, and the Nursing Management Minimum Data Set. This Web site could be helpful to nurse administrators when searching for educational programming, but the information on the site is limited to a very narrow purpose.

4. HCPro

http://www.hcpro.com

HCPro began as many publishing companies do, serving customers in a particular niche market area. Formerly OPUSCOMM Online, HCPro.com is designed to meet customer needs through unique Internet-based solutions. With each HCPro Company having a commercial Web site, HCPro is an example of a "portal" industry that is a highly specialized, content-driven site designed to foster improvement in the health care industry. These portals unite both visitors and advertisers, and deliver content and services through e-Business technology. HCPro's mission is to meet the specialized information, advisory, and education needs of the health care industry and provide services and products to customers to help them achieve success in their organizations.

This supersite considers itself a leader in health care compliance, regulation, and management, to meet the needs of health care professionals in a variety of areas. The site provides access to publications, background checks, and clinical references (*hpCheck,* online learning (*hcprofessor Online Learning*); accreditation information (accreditinfo. com); compliance information (complianceinfor.com); and a health and safety supersite (*heatlhsafetyinfo.com*). As a supersite, the nurse administrator has the opportunity to go to one place for a wide range of resources, information, and assistance. As the role of the nurse administrator expands beyond traditional nursing service to management of other patient services departments, it is important for nursing administrators to expand their knowledge and expertise. One way to quickly obtain information is by accessing Internet sites that provide a wide range of information about the management of health care—beyond the management of nursing.

This Web site, like other supersites, is very easy to use, with rapid response to each of the different areas. For example, the *compliance-info.com* provides valuable information on HIPPA and the *SNFinfo. com* provides easily accessed information on long-term care regulations. Some of the services are for sale, such as the *hpCheck* for background checks, but others just provide important information to a health care administrator. Some of the links provided in this supersite would be particularly helpful to a nurse administrator in a rural hospital, whose responsibilities involve a wide range of health care management, including such areas as management of medical staff and anesthesia services.

5. Joint Commission on Accreditation of Healthcare Organizations

http://www.jcaho.org

The Joint Commission on Accreditation of Healthcare Organizations (JCAHO) is the nation's predominant standards setting and accrediting body in health care. The mission of JCAHO is to improve the safety and quality of care provided to the public through the provision of health care accreditation and related services. The JCAHO evaluates and accredits nearly 18,000 health care organizations and programs in the United States. It is an independent, nonprofit organization that has developed professionally based standards and evaluated the compliance of health care organizations against these benchmarks since 1951. JCAHO's evaluation and accreditation services are provided for general, psychiatric, children's, and rehabilitation hospitals. The JCAHO evaluates and accredits other types of agencies such as health care networks (HMOs), home care organizations, assisted living, and long-term care facilities. In February 1997, JCAHO launched *ORYX: The Next Evolution in Accreditation* to integrate the use of outcomes and other performance measurement data into the accreditation process. Through its nonprofit subsidiary, *Joint Commission Resources* (JCR), JCAHO sponsors a variety of education programs, provides relevant publications for health care professionals, and provides consultation to health care organizations. On its Web site, JCAHO provides a comprehensive guide to help individuals learn more about the safety and quality of JCAHO accredited health care organizations and programs throughout the United States. Quality Check™ includes each organization's name, address, telephone number, accreditation decision, accreditation date, current accreditation status and effective date, and its most recent performance report. The performance report provides detailed information about an organization's performance and how it compares to similar organizations.

Although this Web site is quite complex, it is a complete reference for the nurse administrator to standards, workshops, survey information, and changes anticipated in the accreditation process. The site is user-friendly and information is easy to access with Web links to accreditation for different types of health care organizations. It is very up-to-date and would be a very important resource to the nurse administrator.

6. National Patient Safety Foundation

http://www.npsf.org

The National Patient Safety Foundation was founded by the American Medical Association, CNA HealthPro, 3M, and contributions from the

Schering-Plough Corporation in 1996. The NPSF is an independent, nonprofit organization that is committed to making patient safety a national priority through leadership, research support, and education. It is a partnership of health care practitioners, institutional providers, health product providers, health product manufacturers, researchers, legal advisors, patient/consumer advocates, regulators, and policy-makers committed to making health care safer for patients. The Web site is very user-friendly and comprehensive. It provides access to programs, resources, research, a bibliography, and articles on patient safety. A research database is also available for keyword searches and information on sources of funding, topics, and investigators. It provides information on many different content areas related to patient safety. Workshops and research grants are available and the Web site has a number of important links to other sites related to patient safety including the *Leapfrog Group*, the *Agency for Healthcare Research and Quality* (AHRQ), and the *JCAHO Facts on Patient Safety.*

_____ Chapter **3**

Managed Care and Case Management

Erin V. Messett

_____

Health care today has an ever-changing proactive and systematic approach to providing services. Health policy changes, timely clinical information at the point of care, automated data collection processing tools, electronic communication technology, and third party providers are a few of the complicated issues in a managed care environment. Providing high quality, cost-effective, services across the continuum of care becomes a creative challenge. Case management is a practice framework that helps to negotiate this maze while utilizing evidence-based practice and providing data for outcomes.

Six of the sites reviewed identify their focus as case management. Two of these sites focus on managed care. Some clinical practitioners would see case management under the larger umbrella of managed care. A variety of case management models are reviewed, which provide high quality, cost-effective care and resources across the health care continuum. Common theme sites were reviewed with links to a great deal of information in specialized clinical areas, prevention, health education, and much more.

1. American Association of Managed Care Nurses (AAMCN)

http://www.aamcn.org/

American Association of Managed Care Nurses (AAMCN) reports its mission is "to be recognized as the expert and resource in managed care nursing; to establish standards for managed care nursing practice; to positively impact public policy regarding managed health care delivery and to assist in educating the public on managed care." Membership benefits include networking opportunities, free subscriptions to publications, career counseling, job placement services, membership directories, and registration discounts. This site also provides a home study program for introduction to managed care nursing, and a nursing home program. *The Standards of Practice for Managed Care Nursing* are available for ten dollars a copy. The site provides excellent Web links for managed care resources. It also provides the service of on-site educational programs, and e-discussion groups for any topic dealing with managed care. I found this site clear and easy to navigate.

2. American Case Management Association (ACMA)

http://www.acmaweb.org/

American Case Management Association (ACMA) reports its mission is "to support the evolving collaborative practice of Hospital/Health System Case Management." Included in their goals are professional development services identified as mentoring, educational forums, and resource information. The ACMA's philosophy is based on collaborative practice models. "Educational" and "Annual Meetings" links are available reporting on updated conference material and providing limited minutes on the annual meeting. The "Career" link provides a venue for employers and professionals seeking career opportunities. The "Resource Center" offers an excellent summary of available certification centers in case management. Job descriptions, data collection tools, and organizational charts are available to members for a fee. Overall the site is clear and easy to use. One great feature is the link "Headlines" that offers a U.S. Department of Health and Human Services "Fact Sheet" and a link to all HHS press releases that can be very informative.

3. Anthony and Associates

http://anthony.casemanagement.com

Anthony and Associates is owned and operated by Mary Pat Anthony, RN, CCM. This case management site specializes in worker's compensation. Their services include "medical case management, telephonic case management, vocational placement services, transferable skills analysis, retrospective utilization reviews, IME or second opinions, peer reviews, file analysis, and physical therapy peer/case reviews." This company has a national network of case managers, consultants, and rehab specialists. An "Overview" link reviews the interview, advantages, and other benefits of the service. "Sample Case" link gives a case example in narrative and graphic format. The site provides a map of national service areas. A case management service request form and response is available for a minimum fee and an instant "PayPal" link is available. The site links are appropriate, up-to-date, and clear. The case example was short and concise. This site is very comprehensive and easy to navigate.

4. Case Management Resource Guide

http://www.cmrg.com/

Case Management Resource Guide is a searchable database of over 110,000 specialty health care services covering over forty categories of services. National and regional companies and networks are available on this site. Disease management resources that are listed for specific clinical conditions are comprehensive and clear. *The Case Management Resource Guide Healthcare Directory* is also available in print and can be ordered on this Web site. Over 2,000 listings are included for patient information and support resources. A search engine is available for continuing education programs. The health care information page includes directories, research reports, databases, mailing lists, jobs, products, and related links. One managed care feature is a physician groups and network databases including Independent Practice Associations (IPA), Physician Hospital Organizations (PHO), Physician Practice Management Companies (PPMC), Management Service Organizations (MSO), and physician group practices. The directory identifies the group ownership, addresses, key contacts, affiliations, and contracted and capitated numbers.

5. Case Management Society of America (CMSA)

http://www.cmsa.org/

Case Management Society of America (CMSA) reports their mission is "to promote the growth and value of case management and to support the evolving needs of the case management professional." The "Membership Information" page explains in detail their definition of case management, CMSA member benefits, services, products, publications, conferences, and all other services. On line continuing education units with a list of currently offered classes is available. National chapter conferences with a Web contact address and phone number are listed. The "Resource" page provides clinical information on selected disease-related issues. The disease-related links have excellent organizational Web resources. "News" offers a brief review of current topics with associated Web sites. This also includes a link to Health Insurance Portability and Accountability Act (HIPAA). The CMSA site has links to frequently asked questions, job postings, International Case Management Forum, and e-mail.

*6. Geriatric Care Managers (GCM)

http://www.caremanager.org/

Geriatric Care Managers (GCM) is a national association of practitioners with a goal of providing dignified, cost-effective care for the elderly and their families. One focus is to maximize the independence and autonomy of the individual. GMC services include assistance with care planning, in-home support services, crises intervention, consumer education and advocacy, and a review of financial, legal, and medical issues, to offer referrals and make recommendations. Services can be provided to long distance caregivers and GCM providers are available after hours and on weekends. Benefits of this service include quality

---

*Sites suitable for consumer use.

control, efficiency, and cost control. Association links include all committees with e-mail addresses of chairs for easy contact. Links provide information on membership, benefits, products, chapter and annual conferences, and care manager selection. This site has a link called "Care Management Resources" which provides a variety of Web sites for information, bioethics, products, support services and much more, in a variety of care settings. This link provides good information for both professionals and consumers.

*7.   Health Care Financing Administration (HCFA) Services

http://www.hcfa.gov/siteindex/

Centers for Medicare and Medicaid (CMS) Services

http://www.hcfa.gov/

This site provides information in five major categories "Medicare," "Medicaid," "State Children's Health Insurance Program (SCHIP)," "What's new on hcfa.gov," and a site index. The Medicare.gov home page provides phone numbers, links for nursing homes, prescription drugs, physician directories, Medicare health plan comparison, and medigap comparison search tools. The Medicaid and state operations search wizard includes consumer information, professional and technical information, and national account representatives. The SCHIP page provides information on enrollment, outreach, legislation, and other related links. The site "What's new on hcfa.gov" highlights additions to hcfa.gov within the past 2 months. The site index provides an overabundance of information about the programs, agency, Web site, career opportunities, resources, publications, fraud and abuse, laws and regulations, and much more. It also has a search engine. Health Care Financing Administration (HCFA) has changed its name to Centers for Medicare and Medicaid (CMS) as of July 1, 2001. The new site is also migrating information from the first Web site. The connecting links make it easy to move back and forth between sites. This site offers a wealth of information for consumers and health care providers.

8. The Center for Case Management (CCM)

http://www.cfcm.com/

"The Center for Case Management, Inc. (CCM) is an international health care consulting company founded in 1986 at New England Medical Center Hospitals for the purpose of development and teaching provider/clinical-side strategies for managing care and achieving clinical integration." The CCM home page identifies consultation services and provides consultant biographies. Consult services include clinical audits, case management system evaluation, Utilization-Case Management Initiative (UCMI), Clinical Path/Care Map Assessments, and development of "Data Dashboard" System. This site offers several products including Critical Indicators, Care-Map Tools, staff training manuals/videos, texts, and books. Unfortunately, no online ordering is available; however, purchases can be made via phone. Customers may design a customized workshop for any private location or at CCM's location. An example series is available for review. The publication "New Definition" is available for viewing free on a semi-annual basis. This site offers a "Speakers Bureau" link to meet audience specific needs for a presenter. The "Certification" link reviews information needed for certification for case management administrators. "Partners" discusses business alliances and provides an e-mail contact link. This Web site is clear, concise, and easy to navigate. Each Web page has an update listing. Additionally, for Japanese customers, consultation is offered in Japan through Medical Create. The "Medical Create" link is in Japanese.

Chapter 4

Evidence-Based Practice

Jane H. Barnsteiner and Deborah M. Joers

N urses continually confront questions about the most current approaches to the care of patients and families, knowing how to appraise clinical information and biomedical literature, finding the latest research, knowing whether conclusions of a systematic review are valid and whether clinical practice guideline recommendations are all elements of evidence-based practice. There are several excellent Web sites that assist viewers to advance their skills in incorporating strategies of critical appraisal of the literature, and support evidence-based nursing practice through access to best practices using practice guidelines and protocols. Sites were chosen for accurate and current content, ease of navigation, and frequent updates and credible sponsors.

*1.　Agency for Healthcare Research and Quality (AHRQ)

http://www.ahcpr.gov/clinic/epcix.htm

This is a United States government sponsored clearinghouse of information on evidence-based practice. AHRQ provides evidence-based

---

*Sites suitable for consumer use.

information on health care outcomes, quality and cost, use and access to allow informed decisions and to improve the quality of health care services. The site is sponsored by AHRQ (formerly the Agency for Health Care Policy and Research). The intended audience is health care professionals and consumers. The site is updated frequently although the date of the last update is not apparent. The site author is identified and there is the ability for e-mail correspondence. Features include a drop-down menu to easily click into sections and a "what's new" section to enable the repeat visitor to easily find recently entered information. Evidence-based sections include clinical information, funding opportunities, data and surveys, research findings, and quality assessment information. There are links to related sites on child health, women's health and minority health. The site is in English and some information is also available in Spanish. The site provides the ability to search and browse. It is easy to navigate and all of the links were active.

2. Bandolier

http://www.jr2.ox.ac.uk/bandolier/index.html

Bandolier is both a print and electronic bulletin about evidence-based medicine. The paper and electronic versions are separate. The online site includes access to both. The purpose of the bulletin is to provide a summary of current evidence-based materials to health care providers. The editors of Bandolier search PubMed and Cochrane collections each month and choose those reviews and meta-analysis that they find interesting for publication. Bandolier is produced by the Pain Research staff at Oxford University and receives no-strings-attached funding from a variety of companies, primarily pharmaceuticals. The intended audience is health care practitioners, particularly general practitioners in the National Health Service in England. The information would be of interest to nurses because it is related to current clinical practice, diagnosis, and treatment. Bandolier is updated each month. Web essays, which are focused on a particular topic and more educational than review of research, are published as often as weekly. Each review article is in a standard format: study or review/results/commentary. Keyword searching is available. The online version has 16 regularly updated "resource centers" that have systematic reviews of the literature on a particular topic back to 1994. They are trying to develop

17 others. Bandolier is also available in Spanish. Access to a ".pdf" printout version is 2 months behind the electronic publication. One drawback of the site is that the individual articles are not dated. There are many articles on the site. The information is presented in a conversational tone since that is the tone of the Bandolier paper version. The online site has simple, plain text links and new items are clearly marked.

3. Cochrane Collaboration

http://www.cochrane.org

The Cochrane Collaboration provides systematic reviews of the literature related to a particular clinical topic. They present highly structured reviews of the effects of health care for more than 50 topic areas. The Cochrane Collaboration is an international nonprofit organization with centers in 15 countries that sponsor 50 topic related review groups. The groups hand search the health care literature related to their topic and produce reviews to promote the use of evidence-based care. The reviews are constantly updated as new research becomes available. The library and associated databases are produced and managed by Update Software for the Cochrane Collaboration. The reviews are intended for practicing clinicians. Each review group updates the information as it becomes available. The review groups are comprised of volunteer experts in the content area. The online site provides access to abstracts of all of the collaborative group reviews as they become available. The abstracts and reviews are searchable by keyword, alphabetically or by topic. The abstracts of the reviews follow a consistent structured format that can be printed. Access to the full reviews is by subscription only.

English is the official language of the library but the abstracts are also available in Italian. The centers in the various countries have sites in the native language—Spain, Germany, France, Netherlands, Brazil, Italy, China, South Africa, and more. The site provides links to all of the international centers. There are also informational brochures available in a multitude of languages on the various international sites. There are an extensive number of reviews available in 50 different topic areas. They are very complete and continuously reviewed providing very up-to-date evidence-based information. The Cochrane Collaboration manages some areas of the site. However, when you enter the actual library Update Software manages it. Choosing the homepage may return you to either the main page of the Cochrane Collaboration or the main page of the Update Software Site.

4. EBN Online

http://ebn.bmjjournals.com/

EBN Online is the online version of the quarterly journal *Evidence-Based Nursing,* which is published by British Medical Journal Publishing and the Royal College of Nursing Publishing. Each quarter EBN reviews more than 130 health care journals and selects those articles meeting predefined criteria that report studies and reviews that are relevant to practicing nurses. They summarize the articles in structured abstracts that describe the studies, their methodology, and their conclusions. They add a commentary on the article, the study methods, and the clinical implications. The Royal College of Nursing and British Medical Journal Publishing Companies along with Stanford HighWire Press produce and manage the site. This site is primarily aimed at practicing clinical nurses. The information is published quarterly in conjunction with the publication of the paper version. The site is searchable by the author's name and by words in the title, the abstract, or the article. You can also browse by issue or by topic. All issues back to 1998 are available full text online to subscribers. Printer friendly .pdf downloads of articles are available. One can download to the most popular citation managers like EndNote, Reference Manager, and ProCite. It also links to Medline. The table of contents can be received each quarter by e-mail. After January 14, 2002 only subscribers will have full access. The site is only available in English.

EBN is easy to navigate. The links are either blue ovals or in a column on the right hand side of the article page. The links are consistently placed. Attention has been paid to making graphics small and easy to download. It has a crisp appearance: white background with red and blue lettering and links.

5. The Joanna Briggs Institute

http://www.joannabriggs.edu.au/

This is international research collaboration for the evaluation of research and integration into nursing practice. The purposes are to identify practice arenas that require summarized evidence, conduct systematic reviews, and design, conduct, and promote broad dissemination activities. The Royal Adelaide Hospital and Adelaide University in Australia sponsor the site. Information about the evolution of the

Institute and participating members is provided. The intended audience is nurses in research, education, and practice. The information is current and the last update was within a week. The site includes information about the Institute and Evidence-Based Nursing. Best Practice Information Sheets and Executive Summaries of reviews are available free online. Full research synthesis reviews and a Nursing Practice Manual are available for purchase. English is the only language available. The site is easy to navigate, the icons are useful, and there is no advertising.

6. McMaster University Evidence-Based Health Care Resources

http://www.cochrane.mcmaster.ca/evidence-based.htm

This is a directory of Canadian and International Web sites that specialize in evidence-based health information. It provides links to almost 50 evidence-based–care Web sites throughout Canada and the world. McMaster University Health Information Research Unit produces it. The site is aimed at health care clinicians interested in evidence-based care. No information was available to determine when the last update occurred; however, at the time of this review, all links were current. All of the sites are related to evidence-based care and have hyperlinks. Canadian sites are the predominant focus of the Web sites. There are no reviews of research available on this site. The Web page is a directory of sites that focus on evidence-based care. The site is easy to use as sites are listed alphabetically in English.

7. National Guideline Clearinghouse

http://www.guideline.gov/index.asp

This site is a United States government database for evidence-based clinical practice guidelines and related documents. Evidence-based clinical practice guidelines and related documents produced by the Agency for Health Care Research and Quality (AHRQ) and by other clinical organizations can be obtained through this site. AHRQ, the American Medical Association, and the American Association of Health Plans sponsor the site. The site is intended for use by nurses, physicians, other health care professionals, and consumers. The site is updated weekly. Structured abstracts, synthesis of guidelines, annotated bibliographies, and links to full text guidelines are provided through the site. Some guidelines can be downloaded to handheld computers. An electronic forum is available for information exchange. Criteria for development and submission of guidelines are listed. All guidelines are current within 5 years and the date of last review is listed. A Frequently Asked Question section contains helpful information for infrequent or first time site visitors. English is the only language available. The site is easy to navigate. There are multiple options for searching, for example, by disease, treatment or organization.

8. Sarah Cole Hirsh Institute

http://www.hirshinstitute.com/default.htm

This is a Nursing Institute that offers state of evidence reviews, a certificate program on *Implementing Best Nursing Practices,* and consulting services. The purpose is to build a repository of best nursing practices through integration of research and practice. The goal is to stimulate use of research-based nursing practices to improve care, direct research, and provide standards for nursing education and practice. The Frances Payne Bolton School of Nursing at Case Western Reserve University sponsors the site. Information about the school and the evolution of the Institute is provided. The site is intended for use by nurses in education, practice, and research. Date of the last update is not apparent. However, information is current. The site author is not identified. The site includes best of evidence reviews, abstracts of current reviews, information about the certificate program, and the ability to register online to attend the program. Screens related to institute personnel need updating. Full-length reviews are available for purchase. English is the only language available. The site is easy to navigate and user-friendly. All links are active.

9. University of York Centre for Evidence-Based Nursing (EBN)

http://www.york.ac.uk/depts/hstd/centres/evidence/ev-intro.htm

This is a British Web site that describes the activities of the Centre for EBN and provides links to EBN education and practice resources. The Centre exists to further EBN through education, research, and development. This is one of a few EBN sites. The Department of Health

Studies at the University of York sponsors it. The intended audience is nurses and other health care disciplines. The information is current. The site was updated within the previous 2 weeks. The site author is identified and there is the ability to communicate by e-mail. The site lists titles in the EBN Journal and the Cochrane Database of Systematic Reviews. It provides links to a variety of resources such as *Effective Healthcare*. The site provides updates for EBN teaching and practice including online links, teaching resources, and training and development opportunities. There are opportunities to interact with the site hosts and there is an online discussion of EBN topics. The site is user-friendly and easy to navigate. Icons are useful.

10. University of Rochester Center for Nursing

http://www.urmc.rochester.edu/son/research/crebp.html

The University of Rochester Center for Nursing and Evidenced Based Practice facilitates evidence-based practice at the School of Nursing and in the clinical setting. It provides a model for academia to work with a University Medical Center. The Center for Nursing also houses two Centers of Research Excellence. These are the Centers on High-Risk Children and Youth and the Center for Clinical Research on Aging. Together they provide support for research at the School of Nursing and with advanced practice nurses at the University Medical Center. The University of Rochester School of Nursing sponsors the site. Two newly established centers featured on the site work in close collaboration with the University Medical Center. These are the Center for Clinical Trials and Medical Device Evaluation and the Center for Advancing Research and Clinical practice through close Collaboration (ARCC). This site provides valuable information to those who are looking to foster evidence for a clinical practice setting to foster research.

The Center for Clinical Research on Aging section of the site provides information on completed and research in progress. Numerous links are provided to featured researchers. Since the Center is fairly new, much of the research is still in progress. English is the only language available. This is a site worth watching as the collaborative model that they have developed begins to produce results.

_____ Chapter **5**

Culturally Competent Care

Antonia M. Villarruel

_____

Cultural competency is the capacity to work effectively in cross-cultural situations. Recently, cultural competency has taken on increased significance. Trends have highlighted the need for nurses to develop the requisite knowledge, skills, and abilities to work with persons from diverse racial and ethnic backgrounds as well as those whose dominant language is something other than English. The continued growth rates of minority groups in the United States, the significant numbers of limited English proficient persons, the lack of diversity within the nursing force, and recent federal law and state, local, and health care regulations are some of these trends.

*1. The Cross Cultural Health Care Program (CCHP)

http://www.Xculture.org

The CCHCP was funded in 1992 with a grant from the W.K. Kellogg Foundation in order to meet the diverse health care needs of the Seattle

_____

*Sites suitable for consumer use.

population. A second grant from the Foundation was directed toward dissemination of products and programs at the national level. The CCHCP serves as a bridge between communities and health care institutions to ensure full access to quality health care that is culturally and linguistically appropriate. Health care providers and consumers are the intended audience. This Web site provides access and links to a number of important resources in dealing with issues of cultural and language diversity in health settings. One important feature of the Web site is its community profiles of 12 ethnic groups, including Arab, Samoan, Soviet Jews, and Ukrainian. Although the profiles were developed in 1996 and have context-specific information related to the Seattle area, they provide a great deal of user-friendly information to assist providers. Another useful resource is a bibliography related to cultural assessment. Many of the other resources listed, including videos and reports, must be purchased. However, purchase can be done easily through the Web site. One particular video, "Working with a Medical Interpreter," is excellent in portraying issues and strategies in working with interpreters and how the need for an interpreter impacts the delivery of care. While the site is relatively easy to navigate, it does take time to determine what resources are available online and what needs to be purchased. The level of information is average, with more detailed information available through another source.

*2.   Diversity Rx

http://www.DiversityRx.org

The Web site is a clearinghouse of information on how to meet the language and cultural needs of ethnic minorities, immigrants, refugees, and other diverse populations seeking health care. It includes specific information on model programs, policies, and legal issues related to cross-cultural health, and limited English Proficiency. Listed sponsors include The National Conference of State Legislatures (NCSL), Resources for Cross Cultural Health Care (RCCHC), and the Henry J. Kaiser Family Foundation. The editor of the Web site, Julia Puebla Fortier, is a recognized expert in the area of policy and cultural and linguistic standards in health care. Health care providers, policymakers and legislators, and consumers are the site's intended audience. This site would be most helpful to nurses who want to know more about the legal and policy issues regarding culturally competent health care, as well as specifics related to the use of interpreters in health care settings.

This is a comprehensive Web site that includes essential information on the importance of language and culture in health care, models and practices of cultural and linguistic competence, policies, legal issues, and current information. The site provides opportunities for networking and there are important links for additional policy information, programs, and resources. The information appears current, although a number of content areas listed are under construction. The site does best in providing information about interpreter services, guidelines, training, and curriculum. It also does well in providing information about culture and linguistic standards, laws, and policies. There is less specific information about particular racial/ethnic/cultural groups. The level of information overall is average to high. The Web site is easy to navigate, and includes a section "Getting the most out of Diversity Rx." A glossary of terms is included which adds to the ease and helpfulness of this site.

3. EthnoMed

http://www.ethnomed.org

The purpose of the EthnoMed site is to provide health care providers with the information about cultural beliefs, health care issues, and other related issues pertinent to the health care of recent immigrants to Seattle, WA. The University of Washington Harborview Medical Center sponsors the site. Health care providers, especially those in direct practice, are the intended audience. This Web site provides a wide array of information for health care providers as well as resources readily available for patient use. Information is provided about the background, cultural beliefs, health practices, and remedies for 10 population groups in the Seattle area. These groups include Amharics, Cambodians, Eritreans, Mexicans, and Somalians. The information provided is not provided with the same depth and breadth across the listed groups. However, the resources provided are easy to navigate and accessible. A major strength of this site is the availability of patient education information in different languages. For example, for each group there is a section on "Patient Information." There are translated materials available regarding common health issues such as fever, tuberculosis, and cancer screening. Some of these materials have been developed by federal organizations, such as the Centers for Disease Control. In the site pertaining to Chinese, there is even a video available in Chinese, "A New Pathway to Women's Health," designed to promote cervical cancer screening.

In addition to ethnic specific information, there are several articles, including research reports, and resources available to health care providers regarding specific topics. Links are provided for other organizations dealing with specific ethnic groups as well as those dealing with cultural and linguistic issues. The ready availability of materials for patient use and for practitioner reference is a major strength. The information appears current and is at an average to high level, depending primarily on whether the information is for providers or patients.

*4. Office of Minority Health, Department of Health and Human Services

http://www.omh.gov

The mission of the Office of Minority Health (OMH) is to improve the health of racial and ethnic populations through the development of effective health policies and programs that help to eliminate disparities in health. OMH has a role in the development and coordination of federal health policy by addressing minority health concerns and making progress to eliminate health disparities. Health care providers, policymakers, and consumers are the intended audience. This Web site is one portal of entry to the vast resources of the federal government available to understand and address the health care needs of diverse populations. Major links include information about conferences, publications, data and statistics, federal clearinghouses, and health links for consumers. Some links provide general information while others provide more specific information about minority health. One of the most helpful aspects of this site is that it provides important access to the Office of Minority Health Resource Center, a site where you can request specific information by topic and racial/ethnic group. The OMH Web site also provides important links to major and recent policy initiatives from the Department of Health and Human Services (HHS), initiatives regarding minority health, such as the Hispanic Health Agenda, and the *Asian American and Pacific Islander Action Agenda*. Links are also provided to regional Offices of Minority Health, where specific information regarding funding opportunities can be further explored. While the site is easy to navigate, effort is required to access the specific information one may be seeking, especially if one is in search of specific vs. general information. The level of information provided is average to high, depending on whether you are requesting patient information or policy relevant information.

5. Opening Doors

http://www.opening-doors.org

Opening Doors: Reducing Sociocultural Barriers to Health Care is a national program that supports service and research projects to identify and break down nonfinancial, culturally based barriers to health care. Robert Wood Johnson Foundation and Henry J. Kaiser Family Foundation sponsor the site. Health care providers and administrators are the intended audience. This site would also be useful to educators.

This Web site provides a mechanism for dissemination of research and demonstration projects funded by the Opening Doors initiative. While grant recipients and contact information are presented, there is little information about the nature of their funded activities. References for articles and published articles are provided, but none is accessible through the Internet. Interested persons must purchase or contact the grant recipients for further information. The best features of this Web site are the sections entitled "The Changing Face of America" and "Sociocultural Barriers to Health Care." These sections, while brief, provide health care providers with an overview of the importance of addressing diversity issues in the delivery of health care. The section on sociocultural barriers briefly outlines issues of language and nonverbal communication, role of the family, and knowledge and expectations of patients. The short vignettes that are provided bring to life the issues and serve as a starting point for further discussion or case study development. The section on "lessons learned" by grantees and program offices about sociocultural barriers, strategies to reduce them, and as a result of research are also useful.

The Web site does not appear current. A networking and conferencing feature that was to by running by February of 1999 was not functional. The level of information provided here could be considered simple to average. The site was relatively easy to navigate.

6. Voices for Health

http://www.voicesforhealth.org

The mission of Voices for Health is to help the health care industry address the linguistic and cultural needs of communities so that access to services may be improved. The Web site provides access to services that include translating and editing, interpretation, Spanish courses, research assistance, provider seminars, and interpreter education. The site is sponsored by Voices For Health, Inc., which was founded in 1997 by a registered nurse and is owned and operated by health care providers who are bilingual and experienced in caring for clients of culturally diverse communities. Health care providers, organizations, and researchers are the intended audience.

The purpose of this site is to promote services of Voices for America, which includes both translation and interpretation. The strength of this Web site is that it provides information about actual services that might be needed for practice and research. For example, interpretation is provided for over 40 languages 24 hours a day, 7 days a week. Languages include Daria, Farsi, Spanish, Thai, and over 5 dialects of Chinese. Interpreters are trained and both promote and follow the Standards of Practice and Code of Ethics of the Massachusetts Medical Interpreters Association. Translators are available from many disciplines and a bilingual registered nurse supervises each project. Translation services are available for patient education, consent forms and legal documents, as well as research instruments. Back-translation services are also available. In addition to services, there are links to various interpreter and translation associations as well as general cultural resources. The Web site is easy to access and navigate.

Chapter 6

Nursing Informatics

Sarah Farrell and David A. Conner

N ursing informatics is an emerging specialty in health care information management. It combines computer science, information science, and nursing science to facilitate the management and processing of nursing data, information, and knowledge that support nursing practice and the delivery of patient care. Nursing informatics was first recognized as a specialty of advanced practice nursing by the American Nurses Association in 1992, and a certification in this area was offered. Nursing informatics specialists identify clinical information management problems, design information system solutions, evaluate and select appropriate technology products, supervise the implementation process, train system users, test systems, and support systems by developing and implementing improvements.

1. American Medical Informatics Association (AMIA)

http://www.amia.org/

The American Medical Informatics Association is the official representative organization to the International Medical Informatics Association. AMIA is a nonprofit organization with individual, institution, and corporate members committed to the development and use of information technologies to enhance the delivery of health care services. Members of AMIA include physicians, nurses, computer and information scientists, biomedical engineers, medical librarians, and academic researchers and educators. This site includes information about the AMIA Annual Symposium and the AMIA Spring Congress. There are links to the *Journal of the American Medical Informatics Association* and specific informatics workgroups including the AMIA Nursing Informatics Workgroup. Members use these workgroups to research and exchange information with colleagues on a particular area of medical informatics. In addition, the site includes information on public policy concerning informatics, a virtual resource center for medical informatics, and information on job opportunities in the health care informatics field. The Web site is colorful, comprehensive, and easy to navigate. Information is current and accurate. The design of the home page includes a table of contents listed on the left-hand side of the page. It provides easy access to the site's content.

The Nursing Informatics Working Group of the AMIA *http:// www.amia-niwg.org/* supports the AIMA mission of promoting the advancement and integration of NI into the broader context of health care. NIWG will assist in advancing the field of NI by fostering innovation and scientific exchange, education of professionals and the public, and influencing decision makers and policymakers regarding the use of information in nursing and health care. Starting with 35 members in 1990, the working group currently has 294 members and a strong Web site to share resources with its membership. The Web site's audience is for members and potential members. The content seems to be updated regularly. A site map or structure for the site is not provided. The content appears to be accurate, although the site does not subscribe to "Health on the Net" or other sources of credibility for health care sites. The content may be inclusive, but the site's design needs some work. There is a waving flag at the top and a whole frame on the right with nothing except blue color, both distracting. The seven bullets seen on this day could be very well moved by tomorrow, since the bullets do not appear to be permanent icons or placements. This makes the site rather difficult to navigate, but could be easily improved. Too many different styles of fonts and color are also distracting.

2. American Nurses Association (ANA)

http://www.ana.org

The ANA site includes ANCC site where nurses interested in obtaining information on certification for nursing informatics can find information.

In addition, documents can be ordered. These include government documents such as *Scope of Practice for Nursing Informatics and the Standards of Practice for Nursing Informatics.*

3. American Nursing Informatics Association (ANIA)

http://www.ania.org/

Established in 1992, the American Nursing Informatics Association is a nonprofit organization that supports professional nursing informatics specialists who design, implement and manage information technology and systems that enhance clinical practice, nursing education and research through professional activities, networking, and education that focuses on a variety of nursing informatics interests. The ANIA Web site includes information about the organization, the profession of nursing informatics, and ANIA conferences and other meetings of interest to nursing informatics. The site also contains an extensive resource links section indexed into subcategories including career resources, education resources, health care informatics groups, nursing informatics groups/organizations, and other nursing resources, with 238 links in total. While the ANIA's Web site is a great resource engine for online information of interest to nursing informatics, the site itself is limited by the lack of detailed information or discussion about current events and subjects specific to nursing informatics. The design of the site is simple and pleasing to the eye with an index of sections located to the left-hand side of the home page. The index allows easy navigation of the various aspects of the site.

4. Computers in Nursing

http://www.nursingcenter.com/journals

Computers in Nursing is published bimonthly by Lippincott, Williams, and Wilkins, Inc., at 16522 Hunters Green Parkway, Hagerstown, MD 21740-2116. Leslie H. Nicoll, PhD, MBA, RN, is the Editor-in-Chief. The intended audience is for the range of nurses interested in computers, from novice to expert. Original full text articles include topics such as ways the computer can help save time and money and solve practical nursing problems. Columns and original articles intend to provide practical step-by-step methods for increasing productivity with computers.

The site is easy to navigate and functional without a lot of bells and whistles. The site is in English only.

5. Healthcare Informatics

http://www.healthcare-informatics.com/

The first issue of this magazine was published in 1984, under the title *Healthcare Computing and Communications*. It then evolved into *U.S. Healthcare Computing and Communications*, as the owner had international expansion aspirations and in fact launched *Healthcare Computing and Communications-Canada*, which still publishes today. Soon it was shortened to *U.S. Healthcare*, though trademark issues soon forced a change to its current title.

6. Health Information Management Systems Society (HIMSS)

http://www.himss.org/

The Health Information Management Systems Society is a nonprofit membership organization that provides leadership to health care informatics professionals for the management of clinical, information, and telecommunication systems. It accomplishes this through annual conferences, publications, educational opportunities, and member services. HIMSS members are responsible for developing many of today's key innovations in health care delivery including telemedicine, computer-based patient records, community health information networks, and portable/wireless health care computing. The HIMSS Web site is a dynamic directory of industry news and current events, HIMSS announcements, publications, conference calendars and curricula, and solutions including vendor products and services. Career resources include postings for job opportunities specific to health care information technologists and learning opportunities via HIMSS WebU (i.e., a distance learning initiative that uses Web seminars, CD-ROM, and partnerships with academic institutions). The Web page provides current, extensive, and relevant information for system managers and leaders in health care informatics. Various sections of the page may be accessed from the list of contents on the home page. A contact section lists addresses and phone numbers to different departments within the HIMSS.

7. Nursing Informatics.com

http://www.nursing-informatics.com/

Nursing Informatics.com is a creative and entrepreneurial Web site developed and maintained by June Kaminski, RN, MSN. The site is intended to be an online "mecca" for nurses who are enthusiastic about all aspects of nursing informatics. Created to offer unique comprehensive resources for nurses interested in developing related knowledge and applicable skills, the site is clearly evolving as a distinct site from .net and .orgs. Future components include articles, tutorials, a discussion board, a newsletter, distance ed courses, books, links, workshops, and consultant services. The strongest aspect of the site is the professional design, obviously not a personal page. The weakest aspect is the fact that the site is not tied to an organization or group, and it remains to be seen if the site develops to its full potential. At this point, the site, created in Canada, tends to be oriented toward Canada rather than globally. That could change with more contributions and activity. The site seems to be for the purpose of establishing a dot com business and the future of any such site remains to be seen and tested. The site is in English only.

8. Nursing Informatics.net

http://www.lemmus.demon.co.uk/inf_main.htm

Peter Murray, a nurse informaticist has re-launched this site as of January 2002 with the purpose of providing an index, global resources, a news service, and original content. The United Kingdom is home for the site. The site is divided into 4 sections: organizations, journals, defining, and studying. The site is intended for nurses interested in informatics, to serve as a network, not just for specialists in informatics. Informatics is, or should be, at the heart of all nursing. All nurses make use of information every second of every day—*so informatics is for **all*** *nurses.* The site provides easy access to a listserv for the purpose of dialogue. The content will be updated regularly and should be accurate.

9. Systematized Nomenclature of Medicine (SNOMED)

http://www.snomed.org/

Nursing informatics specialists, educators, and students interested in the most comprehensive reference terminology in existence today for the clinical environment are encouraged to visit the SNOMED Web site. Maintained by the College of American Pathologists, SNOMED allows for consistent gathering of detailed clinical information, thus enabling providers of various specialties, researchers, and even patients to share common understanding of health concepts across sites of care and computer systems. SNOMED is used in many institutions and clinical information systems throughout the world and is an ANA recognized nomenclature. This is an excellently designed Web site that functions as an online guide and newsletter for SNOMED. A brief history and description of SNOMED is provided along with press releases on the product, announcement of conferences, presentations, and an extensive list of uses for SNOMED. Links to related Web sites are provided such as AMIA and HL7. A special contact section enables readers and Internet navigators to send inquiries to staff of SNOMED International. Some select information is also presented in Spanish.

_____ Chapter 7

Nursing Education

Kristen S. Montgomery and Laree J. Schoolmeesters

N urse educators are responsible for teaching in a variety of settings and therefore have diverse needs. Nurses teach as a part of their normal day-to-day practice as well as in formal and informal settings. The Internet has excellent resources to research the content of topic areas as well as the tools to empower teaching. Online publications, resources, and chat rooms are invaluable aids for the educator to attain expertise and to mentor others. Available sites can provide access to test construction and evaluation, the ability to teach students directly on the Web, the latest information related to issues and trends in nursing education, and the ability to communicate with other nurse educators to enhance support. These tools enable the professional to stay at the forefront of the ever-changing educational environment.

1. American Association of Colleges of Nursing (AACN)

http://www.aacn.nche.edu

The purpose of the AACN and its Web site is to help schools of nursing in managing and staying abreast about the changes in health care.

For nonmembers there are eight sections to explore: What's New, the Education Center, the Data Center, Government Affairs, Conferences, Commission on Collegiate Nursing Education (CCNE) accreditation, Colleagues for Caring, and End-of-Life Care. The What's New section aims to keep educators up to date on latest issues. The Education Center identifies AACN's curriculum standards, position statements, and other educational resources. The Data Center reports annually data regarding nursing education, for example, student enrollment, graduations, and faculty salaries. Other services include customized data reports to a school's specification and benchmarking data on best financial practices for nursing schools. Government affairs explains AACN's issue briefs, testimony, and advocacy regarding funding programs and regulatory policies that support nursing education programs, students, and nursing research and practice. CCNE accreditation provides information on standards and procedures for nursing education programs and improvement of collegiate education. Colleagues in Caring and End-of-Life Care are national grant programs funded by *The Robert Wood Johnson Foundation.* The purpose of Colleagues in Caring is to assist in health care workforce development at a state and regional level based on population demographics and the employment market. The End-of-Life project goals are to develop a core of expert nurse educators and to coordinate national nursing education efforts in end-of-life care. The site is in English with average to above average reading ability required. The site is easy to navigate. The Web site is a comprehensive, concise look at the many facets of nursing education.

2. American Nurses Association (ANA)

http://www.ana.org
http://www.nursingworld.org

The purpose of the ANA and the Web site is to represent and advance the nation's Registered Nurses by fostering high standards of nursing practice, promoting the economic and general welfare of nurses in the workplace, projecting a positive and realistic view of nursing, and by lobbying the Congress and regulatory agencies on health care issues affecting nurses and the public. The site has 3 basic arenas, Nursing Insider (up-to-date information), Nursing World (major organizations and journals), and Nursing Mall. The site is not just comprehensive, but a bit overwhelming with the amount of information it offers. Check out the index or use the pull down menus to explore this large site.

There are a few areas on this large Web site that educators may find of interest: Continuing Education (CE) online, Nursing Links, RN = Real News, Safety and Health, and Safety and Quality. CE online has an alphabetical topical listing of online free and for fee CE credits. Check out a great educational tool on becoming more politically active in the RN = Real News. Click on the nurse's toolkit to find out great tips and samples about writing letters to the editor. Safety and Health is a conglomeration of occupational health issues including health concerns, selected articles from *The American Nurse*, and links to other occupational health resources. Safety and Quality has four subcategories: education, research, policy and legislation, and other links. Education has pertinent information from various sections of the Web site. For example, *Professional CE Programs* including Educating Staff Nurses About Quality Indicators and *Staffing/Skill Mix*, Skill Mix and Outcome Analysis with a brochure *Principles for Nurse Staffing,* that can be read online or purchased. The Research subcategory has information on (a) Acute Care Indicators Refinement, (b) Community-Based Non-Acute Care Indicators, (c) *Costing of Nursing Quality Indicators,* and (d) a *Fact Sheet: Nursing Sensitive Quality Indicators for Acute Care Settings.*

The Online Journal of Issues in Nursing is a peer reviewed electronic journal published by Kent State University College of Nursing that is available free online. Nursing links include academic organizations, general health, general nursing practice, government resources, grant information, informatics and technology, international organizations, listservs, and newsgroups, maternal-child health, publications and references, specific health conditions, specialty practices, state boards of nursing index, tutorials, and online learning. All information is in English with French and Spanish Web sites available for the International Council of Nursing section. This site is huge and easy to navigate with an extensive index and a search feature, although at times you end up on a page without a link to the homepage.

3. Bandido Books

http://www.bandidobooks.com

Bandido Books is a commercial Web site that provides some interactive puzzles that are most appropriate for undergraduate students. The main purpose of the site is to sell books and other products developed for nurses and nursing students; however, the interactive puzzles on nursing theory and different body systems can be a useful tool to help undergraduates learn the content in a fun way. Additionally, the site (and company) offers nursing student fundraising opportunities and quotes and pictures of interest to nurses. E-mail contact is provided for questions and comments on the Web site. Content is presented at a simple level in English.

4. Blackboard

http://www.blackboard.com

Washington, D.C.-based Blackboard Inc. was founded to transform the Internet into a powerful environment for teaching and learning. Blackboard traces its technology roots to Cornell University. Blackboard delivers software products and services that power a total "e-Education Infrastructure" for schools, colleges, universities, and other education providers. Blackboard solutions deliver the promise of the Internet for online teaching and learning, campus communities, auxiliary services, and integration of Web-enabled student services and back office systems. In the Resource Center, nurses can look under categories for medicine and health. Additionally, disciplines from biologic chemistry to physical education may be useful. Nurses may find medicine, neurobiology, disease, drugs, nutrition, and pharmacology most pertinent to their needs. The Instructor Training Center has featured tutorials (blackboard basics and designing an online course) and general tips sheets that can be downloaded and include 13 practical areas to increase you knowledge about online teaching. Topics include titles such as "10 easy steps to creating your online course" and "educational benefits of online teaching." Blackboard has a variety of areas for teaching in conjunction with blackboard.com. Course Cartridge has two topical areas that may be of interest: Education, and Medicine and Allied Health. There are 10 cartridges specific to nursing, although the information is limited to the topic publisher and the size of the cartridge. The site is in English, however, users from selected countries can subscribe to the client-sponsored Blackboard Foreign Language Users' Group Discussion Boards. The site may be a bit confusing for those who have limited e-technology experience.

5. Education World

http://www.education-world.com

Education World was begun in 1996 and was designed to be a site specifically for educators. The site is not directly geared toward nursing educators or even higher education, but is more suited toward K-12 educators. However, the site provides information that can be easily modified for use in collegiate educational settings. The site provides message boards, an online resource guide for lesson plans and curriculum, and research materials. The search engine is limited to only educational sites. Using the advanced search mode, it is possible to carefully narrow a search to retrieve specific topics, target audience, or age of the document. A private company funds the site and there are small ads placed on each page. These are somewhat busy and some blink, which can be distracting. Otherwise, the site is colorful and well planned. There is a column of links on each page that allows the user to move from one topic area to another with minimal difficulty. Education World is easy to use and provides a supportive environment for educators to search and retrieve useful data. The text is presented in English at a simple level.

6. Internet Resources for Nurse Practitioner Students

http://nurseweb.ucsf.edu/www.arwwebpg.htm

This is a list of Web sites compiled to assist NP students but it is also useful for practicing NPs and other APNs. A nursing student at the University of California, San Francisco (UCSF), compiled it. She includes links organized under the following categories: health information gateways, nursing resources, clinical practice guidelines, case studies and interactive tutorials, evidence-based health care, government agencies, and pharmacology. She also includes sections for various specialties including primary care, pediatrics, adolescent health, school-based health, women's health, HIV/AIDS, and complementary and alternative therapy. This site is linked to the UCSF School of Nursing. This is an extremely well developed list of links. Although the site contains little information and has not been updated since July 1999, it is still useful. The site is well organized and contains applicable links. A short description of each link might make this a better site. The site is available in English at a simple level.

7. National Council of State Boards of Nursing (NCSBN)

http://www.ncsbn.org

The National Council has several sites that provide a wealth of information, support, and resources. The National Council of State Boards of

Nursing provides a database that will search one section, the entire site, or the archives within the National Council. The focus is on policy analysis, regulation of nursing practice, and data related to nurse licensure. Information on career opportunities at the NCSBN is also available. The NCSBN also sponsors nclex.com, which provides access to online courses for students, nurses, and educators. Some of the courses are free and others require a fee. There is an online course for test development and item writing for educators and there is a tour of the site before registering. Free study tools and a weekly practice question are also provided. These two sites are clearly written and sufficiently narrow in scope. There are no advertisements and the arrangement of the text is easy to read. The announcement section is up to date and provides relevant information. This is a free site with a registration area for members. A good portion of the site's content is only available to members. Text is provided in English at an average level.

8.   National League for Nursing (NLN)

http://www.nln.org

This site contains information on NLN membership, organizational goals, accreditation, testing services, and publications. Additionally, there are sections on job opportunities, references, councils, current events, and the NLN journal *Nursing Education Perspectives*. The left side of the home page features the main sections of the Web site and the mechanism to subscribe to the free NLN update and CEO e-mail letter. The center section contains highlights of new events in a variety of NLN-related areas. Highlights of new NLN initiatives include the faculty development institutes, online courses, and a certification program for nurse educators, which is a strategic alliance with Indiana University School of Nursing. The right-hand side includes information on the Annual Education Summit and the NLN mission statement. The "about NLN" section contains information on the organization, members, constituent leagues, accreditation and testing, a health care information resource section, and information on the Community Health Accreditation Program, Inc. (CHAP). The "membership" section contains information on the mission and goals of the organization, strategic directions, opportunities for members, and membership categories including cost. The Council for Constituent Leagues describes the purpose, functions, goals, and objectives of the constituent leagues. The NLN Web site is well organized and easy to navigate. Descriptions of the different programs and services are clearly articulated in the text. Overall, this is a very good Web site. Text is provided in English at an average level.

9. National Student Nurses Association (NSNA)

http://www.nsna.org

NSNA is the national organization for undergraduate nursing students. Thomson-Delmar Learning sponsors the site. Information is provided on membership, the annual convention, careers in nursing, publications, news, ways to be involved, and faculty consultants. The faculty consultant section contains information on student recruitment (including a video and pamphlets), handouts from previous conventions, and a code of academic and clinical conduct. The "get involved" section includes links to local chapters, call for convention posters, and information on the roles and responsibilities of elected NSNA officials. Overall, this is a great site for undergraduate students with some useful resources for faculty. The site is presented at an average level in English. Navigation is easy.

Chapter 8

Returning to School:
Graduate School Resources

Maria Donovan Fitzpatrick and Joyce J. Fitzpatrick

The Internet is a valuable resource for those who wish to pursue additional education, including many opportunities for e-learning and many other variations of Web-based or Web-enhanced programs. The sites below are organized into two separate categories. First, the best general sites were selected, including those that have basic information on undergraduate and graduate programs in nursing and other professional and academic disciplines. These include sites offered through leading educational information companies such as Peterson's, which produces the Peterson Guide, and U.S. News and World Report, which is well-known for its annual rankings of colleges and universities. The second set of sites includes those that are related to graduate school but are not sites that include discipline-specific program descriptions. Rather, they are sites that provide information about testing, such as the Graduate Record Examination and Miller's Analogy Test, both of which are frequently required for graduate school admission, and financial aid resources. The sites are presented alphabetically within these two subcategories.

1. Graduate Schools

http://www.gradschools.com

This Web site includes over 50,000 graduate program listings in nursing (including midwifery) and other disciplines. It has links to most of the schools included in the directories. One of the special features of the Web site is that it offers information on a broad range of schools in other countries, including programs in Canada, Europe, Japan, Australia, and New Zealand. It also contains links on how to register to be recruited to one of the nursing programs, an online graduate school fair, and certificate programs in a range of subject areas. There is a discussion/chat room, open 24 hours 7 days per week, free to potential students and recruiters. This site is a little less glamorous than other graduate school Web sites, but useful just the same. Although it offers details about schools in other countries, these international listings are limited and the content is in English only.

2. Peterson's

http://www.petersons.com

Peterson's, owned by Thompson Learning, offers information about graduate programs in nursing as well as programs in other disciplines. Thus, nurses interested in graduate school in a wide range of disciplines will find this site useful. In addition to the basic information about career opportunities through graduate degrees, several other categories are included on this Web site, such as financing one's education, distance learning, career guidance, summer opportunities, and study abroad. The site includes a list of about 100 schools that have provided links and detailed information about their nursing programs. (There is, of course, variation in the level of detail provided by each school, as Peterson's does not control the information provided through these independent resources, but only provides the link.) There are also links to financial aid information ($4 billion worth) and opportunities for distance learners as well as a chance to glean advice from college graduates. Major strengths of this site are that it is straightforward and easy to navigate and includes a wealth of information regarding financial aid. The content is more focused on undergraduate study, but there is still plenty of information for students interested in graduate programs in nursing and other disciplines. Content is only offered in English.

3. U.S. News and World Report

http://www.usnews.com

This Web site is sponsored by *U.S. News and World Report*, a magazine owned by Mortimer B. Zuckerman. Since 1983, *U.S. News and World Report* magazine had conducted rankings of colleges and universities. Since 1995 these rankings have been posted on the Web site. Included are rankings of America's Best Nursing Schools and America's Best Hospitals. In addition the rankings of the top ten specialty programs in nurse midwifery, nurse anesthesia, and several nurse practitioner program specialties (gerontology, primary care, family, pediatric nursing) are included. The *U.S. News and World Report* Web site also provides links to the Web pages of the schools and hospitals as well as helpful articles pertaining to the graduate school process. For those interested in distance education, rankings of the best online graduate degree programs are provided. And, for those who are not yet certain of the focus they want to pursue in graduate school, a Career Guide is provided. Several other interactive directories are easy to access from this *U.S. News and World Report* Web site, notably a link to over 600,000 scholarship listings and a College Step-by-Step guide. For nurses pursuing the undergraduate degree there are several useful linkages through this comprehensive Web site. The directories included here are colleges (over 1400 schools), graduate schools (over 1000 programs), community colleges (over 1200 colleges), Internet courses and degrees (over 1000 institutions), and corporate e-learning opportunities (over 600 providers). One of the major advantages of this Web site is the fact that the programs in a range of disciplines are included; nursing is just one of the many graduate degrees that the professional nurse can pursue. The strengths of this Web site are its plethora of content, the ease of navigation, and the accuracy and inclusiveness of the information. There are no major weaknesses and the site is only available in English.

4. Financial Aid

http://www.finaid.org

This site includes information on many types of financial aid, from the traditional sources such as scholarships and loans to more innovative funding sources, including military sources of support, scholarship lotteries, student profile-based aid, aid for specific activities, and college-controlled aid. Sources of federal and state government support are included as well as specific aid programs for graduate and professional schools such as nursing and health professions schools. The site includes many subcategories so that the reader can target aid to both their own background and their future career interests. Contests that offer the winners financial support are included as is information related to sports and student athlete scholarship and aid. There is a section that lists sources of support for domestic exchange programs and study abroad programs. This site includes a great deal of information; it is a comprehensive report of financial resources for the potential graduate student. It is easy to navigate, but is dense in the content. Much detail is included. There are links to financial aid applications and a guide to calculating the expenses associated with graduate school. Thus, the reader is able to project his or her own financial need and eligibility for scholarships and loans. The site is in English only.

5. Graduate Record Examination

http://www.gre.org

This site includes a wide range of information about the GRE (Graduate Record Exam) which is an exam sponsored by the Educational Testing Service (ETS). Included on the site is information pertaining to exam content, including practice software and practice tests. There is a link to test registration online and a diagnostic service to determine one's general test skills. Anyone who has not previously taken any standardized tests for entrance to college or universities should review this site. It is important that potential GRE applicants know that at this time the test is only offered on the computer. One has to go to an authorized test site. The benefit of this computerized testing is that you can take the test at any time (there are not designated days) but this may present a challenge to those not oriented to computerized testing. There also is a link to graduate schools from this GRE Web site. The site offers advice on preparing for the test as well as information about interpreting your scores. This a comprehensive Web site, user-friendly and accurate in the information provided. The GRE is only offered in English, and this Web site is in English only.

6. Kaplan Educational Centers

http://www.kaplan.com

This site offers courses and services aimed at helping GRE test takers understand the format and structure of the exam in order to help them improve their scores. The courses offered include classroom sessions, online sessions, individual tutoring, books and software as well as international options. This site is owned by Kaplan, a well-known testing service; there is a fee associated with most of the services available through this site. Nursing testing information that is provided includes NCLEX exam information and the CGFNS. Links are provided to career information and products and services such as books and software guides for testing. Test registration links also are available. Kaplan is a recognized name in test preparation and the site is commercial. Nevertheless it offers valuable information for those who are interested in basic orientations to test taking. The site is easy to read and navigate. It is offered in English only.

7. The Psychological Corporation

http://www.tcpweb.com

This site has information about the Miller Analogies Test (MAT), one that is frequently required for admission to graduate programs in nursing. The site is sponsored by The Psychological Corporation (TPC), the oldest commercial test publisher in the world. TPC publishes and therefore controls the MAT. TPC is a subsidiary of Harcourt General, one of the world's leading educational publishers. The site is very straightforward; there is not a great deal of design to the content, rather there is a listing of content areas. These include fees and services, application procedures, guidelines for test taking, scoring information, and score reporting information. In addition, sample analogies are included with annotated answers to familiarize readers with the basic structure of the MAT. There are four appendices, including one with test sites and one that allows the reader to convert the raw score to a percentile score. One of the weaknesses of the site is that there is dense content, rather than content presented in diverse styles. The site is available in English only.

_____ Chapter **9**

Government Resources

Trudy Johnson

_____

G overnment agency Web sites provide the public with access to the work of government agencies and publications related to guidelines, regulations, or laws, and facilitate communication with these agencies and legal bodies. There are numerous government agencies whose primary mission is health related such as the Centers for Disease Control, whereas other agencies include health care as a facet of their work (i.e., Environmental Protection Agency). In addition, agency Web sites offer the public direct access to communicate via e-mail with related agencies or governmental bodies (e.g., House of Representatives, Senate, or the White House).

The publications and documents available provide a wealth of information for the clinician, researcher, administrator, or educator. In the past, access to this information was not always readily known or obtaining copies was not as easy as the current process of logging onto the Internet to print a current guideline or publication. On the other hand, not all information is free since there are costs associated with compiling documents that are long in length for publication on the Web. Rapid, timely access to information facilitates knowledge validation and research of public policy issues.

When nurses are active in public policy, the use of government Web sites is crucial in obtaining the most current information regarding legislation and communicating online with legislators and senators. Additionally, important regulatory information is published on the Web to ensure access to all organizations governed by health care regulations and laws. Often individuals receive notification of updates to important sites via e-mail by subscribing to listservs associated with regulatory or accrediting agencies. When government sites hyperlink to the U.S. Congress it enhances the likelihood that nurses will advocate for consumers by writing via e-mail to congressional representatives or senators regarding their opinions about public health and health policy.

Many search engines lack a specialty heading for *Government.* Yahoo has the best search engine for government. It takes the user to hyperlinks for the branches of government that are subdivided by executive, judicial, and legislative. Another possible selection for hyperlink is by agencies and statistics that facilitate finding government-related health care agencies and data. Yahoo's search engine functions at sufficient speed to satisfy users who frequently conduct database searches. The review of government sites below is in alphabetical order and provides diverse information for many specialties and roles.

*1.   Agency for Health Care Research and Quality (AHRQ)

http://www.ahrq.gov

AHRQ is under the auspices of the Department of Health and Human Services. It is the lead agency that supports research, evidence-based practice, improving quality health care, and reducing the cost of health care. The site is useful for health care professionals and consumers alike. In the past, professionals and consumers requested copies of the clinical practice guidelines by mail or telephone. The 19 AHRQ clinical practice guidelines are now available to download directly from the Web. Consumer and professional versions are available in English and Spanish. Additionally, other online documents include Evidence Reports (e.g., Criteria for Weaning from Mechanical Ventilation) or the Surgeon General's Reports. The design of the homepage readily distinguishes the consumer link, making access to information on dis-

---

*Sites suitable for consumer use.

eases, health plans, wellness, smoking, and surgery easy to retrieve. Consumer information is also available in Spanish. For professionals, some of the benefits of the site include the online guidelines, funding opportunities and research findings, and quality measurement data about health care. The *Quality Assessment* section contains many useful sections for all audiences. The page on "Medical Errors and Patient Safety" includes several guidelines that are readable by consumers and valuable for professional work. The document *Quality of Health Information on the Internet: Enabling Consumers to Tell Fact From Fraud* (*http://ahrq.gov/qual/hiirpt.htm*) is worthwhile for all readers of this book.

2. U.S. Department of Health and Human Services (DHHS)

http://www.dhhs.gov

The Department of Health and Human Services is the principal government agency to promote health and provide human services for all persons. There are a wide array of programs addressing health care research, insurance, and community-based care for all ages of the population. From the *Agencies* link in the left frame of the homepage one can connect to the Web sites for all the agencies under DHHS, including the AHRQ and FDA Web sites that are also reviewed in this chapter. Data and information from the latest headlines to "Fact Sheets on Health" are available from the homepage. The "Get Information" search field at the top of the page allows selections of topics from A–Z (aging to women's health). The *Firstgov* hyperlink on the homepage connects to the *http://firstgov.gov*, a site that has a wealth of information including bioterrorism. The *Health* link takes the user to *http://healthfinder.gov*, a site that includes a health library, directory of important organizations, current health news, and "just for you" guidelines that can be used by consumers or professionals. "Just for you" uniquely focuses on different age groups as well as different social/ethnic groups. This Web site is designed for persons who may have less than a 12th grade education.

*3. Federal Drug Administration

http://www.fda.gov

This site covers all products regulated by the FDA including human drugs, foods, biologics, animal drugs, cosmetics, medical devices, radiation-emitting devices, and related research. The site provides a selection for consumers and professionals that describe what is available on the site. For consumers, there is information about approved drugs and current news related to various health care topics (e.g., HIV, cancer, special populations). The section for professionals provides special alerts for patient safety and online reporting such as MEDWATCH, for medical devices. The *Reference Room* provides useful links to the Federal Register, laws enforced by the FDA, and information on manuals and publications that are produced by the FDA. The drug link from the homepage links to the *Center for Drug Evaluation and Research,* which is equally valuable for consumer drug information and professional use, and includes a valuable page on "medication errors" that links to current reports and articles. MEDWATCH safety alerts are also posted from this page. The material is kept current, making it useful for clinicians who want to implement new devices, and organizations that need information to ensure compliance with the FDA.

*4. Center for Medicare and Medicaid Services (formerly Health Care Financing Administration)

http://www.cms.hhs.gov

This federal agency administers Medicare, Medicaid and the Child Health Insurance Programs and changed the agency's name to the Center for Medicare and Medicaid Services during the 2001 calendar year. The hcfa.gov Web site is still active, however, one can also access *http://cms.hhs.gov*, which brings the user to a different homepage. This page can also be selected from the hcfa.gov homepage. The new *http://cms.hhs.gov* homepage has three distinct selections at the top of the page: for consumers, professionals, and public affairs. CMS serves as the regulatory body to ensure federal laws and regulations related to these programs are appropriately administered by the states. The Web site covers the initiatives related to HIPAA (Health Insurance Portability and Accountability Act) compliance; insurance fraud and abuse; policy updates on Medicare statistics; NEWS on topics such as insurance reform, laws and regulations; and data regarding defined quality indicators. The site is easy to use and will probably change more over the next year as they merge the original hcfa.gov site with the design of the newer CMS.gov site. From the professionals section on the CMS.gov page the *Researchers* selection provides numerous valuable options including the HCFA Newsletter. The newsletter is useful to keep professionals informed of new regulations governing patient care. The *Public Affairs* section is particularly useful to professionals who want to keep current with public testimony, press releases, and fact sheets related to Medicare and Medicaid.

5. Library of Congress

http://www.loc.gov

THOMAS Legislative Information

http://www.thomas.loc.gov

The Library of Congress is the resource for copyright applications, legal documents, and the U.S. Congress. Any entrepreneurial nurse is familiar with the need for copyright protection of unique work. Definition of the different types of copyright is available online and the necessary forms may be downloaded using Adobe Acrobat in PDF format. The most significant benefit of the Library of Congress site is related to public policy advocacy. The *THOMAS Legislative Information* (*http://www.thomas.loc.gov*) provides the headings of *Legislation, Congressional Record*, and *Committee Information. THOMAS* provides links to the text of bills, records of congressional action, committee reports, and roll call from the House and Senate. One can enter a bill number and print out the full text for review and dissemination at professional meetings where health policy and advocacy is discussed. *Bills in the News* on the homepage of *http://www.thomas.loc.gov* is an alphabetical listing that one can easily scroll through and see what is new regarding Medicare or other common topics related to health (e.g., abortion, child health insurance, tobacco).

6. National Archives and Records Administration

http://www.nara.gov

The Federal Register

http://www.nara.gov/fedreg/

The National Archives and Records Administration is not health care specific but anyone interested in related government archives can use this database to locate important government and library materials when interested in public health and health policy. Most valuable of these printed documents is the *Federal Register*. The Office of the Federal Register provides public access to the rules, proposed rules, and notices from federal agencies and organizations. This includes information such as "Conditions of Participation for Medicare" that regulate how health care must be provided for continuing reimbursement as a Medicare provider. The link for the *Federal Register* in the left frame connects to the U.S. Government Printing Office Access site. It allows you to browse the Table of Contents, conduct searches for different years in the database, and select the codes to search (the code for example would be rules, proposed rules, notices, etc.). It is important to complete as much information as possible to narrow the search since this is a large database. The ideal search can be done if you know the actual date of issue. When viewing or printing from the *Federal Register* you can do it in text or PDF (using Adobe Acrobat); it is highly recommended to print the PDF format for briefer documents that are easier to review and share.

7. National Guideline Clearinghouse (NGC)

http://www.guidelines.gov

This is one of the superior compilations of evidence-based literature summaries available. The sponsors are the Agency for Health Care Research and Quality in collaboration with the American Medical Association and the American Association of Health Plans. The intent of this site is to readily provide health care professionals with abstract and summary information of evidence-based clinical practice guidelines. Searching for a topic of interest is simply done by performing a keyword search to compile a list of sources that can be viewed in summary format or complete text. The list of options will meet the broad needs of numerous clinical specialties and the different perspectives for researchers or advanced practice nurses. Every clinical specialty is covered extensively and the site can also be accessed directly from the *http://www.ahcpr.gov* site. Many of the documents on this site are from other health care or professional organizations such as the guideline on Asthma from University of Michigan Health System. Because this site is designed primarily for health care providers, there are hyperlinks provided through the NGC Resources page to *Patient Resources* links. The links are extensive and also provide clinicians with useful materials for patient education.

*8.   National Institutes of Health (NIH)

http://www.nih.gov

A division of the DHHS, the NIH is the United States' government medical research organization. The mission is to uncover new knowledge, through research, that will lead to better health. The NIH supports the work of some 35,000 research projects nationwide, covering the spectrum of diseases. The NIH site has a wealth of general health information clearly linked for consumers and professionals including links for MEDLINE for drug information and the HEALTHFINDER® site previously mentioned under *http://www.dhhs.gov*. Additionally there is information on clinical trials, which is particularly valuable for consumers who may be considering participating in a clinical trial. The *News and Events* is most valuable for professionals who want to remain abreast of information about new funding or research findings. The selection options are extensive on this site and are primarily useful for professionals and highly educated consumers.

Chapter 10

Health Policy

Stephen J. Cavanagh and Barbara K. Redman

The current health care cost crisis, as well as the nursing shortage, are key areas for nurse involvement in health policy. Nurses can be politically active as individuals or through other organizations such as the American Nurses Association or state nurses associations. Additionally, other professional organizations (e.g., National League for Nursing) and Specialty Organizations (e.g., Association for Women's Health, Obstetric, and Neonatal Nurses) provide members with resources to keep abreast of current legislation related to nursing and health care. The sites below provide nurses with information and resources regarding health policy in the United States.

1. American Nurses Association

http://www.ana.org/

This is the home page of the American Nurses Association. The site is primarily aimed at giving professional nurses a simple way of obtaining information about the ANA and to showcase a number of the Association's activities, for example, monitoring health policy as it relates to nurses and detailing a number of ethics and human rights issues such as end-of-life considerations. Professional nurses are the intended primary audience for this site. Information appears to be current in terms of recent legislation. The content also includes debates on current issues such as genetic engineering. Many of the link pages have not been updated for a year. The strength of this site is its concern for workplace issues for nurses. It brings together a great deal of information about staffing issues, health and safety, and collective bargaining policy. The collection of ANA position statements is an important contribution to nursing and health policy. The nursing links section is a very comprehensive collection of further reading and information. Current events and links to journal articles can quickly identify many sources of information. From a policy perspective the intent of the site is to look specifically at nurses and their practices. Health policy encompasses much more than this and global issues are generally not covered by this site. English is the only language available on the site. This site provides an average level of information. Many issues are in a simple and readily available format; other material such as the policy statements offer more substantive reading. The site is easy to navigate through although much of the material is offered in list format that requires extensive scrolling. The electronic links were extant and took the reader to the intended sites; the site has an effective search engine.

2. Duke Health Policy CyberExchange

http://www.hpolicy.duke.edu/cyberexchange/

This site offers an introduction to health policy and a portal to international and national health information sites and specific health policy issues such as health expenditure. The purpose of the site is to disseminate research findings on health policy issues to those who have an interest in, or who are making, health policy decisions. The site is part of Duke University's Center for Health Policy, Law and Management. The site is aimed at an eclectic audience. It contains many areas of relevance to nursing including health promotion and public health. The site contains many recent papers and analyses and appears to be updated on a very regular basis. The most important features of this site are the links provided in the "What's What in Health Policy" section and the content of the "Key Health Policy Issues" pages. From these sections it is very easy to generate many sources of health policy information and quickly find current policy papers on a number of issues relevant to nursing. Many of the policy issues relevant to nursing and nurses must be accessed through the search engine, as there are no direct links to this information. Fortunately, the search facility is simple to use and yields a number of nursing-specific policy issues such as cost-containment. The site is in English only. The information on this site has a high level of content and analysis. Some of the documents are long and some can be downloaded. This is a well-designed site where the links really work. The text is presented in a clear, uncluttered way, making navigation simple. Extensive scrolling is avoided making it easy to click between pages.

3. Electronic Policy Network

http://www.epn.org/

"(The) Electronic Policy Network provides timely information and leading ideas about the policies and politics that shape our world." This site is aimed at offering a quick and accessible look at policy, primarily from the American perspective but includes world issues. EPN's goal is to offer policy analysis to all and to communicate up-to-date information. EPN consists of a consortium of major policy and advocacy groups who want to communicate their ideas to a wider audience in a timely manner. This site has information for almost everyone. Health policy is as major component of EPN. While not addressing nursing specifically, policy related to nursing is well documented. If there is a relevant nursing issue it will be reported. Information is offered on a daily basis and sometimes hour-to-hour reporting. The strengths of this site are its comprehensiveness and timeliness. The reports are well written and concise. There is a health policy section that deals with large-scale issues such as health insurance for the recently unemployed. A comprehensive search facility will identify nursing-specific policy issues. These tend to be related to administrative policies and nursing homes. While this is a quality site, the one noted weak point is that there is insufficient nursing representation. While policy issues related to nursing are present, major policymaking organizations for nursing seem not to be represented (medicine is also excluded). This site would benefit from a greater nursing input. This is an English language only site. This is a high-level site in terms of the content of material and the level of analysis. This is a high-quality site that offers a great deal of information for nurses interested in health policy. The site is well constructed allowing for easy navigation between the many sections of the site. The search facility is excellent and policy updates can be received via e-mail without charge.

4. Health Resources and Services Administration (HRSA)

http://www.hrsa.gov/

This is the home page of the Health Resources and Service Administration for the Department of Health and Human Services. The site aims to document the activities of HRSA and its mission of improving the nation's health by assuring equal access to comprehensive, culturally competent, quality health care for all. The site will be of interest to both professionals and nonprofessionals. There are many health policy issues found on this site relevant to nurses, including Rural Health Policy. The information contained on this site is current and accurate. It appears to be updated on a regular basis. The site contains a wealth of information about health professions, primary health care, maternal and child health initiatives, and rural health issues. There is much on the site related to health policy and regulation that will be of interest to nurses. As with other sites reviewed, the search engine is often the quickest way to access the vast amounts of information available using the appropriate keywords to limit the size of the results. This site offers a simple way of obtaining individual state information through the "State Profiles" links. The policy aspects of HRSA links do not always work. This necessitates the use of the search engine. More policy links would make the site easier to use for those looking for this material. The site is written in English and contains information aimed at many levels. There is an informational level that makes available health information widely accessible, while detailed policy analysis is also presented. The site contains a voluminous amount of information that is relatively easy to navigate through. Some scrolling is required to move from the top to the bottom of the site. The search engine works efficiently, and the links identified were functioning. The site was a 2001 winner of a World Wide Web Health Award.

5. International Council of Nurses (ICN)

http://www.icn.ch/

This site is the home of the International Council of Nurses whose aim is to advance nursing worldwide, to bring nursing together worldwide, and to influence health policy. The site provides detailed information about the ICN organization and its program areas. There are many nursing policies and fact sheets described that give the ICN position on world nursing issues such as tuberculosis and occupational stress. There is a newsroom that provides a source of international policy information relevant to nurses, and a bookshop where publications can be purchased on-line. Nurses are the primary audience. The site is updated regularly and has news events relevant to nursing reported quickly. ICN fact sheets are drawn from current published reports and some ICN policies have been revised recently. Future conference dates are advertised. This site makes available many informative documents and advances a number of key issues for nursing. All are well written and researched. It is the only site that takes a truly global nursing perspective. The content in this site is aimed at large policy issues. It is not the intention to produce country-specific policy, although much is pertinent to all countries, particularly the policy paper on nursing and disaster preparedness and resources for coping with terrorism. Links to French and Spanish translations exist on the home page. Information presented is of high relevance to nursing and of high content quality. This site is a major source of information for all nurses. It is a well-constructed site with navigation buttons to guide the reader. It has a well-functioning search facility as well as FAQ aimed primarily at membership and the workings of the ICN.

*6. Kaisernetwork.org Health Policy As it Happens

http://www.kaisernetwork.org/

This site is primarily concerned with U.S. health policy issues. The site aims to " . . . provide timely, reliable, and non-partisan information on national health issues to policymakers, the media, and the general

---

*Sites suitable for consumer use.

public." The Kaiser Foundation produces and sponsors this site in its entirety. Anyone with an interest in health policy will find this site informative. Nurses will find many of the important health policy issues, such as the nursing shortage, easy to find. The site is very comprehensive and nurses wanting to examine individual state health policy issues can do so. The site is updated on a daily basis. Information is current and timely. Almost all of the major health policy issues are covered. This is a comprehensive site that offers both information and analysis in an accessible way. Nurses will find much of relevance to them on this site. Through features such as AdWatch and e-mailed health policy highlights, nurses can obtain up-to-the hour information. Key policy issues including patient rights, stem cell research, and bioterrorism are discussed. The site would benefit nurses by having specific links to nursing issues. The site is English language only. This site offers a high level of information and analysis making it a good current source of materials for nurses. This is a very good example of what a site should look like. Uncluttered and clear pages are easy to follow. A good search engine and information via e-mail make this is a very friendly site for nurses to use.

7. National Academy for State Health Policy

http://www.nashp.org/

This is the home page of the National Academy for State Health Policy. This site is a vehicle for the dissemination of health policy information to states, as well as offering support in developing " . . . practical and innovative solutions to complex health policy issues." The site is produced by NASHP, whose activities are funded through grants and sponsored projects. The site is aimed at policymakers and users, including governors and state legislators. Nurse practitioners will find the NASHPs work on State Children's Health Program informative. The site provides accurate information but is not intended to present a rapid news reporting service. This site offers information about health policy at the state level. It provides an accurate account of many policy issues and reports a number of surveys from its members, information that is difficult to find from other sources. NASHP could strengthen their site by having a state-by-state breakdown of health policy issues. This would facilitate dissemination of information and research. Absence of a comprehensive search facility can make the site slow to use. Additional information and links would make this site more useful for practitioners and researchers. This is an English-only Web site. This site offers a high level of detailed information making it excellent for research. Many documents can easily be downloaded from the site. The site is relatively small in terms of pages and these are clear to follow and navigate.

8. National Institutes of Health (NIH)

http://www.nih.gov/

This site is the main portal into the activities of the NIH, including research and health policy. This site offers information on the main activities of the NIH, including health information, grants and funding, news and events, scientific resources and information about the individual centers comprising the NIH. This is a Web site supported by the U.S. government. The audience will be anybody interested in research and health policy issues. Nurses will find key sources of information on research and policy. The site is regularly updated and materials are current. The site is the stepping-off point for federally supported research; it's the first port of call for this information. There is, however, much more available on the site than just research. A cursory search of the terms 'health policy' and 'nursing' identified over 1000 information links, mostly directed at research. This site is a major source of policy information for nurses. Health policy and nursing information is accessed primarily through the search engine. As large numbers of 'hits' are produced the advanced search engine must be used. Narrowing down search criteria can be time-consuming but generally yields pertinent information. This is primarily an English language site with information in Spanish accessible from the home page. This is generally a high-level site for information content and discussion. This is a huge site that is relatively easy to navigate through. The design avoids large amounts of scrolling, instead tabs and hot-links are used to move the reader through the content areas.

ACKNOWLEDGEMENT

We acknowledge the assistance of Sam Felarca and Marija Franetovic in the writing of this chapter.

_____ Chapter **11**

Leadership

Sheila C. Grossman

_____

This section highlights current leadership Web sites. All sites provide average- to high-level information in English only. There is a growing demand for all nurses to assume leadership in our roles as staff nurses, nurse managers, administrators, and educators. This chapter guides nurses in identifying resources to improve communication and negotiation skills, vision development and goal planning, adjustment to change, and flexibility to the chaotic times presently facing the health care system. Leadership training is frequently accessed through Human Resource Departments; therefore, some sites may appear, at first sight, not applicable to staff nurses or even nurse managers. However, there are many possibilities that nursing can adapt from leadership training sessions to further leadership development. Nurses generally have complaints about lack of resources and support from administration, problems with role/job description, and general discontent with the health care system and managed care. Increasing one's ability to be creative with new ideas, learning how to empower oneself and others, and learning to take risks to make a significant difference in health care practice and policy development can benefit most of us. Not all nurses are born leaders; however, we can certainly develop our leadership ability.

1. Army Leadership Development

http://www.army.mil

The United States Army (U.S. Army, Army Public Affairs, Washington, D. C. 20310) is responsible for this (last update = 12/18/01) site which includes exciting links to vision development, the idea that people not equipment are the key to a successful army, and examples of real army leaders. There are a multitude of links from this site that could benefit nurses.One especially helpful link is the summary of the army's project regarding leadership development for commissioned officers at *www.army.mill/altd/default.* Although not specifically for nurses or other health care workers, this site provides many helpful suggestions for leadership development of nurses such as a systems approach to training, a training and leader development model, a management protocol, and commitment to lifelong learning. The process by which this project developed is explained and includes how surveys, focus groups, personal interviews, and independent research were used. The idea of self-development and the whole army development is very applicable to the individual nurse and his/her health care organization's development. The Web site includes many excellent suggestions regarding how to incorporate variables influencing an individual's home/ family situation and improving one's performance at the work setting.

2. Center for Creative Leadership

http://www.ccl.org/capabilities

The Center for Creative Leadership identifies leadership development as the basis of organizational success. For greater than thirty years, its purpose has been to assist with expanding the leadership capabilities of individuals and organizations. Its primary purpose is to generate and publish knowledge about leadership and leadership development. The Center is dedicated to helping people be future-oriented with a focus on thinking differently than ever before and maximizing communication between all workforces of an organization. A variety of leadership development strategies are offered via workshops, journal articles, and conferences (every year greater than 20,000 people attend training conferences). It is considered one of the largest institutions focusing solely on leadership and is ranked #1 by *Business Week*. This site is well maintained and updated.

3. Center for Leadership and Change Management

http://leadership.wharton.upenn.edu

The University of Pennsylvania Wharton School of Business independently manages this site. The purpose of the site is to offer information on leadership and change and to provide ideas on application of these two phenomena. The site links to various resources such as conferences, meetings, program overviews, specific courses, recommended readings, journals, and other Web sites on change and leadership. There is an interesting link to the Wharton Leadership Mentoring Program that presents several founding student organizers of the program who can be accessed for questions about their mentoring experiences with mid-career alumni. Other examples of application of leadership and change can be found in descriptions of student service projects.

4. The Institute for Nursing Healthcare Leadership

http://www.caregroup.org/inhl

The purpose of this site, which is sponsored by Care Group Health System and Harvard Medical School, is to provide a foundation for professional collaboration in addressing the variety of issues challenging today's health care leaders and to advance the leadership role of nurses. The Institute for Nursing Leadership (INL) has three specific programs including the Leadership Assessment and Development Collaborative, the Research Collaborative, and the International Nursing Studies Collaborative. Links to present and past conferences, the academic nursing collaborative, and nursing consortium are available to viewers. Short biographies are presented of the Institute's Resource Team who maintains this site. There are several links to methods of leadership improvement, leadership development, health care delivery system redesign, specialty education, and leadership training for nurses in the international community.

5. Institute for Nursing Leadership (INL)

http://www.nursingworld.org/tan/98julaaug/enhance.htm

In 1996 the American Academy of Nursing and the American Nurses Foundation partnered to develop the INL. Members of the INL represent the American Nurses Association, State Nurse Associations, American Academy of Nursing, American Nurses Foundation, and the health care industry. The general mission is to develop leadership in nurses who have the potential to make significant changes in improving health care in the United States. There are several goals of this institute including the development of plans to implement leadership in nursing curricula, sponsorship of Student Fuld Fellowships, a selective program for undergraduate student nurse leaders, and funding for individual School of Nursing leadership development programs. Another major goal of the institute includes supporting the American Association of Colleges of Nursing (AACN) Leadership for Academic Nursing Programs, which is a development program for Deans and Deans-to-Be of Schools of Nursing. The site provides a detailed explanation of each program, the application process, and information to assist nurses in applying to the programs. Multiple links can be accessed regarding current student fellow activities, descriptions of various funded projects, and some of the planned leadership modules that are to be implemented in nursing curricula. These modules include systems analysis, risk-taking, conflict resolution, consensus building, and advocacy.

6. National Student Nurses Association Leadership University Facilities

http://www.NSNA.leadrshipu.org/library.htm

This site is a link from the NSNA home page and offers excellent resources that are accessible by the Internet. There are approximately one hundred Web sites to assist nurses and student nurses to retrieve information on change, professional topics, conflict management, further education, vision building, goal planning, decision making, and staffing. There are a variety of student and faculty lounges, such as an international lounge and a mentor lounge, available to NSNA members to have discussions on the topic of leadership. There is also a comprehensive listing of Attributes and Competencies Needed by Future Nurse Leaders and Managers that could be helpful to all nurses.

7. Nursing Leadership Forum

http://www.springerjournals.com/nlf/home.htm

This is home page for the journal *Nursing Leadership Forum.* Table of Contents of the journal from 1999 to present can be accessed directly from this site. One can also do an author or subject search for work that has been published in the journal. Volume number and issue are identified for the desired work. Just from reading several of the Tables of Contents it is easy to realize the journal is designed for all types of nurses practicing leadership in all settings. Each issue also has book reviews. In addition, the journal presents a point/counterpoint column in which nursing leaders dialogue regarding timely topics. These discussions are also noted on the site. Author guidelines are available for nurses interested in submitting a manuscript. Subscriptions to the journal may also be purchased online through this site. Harriet Feldman, PhD, RN, FAAN, is the current editor of this journal. The editorial board is comprised of many nursing leaders.

8. Robert Wood Johnson Executive Nurse Leadership Program

http://www.futurehealth.ucsf.edu/rwj.html

This Executive Nurse Fellows Program is sponsored by the Robert Wood Johnson Foundation (RWJF) and directed by Marilyn Chow, DNSc, RN, FAAN, at the Center for the Health Professions at the University of California at San Francisco. All information needed to apply for a fellowship is available at this site. The Executive Nurse Fellows Program focuses on five key leadership competencies that include strategic vision, self-knowledge, risk taking and creativity, interpersonal skills and communication effectiveness, and managing change. The 3-year fellowship involves a core of leadership skills and an individual leadership internship with a senior executive mentor. There is an ongoing group of leader mentors and graduated fellows who are also accessible through this Center via e-mail. Community leadership projects are also funded through the center. The site has multiple links to access proposal applications, determine eligibility, review the proposal process, assess priority funding areas, view frequently asked questions about writing a proposal, and budget guidelines. One can download the Budget Preparation Guideline to assist in preparation of a proposal.

9. Sigma Theta Tau International Leadership Institute

http://www.nursingsociety.org/programs/chiron.html

This link from the home Web site for Sigma Theta Tau International (STTI) describes the Leadership Institute program The Mentor-Fellow Forum called Chiron. (This was originally the Externship Program.) This program offers all active STTI members who are accepted into Chiron an individualized leadership development program. Members may participate in the program as an applicant or mentor. All information regarding the application process, financial resources needed to participate, and the Chiron application is accessible from this site. The STTI Leadership Institute provides opportunity to ask questions regarding the program via an e-mail address. Members from all countries are encouraged to apply, however, strong skills in written and spoken English are required. Each year the Institute offers a mid-year retreat for all Chiron members.
for #9.

_____ Chapter **12**

Nursing Outcomes

Gail L. Ingersoll

_____

W eb-based information concerning the measurement of nursing outcomes is limited. Most Web sites include descriptions of specific activities at local institutions or publications available for purchase. Although several of these provide useful program-specific content, the focus of this chapter is on the identification of sites that contain general discussions of nursing outcomes measurement issues and options for assessment of care delivery outcome.

1. Agency for Healthcare Research and Quality (AHRQ)

http://www.ahrq.gov

The Agency for Healthcare Research and Quality (AHRQ) is the Department of Health and Human Services' primary source for information about research concerning quality of health care and care delivery outcome. The site is targeted for consumers of health care, researchers, and practitioners, although most discussions and listings are of principal interest to researchers and others interested in recently completed, current, or planned research activities. The Web site is comprehensive and consistent with each of the Web sites developed by the federal government. It contains information about the agency's mission and strategic plan and a listing of all currently funded research. It also contains links to descriptions of funding opportunities related to care delivery outcomes and identifies contact persons for individuals interested in submitting outcomes research proposals. An online newsletter provides up-to-date information about recent research findings and information about topics of interest. Several content-specific links are included that facilitate easy access to some of the more common areas of outcomes research.

This site is highly useful for researchers and others interested in outcomes research. It may be somewhat less helpful for clinicians looking for broad discussions of care delivery outcomes and may be overlooked because of its stated focus on the study of health care quality. Reports of completed research, however, are beneficial to all.

2. Center for Clinical Informatics

http://www.clinical-informatics.com/jlarc

Contained at this Web site is a report prepared for the Joint Legislative Audit and Review Committee of the Washington State Legislature (Brown, Burlingame, & Lambert, 2001). This report summarizes findings of performance assessment methods used by managed care companies and state mental health authorities. It also identifies additional sources for information concerning recommended mental health care delivery outcomes. The authors of the report summarize the indicators most commonly used to assess care delivery outcomes across study sites. They also identify a set of collateral outcomes, which they describe as beneficial to consumers and society, but which are rarely investigated in studies of mental health services. Included in the report is a review of the instruments used to measure clinical outcomes and a discussion of the strengths and limitations of each. The information contained in this report is useful for researchers, quality improvement specialists, administrators, and others interested in the outcomes of mental health services. The information contained in the report, although targeted at mental health services, has relevance to a broader population of care providers. Moreover, the outcome indicators assessed in this study are consistent with those recommended by the Joint Commission on Accreditation of Healthcare Organizations (JCAHO), making the information useful for persons interested in determining the potential usefulness of these proposed indicators.

Locating the report is not always easy to do, although it does appear in general Web searches using readily available search engines. The document is in English and may be most useful for readers with an understanding of outcomes measurement data analysis techniques. Nonetheless, several of the segments of the report are of benefit to a broader audience and merit consideration by policymakers, clinicians, and researchers alike.

3. Centers for Medicare and Medicaid Services (CMA) formerly Health Care Financing Administration (HCFA)

http://cms.hhs.gov/

Available at this site is a comprehensive report of a study of the effect of staffing ratios on care delivery outcome (*Report to Congress: Appropriateness of minimum nurse staffing ratios in nursing homes*). Although targeted to long-term care facilities, the information provided has relevance for a broader audience of investigators, clinicians, and policymakers. The report begins with an overview of the ways in which public policy influences staffing decisions in long-term care. It continues with a review of current staffing patterns and stakeholder perceptions about what constitutes adequate staffing. A review of selected studies pertaining to staffing in long-term care is included, followed by a report of the investigation and its findings. The investigators used three approaches to determine the critical staffing threshold required for satisfactory care delivery outcome. First, they reviewed existing studies and reports of national experts. Next, they developed explanatory models based on a representative sample of nursing homes and using variables hypothesized to influence care delivery outcomes. Finally, they conducted a time and motion study of nursing time required to complete the tasks required for quality care to long-term residents. The investigators found a relationship between minimum acceptable staffing ratios and adverse effect on care delivery outcome. They also reported a clear distinction between a preferred minimum and an absolute minimum.

In the preferred minimum, quality of care improved consistently across all measures. The material contained in this Web site provides useful information from a policy, research, and care delivery perspective. The report is easily accessible, broken down into readily identifiable components, and is summarized in a reasonably informative executive summary. The principal limitation of the summary is its overly brief review of study findings, although notations are included that highlight where the information is contained in the full report.

4. Cochrane Database of Systematic Reviews

http://www.update-software.com/Cochrane/default.htm

The Cochrane Database contains a notable collection of reports of comprehensive reviews of the published research literature. The Web site is expanded and updated as new reviews are submitted and approved for inclusion and as previous submissions are revised to incorporate newly published research findings. The principal limitation of the site is its focus on randomized clinical trials and its consequent exclusion of many important studies relevant to nursing practice. In addition, the focus of the reviews is on care delivery outcomes in general, which may or may not be specific to nursing interventions. The measures used to assess outcomes also may not be sensitive to nursing intervention impact. Nurse clinicians, researchers, and educators using the Cochrane Library will need to supplement their reviews with searches of other electronic reference databases. Nevertheless, the reviews contained on the Cochrane Library Web site can be considered an initial step in the search for evidence concerning the measurement of care delivery outcome.

Examples of outcomes-related topics covered in the Cochrane Database include two reviews by Zwarenstein and colleagues—one that has been completed and updated and one that is planned for completion. The first review pertains to the effect of interprofessional education on professional practice and health care outcomes (Zwarenstein et al., 2001); the second addresses the effect of case management on professional practice and health care outcomes (Zwarenstein, Stephenson, & Johnston, 2001). In the first review, nurse care providers are included with other disciplines. Because of the stringent study inclusion criteria, however, none of the studies identified (nursing, medicine or otherwise) were included in the evidence-based review. As a result, the information provided is limited, although reflective of some of the methodologic concerns associated with the investigation of care delivery outcomes.

The second review (Zwarenstein, Stephenson, & Johnston, 2001) is ongoing and also will include studies in which nurses are members of case management teams. Once again, however, the inclusion criteria seriously interfere with the achievement of an understanding of the state of the science concerning nursing care delivery outcomes.

Access to the Cochrane Library is available through university and public libraries. Individuals may obtain Internet or CD-ROM access through paid subscriptions. Information about the cost of subscriptions is available on the update-software Web site.

5.   Division of Nursing, Health Resources and Services Administration

http://www.bhpr.hrsa.gov/dn

Contained in the Division of Nursing's homepage is a report of the impact of hospital nurse staffing on patient outcomes (Needleman, Buerhaus, Mattke, Stewart, & Zelevinsky, 2001). This report provides information relevant to administrators, policymakers, and researchers interested in the effect of nurse staffing ratios on care delivery outcomes. The report contains an executive summary and a comprehensive review of the study, its background, measurement indices, findings, and conclusions.

Three sources of patient discharge and hospital staffing or financial reports were used to determine the effect of nurse staffing ratios on outcome indicators identified by a panel of experts. Patient-related and hospital-related variables likely to influence care delivery outcome were considered during outcome analysis procedures. Significant relationships were noted between nurse staffing ratios and several patient outcomes. Differences were noted for outcomes associated with medical and major surgical patients. The report contained at this Web site is comprehensive and easily accessible. The authors have defined outcome measures clearly and provided ample information about the methods used to collect data and how the data were analyzed. The results have relevance to administrators, researchers, and policymakers and provide preliminary information about possible nurse-sensitive measures of care delivery outcomes.

6. Medical Outcomes Trust

http://www.outcomes-trust.org/instruments.htm

The Medical Outcomes Trust is a nonprofit organization that focuses on facilitating and improving the measurement of care delivery outcomes. A variety of publications are available for purchase through the Trust's homepage. In addition, a useful section of this Web site is its listing of the instruments the Trust has approved for the measurement of care delivery outcome. Some of the instruments are available at no cost to investigators, while others require payment of a fee prior to use. A brief description of each of the instruments is included. Information about any costs associated is noted, although the ease of obtaining this information varies somewhat across descriptions. Instruments included on the Web site address both generic and condition-specific outcomes. The descriptions contain a brief overview of the purpose of the measure and what is contained in the instrument package. A section pertaining to frequently asked questions also is available for each scale. All of the instruments are available in English. Some are available in other languages as well. The information in the section pertaining to approved outcomes measurement instruments is brief and useful for an initial assessment of some of the measures available to assess nursing outcomes. Some of the instruments have been used regularly in nursing research (e.g., Sickness Impact Profile [SIP], SF-36 Health Survey) and some have not. As with most existing outcomes measurement instruments, the scales included were not designed for assessment of nursing care delivery impact. Consequently, their sensitivity to nursing interventions is not specifically mentioned nor understood. This Web site has a limited amount of information available to nurses interested in measuring care delivery outcome. The instruments listed on the site, however, provide an initial exposure to some of the measures used to assess care delivery impact.

7. National Institute of Nursing Research (NINR)

http://www.nih.gov/ninr

This Web site contains the most comprehensive review of nursing outcomes issues and measurement concerns to date (*Patient outcomes research: Examining the effectiveness of nursing practice*). The principal limitation to the material included on this Web site is its timeliness, as the documents provided are over 10 years old. Even so, the breadth of the content warrants its identification as a foundational source for nursing outcomes information. This Web site contains 20 papers presented at a national conference designed to examine the state of the science and the research needed to enhance care delivery outcomes (National Center for Nursing Research, 1991). The authors of the papers discuss the importance of outcomes research in the documentation of nursing impact. They also propose several methods for integrating nursing outcomes assessment into the larger realm of outcomes research and identify outcomes reflective of clinical practice and a strategy for defining and classifying nursing interventions. Other papers describe patient, family, and contextual factors that influence care delivery outcomes and highlight methods and data sources available for measuring each.

The National Institute of Nursing Research (NINR) developed this Web site as part of its mission to disseminate state of the science information to researchers, practitioners, students, and others interested in the investigation of nursing issues. The site is available in English and is relatively easy to access. It is referenced in several World Wide Web search engines and is retrievable through the NINR's homepage. The level of information contained in this site is high and developed by some of the nation's leading experts in the measurement of nursing outcomes. Because hard copy publications of the papers included in this Web site are no longer available, this is the sole site for access to this information.

REFERENCES

Brown, J., Burlingame, G., & Lambert, M. (2001). *Behavioral healthcare performance and outcomes management: A survey of best practices.* Available at *http://www.clinical-information.com/jlarc/Review% 20of%20best%20practices.pdf.* Accessed 12/24/01.

Feuerberg, M. (2000). *Report to Congress: Appropriateness of minimum nurse staffing ratios in nursing homes.* Available at *http://www.hcfa.gov/ medicaid/reports/rp700hmp.htm.* Accessed 12/19/01.

Needleman, J., Buerhaus, P. I., Mattke, S., Stewart, M., & Zelevinsky, K. (2001). *Nurse staffing and patient outcomes in hospitals.* Available at *http://www.bhpr.hrsa.gov/dn/staffstudy.htm.* Accessed 12/24/01.

National Center for Nursing Research. (1991). *Patient outcomes research: Examining the effectiveness of nursing practice.* Available at *http:// www.nih.gov/ninr/news-info/pubs/porcontents.htm.* Accessed 12/19/01.

Zwarenstein, M., Stephenson, B., & Johnston, L. (2001). Case management: Effects on professional practice and health care outcomes [Protocol]. *The Cochrane Library, 4.* Accessed 12/19/01.

Zwarenstein, M., Reeves, S., Barr, H., Hammick, M., Koppel, I., & Atkins, J. (2001). Interprofessional education: Effects on professional practice and health care outcomes (Cochrane Review). *The Cochrane Library, 4.* Accessed 12/19/01.

_____ Chapter **13**

Research and Grant Resources

Kristen S. Montgomery

_____

This section highlights research and grant-related resource Web
sites for nurses. With an ever-increasing emphasis on evidence-
based practice and outcomes, this section provides a guide for
nurses to begin research projects and implement current findings into
their practice. Additionally, these sites provide services to help the
nurse researcher at every step along the way. An important step in a
research project is obtaining funding for the research. The sites listed
represent the best sites to help one achieve this ambitious goal.

1. American Nurses Foundation (ANF) Research Grants Program

http://www.ana.org/anf/inc/index.htm

ANF is the national philanthropic organization that promotes the continued growth and development of nurses and services to advance the
work of the nursing profession. The American Nurses Association sponsors the site. The most significant feature of this site is the information

on the research grants program offered by ANF. Research grants are available in a variety of areas for both new and experienced researchers. Applications are available in January for a May 1 submission date. Candidates are notified of awards on October 1. Application packets can be downloaded from this site. Additional information is provided on the mission of ANF, its history, board of directors, and staff. The site is simple to use and organized in a clear manner. Text is provided in English at an average level.

2. Canadian-International Nurse Researcher Database

http://www.nurseresearcher.com

This database is a free, must-register service sponsored by the support of individuals and organizations through outright donations; it is not sponsored by any professional organization. This is a large interactive database linking the user with resources and contact information to help with the research process. Services include assistance with methodology problems, locating expert reviewers (both editorial and grant format), research networks, expert clinicians, and consultation to policymakers who want to make evidence-based decisions. The Web site is also available in French, and one has the opportunity to create a personal profile to be added to the database. The Canadian-International Nurse Research Database represents an excellent idea and service for the advancement of nursing research worldwide. However, the mechanism for searching is overcomplicated and difficult to understand without a considerable amount of reading and trial and error. Help pages are offered. Once you get to the actual information, the content is quite helpful. The "About CRND" section is quite comprehensive and informative. Included in this section are frequently asked questions, objectives of the organization, and background information on how the organization was started. Text is provided at an average to high level.

3. The Midwest Nursing Research Society (MNRS)

http://www.mnrs.org

The Midwest Nursing Research Society is a membership organization that promotes the conduct of nursing research in the region and facilitates networking among nurse researchers. The site features the benefits of membership and information on the annual conference. Also included is information on publications, officers, governing board, committee membership, and research and grants information. The homepage also contains contact information for the current president and the executive director of MNRS. The MNRS Web site is colorful and easy to use. The main categories of the site are all clearly listed on the homepage. Text is presented at a simple level in English.

4.　National Institute of Nursing Research (NINR)

http://www.nih.gov/ninr

The National Institute of Nursing Research (NINR) is the nursing research section of the National Institutes of Health (NIH). The site contains general information on NINR funding and activities and events sponsored by the Institute. Descriptions of different types of NINR-funded awards and who to contact within the Institute are also available. The site includes the history of the NINR, employment opportunities (both NINR and NIH), conferences, publications, speeches, a legislative activities section, and information on grants and funding. The "Research Program" section also includes separate sections for intramural and extramural research. The "Extramural" section includes links to the NIH, including training opportunities, CRISP (Computer Retrieval of Information on Scientific Projects—a searchable database of biomedical research projects funded by NIH) and NIH Grants Information, and Guide to Grants and Contracts. There is a small section on the collaborative activities between NINR and NIH. The application process is described along with current funded NINR grants, care centers, and institutional training programs. The NINR Web page also features areas of research opportunity for future fiscal years. The "Scientific Advances" section features highlights and outcomes of current nursing research and health information. The NINR Web page also features the strategic plan, with a mechanism to provide feedback to the NINR director. The NINR Web page is comprehensive, well organized, and easy to navigate. The color scheme enhances ease of use and organization. The text provides clear, succinct information at an average to high level in English.

5. Research! America

http://www.researchamerica.org

Research! America's mission is to make medical and health research a much higher national priority. It is a national nonprofit, membership-supported, public education and advocacy alliance, founded in 1989. The Web site provides general health research information for nurses, physicians, and other health care providers. Highlights include legislative links and an advocacy center. The homepage features a brief description of the organization's mission, links for Research! America's polls, goals and initiatives of the organization, facts on medical research, and newsworthy events. The "Get Involved" section features information on how to contact Congress, including talking points and a mechanism to send a message to congress via e-mail; and the "Legislative Branch" section includes a mechanism to search for one's congressional representative by zip code. The "Executive and Judiciary Branch" section focuses on links to departments and agencies, and to searching the status of federal bills. There is also an option to search for information on federal bills by certain categories, for example, AIDS-related bills. Letter drafts, e-mail postcards, and a "Why Me?" section are also included. The "Medical Links" section is sorted by federal agencies, councils/think tanks, medical/science education, science policy, and international health policy. Lastly, there is a members only section that is password protected. A site map is also available.

Colors on the site are well coordinated and feature red, white, and blue. Navigation through the site is easy. The design and layout of the site have been updated since the previous edition of this book. Text is presented at an average level in English.

6. Royal College of Nursing's Research and Development Co-ordinating Centre

http://www.man.ac.uk/rcn

The Royal College of Nursing is the professional organization representing individual nurses in the United Kingdom. The RCN Research and Development Co-ordinating Centre houses the RCN Research Society, which has 11,500 members. One can link to a wide variety of different databases, including academic departments within the UK that offer a health-related course; the British Nursing Index which contains references to over 220 nursing and allied health journals; cancer registries for Northern Ireland, East Anglia, Trent, Yorkshire, Europe, and International; CHAIN-Contact, Help, Advice and Information Network for evidence-based health care; CINAHL; The Cochrane Collection; English National Board for Nursing, Midwifery, and Health Visiting; European Database on AIDS; evidence-based health resources; online nursing research journals; MEDLINE; National Co-ordinating Centre for Health Technology Assessment; National Research Registrar; National Health Services (NHS) Research and Development Outputs Database; RCN Library and Information Services Online Database; RD Info, a digest of health-related funding opportunities; and REGARD—a searchable bibliographic database funded by the Economic and Social Research Council (ESRC). This is a fully interactive Web site. Job listings are also available. The RCN Research and Development Co-ordinating Centre provides high-quality information for nurses interested in the specific areas of expertise that are offered. While the information is good, the organization could be improved. As it stands, the information is somewhat disjointed. Text is provided in English at an average level.

7. The Royal Windsor Society for Nursing Research

http://www.windsor.igs.net/~nhodgins

The society is a nonprofit association of nurse researchers living throughout the world and sharing an interest in nursing research; membership is free. This group is an Internet-based group, not related to any other professional nursing organization. The Web site contains information on nursing research conferences, centers of excellence, and international research institutions. In addition, the "Research Retrospective" section contains reports from history (such as "Childbed Fever in 19th Century Vienna"). There are also online workshops on topics such as literature search; and study design, analysis, reliability, and validity; with links to dictionaries (both multilingual and crosslingual). There is a section titled "Considerations in Study Design" which includes sections on informed consent, treatment of gender groups, self-reporting, and much more. Finally, there is a nurse-to-nurse section that includes an online journal club with virtual peer review, news-groups, and classified announcements. In the fun and games section, there is an opportunity to play Research Jeopardy. The Royal Windsor Society for Nursing Research Web site is well organized and colorful. The main sections are listed on the home page. The site offers many opportunities for discovering information. Text is provided at an average level in English.

8. Southern Nursing Research Society (SNRS)

http://www.snrs.org

The Southern Nursing Research Society Web site details resources that are available in the southern United States and includes information on membership in the society. The site also provides information on employment and training opportunities and the annual conference. You must be a member to access the research interest groups, *Southern Online Journal of Nursing Research,* newsletters, abstracts, and the membership directory. Overall, this is a very good site. All information is categorized on the homepage for easy access. Organization is logical and clear. The site is in color, easy to navigate, and presented at an average level in English.

9. World Wide Nurse: Nursing Research Funding

http://www.wwnurse.com/nursing/research-funding.shtml

Highlights of the World Wide Nurse: Nursing Research Funding infor-mation Web page include a list of funding/grant resources with links to their respective pages, and a free nursing research chat room. A brief description of each section is provided. The Foundation Center, funding information from the Bureau of Health Professions' Grant Files, a Funding Opportunities Database, grant and contact information from the NIH, the Fulbright Scholar Program, and the Robert Wood Johnson Foundation are featured. Advertising supports World Wide Nurse. Brian Short, a nurse based in Minnesota, produces it. Overall, this is a helpful

Web site. The list of resources and the brief descriptions that accompany them are useful. Additionally, all of the information is provided in one location, which facilitates timely access. There is no apparent order to the listings, however. Also, the site features some blinking advertisements that are distracting.

_____ Chapter **14**

Nursing Theory

Lucinda Farina and Joyce J. Fitzpatrick

N ursing theory is an integral part of the development of the scientific enterprise. Nursing theory is used as a guide to education, practice, and research. There are three basic levels of theory addressed in the nursing literature: grand, middle range, and practice level. Grand theory articulates the philosophical beliefs and goals of the profession; middle range theory includes testable hypotheses; practice level theory addresses practice issues and, through an inductive process, builds theory. As practicing nurses search for understanding of why we do what we do as nurses, nursing theory offers explanation and definition of who we are and what we do. Yet, there are few Web sites that detail specific nursing theories; most of the Web sites available are devoted to grand theories.

The Web sites chosen for review were selected for their potential to assist the practicing nurse in identifying nursing theories, including middle range and grand theories. Two of the reviewed Web sites have a link that details how to conduct a literature search for middle range theory specific to a practice issue. Additionally, two theory sites, one grand theory and one middle range theory, both of which provide an excellent example of nursing theory Web pages, are included in this review.

1. The Comfort Line

http://www.uakron.edu/comfort/

This seven page Web site is devoted to describing and explaining middle range theory developed by Kathy Kolcaba, PhD, RN, C, nursing faculty at the University of Akron. The Comfort Theory and its use for practice and research are well articulated and diagrammed for professional caregivers and researchers. Health care administrators will be interested in how the Comfort Theory impacts institutional integrity. Dr. Kolcaba's telephone number and e-mail address are listed on the Web page and interested parties are encouraged to contact her with questions for either practice or research. Kolcaba has created sections within the Web page to address specific application of the Comfort Theory to practice and to research. The research instrument, the General Comfort Questionnaire, is included on the Web page. References are provided to Kolcaba's work and to pertinent works of other authors. The section on development of the Comfort Theory discusses the grand theories that guided the development of the theory. Easy to navigate, recently updated and available in English only, this Web site is an excellent source for nurses learning to build middle range theory because the process of theory building is clearly modeled.

2. Nursing Around the World

http://world-nurse.com/
http://world-nurse.com/Nursing_Resources/Nursing_Theory

Nursing Around the World is a Danish Web site begun in 1996 by nurse Jim Carlson as an effort to assist Danish nurses in using online resources. The site has developed into an international Web site devoted to encouraging the exchange of knowledge internationally with the goal of supporting the work of caregivers. The site's database contains 885 links to a broad variety of nursing topics. The topic of Nursing Theory is located under Nursing Resources. Within the page are links to 11 U.S. contemporary theorists, 1 British theorist, and Nightingale's model of nursing. There is also a link to nursenet, a global forum for nursing issues, and a Web site devoted to philosophical ideas of energy, health, and healing. The Nursing Theory page provides a list of theorists and their links; it does not attempt to describe or discuss the theories themselves. Available in English only, the site has been recently updated, is easy to navigate, and includes links to emerging nursing theorists who may not yet be well-known, as well as to some of the grand theorists, who are well-known. One unique feature of the site is the opportunity for site visitors to provide feedback ranking the usefulness of each of the individual linked sites. This site provides a starting point for nurses interested in exploring nursing theories or in locating a particular theorist.

3. NurseScribe

http://www.enursescribe.com/link.htm

NurseScribe is a Web site providing multiple clinical and professional resources for nurses. A list of twenty contemporary U.S. theorists and Nightingale, and links to sites about their work are included as one of the resources offered. The site, which is maintained by Becky Sisk, PhD, RN, is available in English only. The site has been recently updated, presents information clearly, and is easy to navigate. Most importantly, the links worked when tested. Nurse theorists are categorized clearly according to their theories, and include early nurse theorists, such as Peplau and Henderson, well-known grand theorists, and middle range theorists. Also included are links to university-based theory pages that list nursing theorists and links to individual Web pages.

4. Nursing Theory Link Page

http://healthsci.clayton.edu/eichelberger/nursing.htm

This Web site began as a student effort at Clayton College and State University in 1996. Now maintained by a nursing faculty member, Lisa Eichelberger, DSN, RN, the site presents a list of thirty nursing theorists and the names of their theories. This site does include a few theorists not included in other sites reviewed. The intent of this site is to provide quick access to information with the minimum amount of surfing required. Links provided for theorists vary in content. Only some of the listed theorists have links which provide an overview of their theory, some have links for bibliographical information, tributes of organizations such as Sigma Theta Tau, lists of publications by the theorists, reviews of theory by graduate students, and nursing theory conferences. Also included in this site is a list of nursing theory books maintained by the Transcultural Nursing Society, a link to an article by Margaret Allen that outlines advice for CINAHL and MEDLINE searches for nursing theory information, and a link to electronic nursing resources from the Hardin Library for Health Sciences. This site is available in English only and is easy to navigate. Eichelberger's e-mail address and telephone number are available on the site and site visitors are encouraged to contribute feedback.

5.   The Nursing Theory Page

http://www.ualberta.ca/~jrnorris/nt/theory.html

This site lists 24 nursing theorists and frequently provides multiple links for an individual theorist. Also included on this Web site are links to other nursing theory list sites, nursing theory conferences, literature search tips located under "Dear Student," resources in French and English, and teaching tools. A list of links to related resources includes nursing theorists not included on the main list. Why this distinction has been made is not identified on the Web site. This collaborative effort by an international group was begun in 1996 and identifies itself as always a work in progress. The site is maintained by Judy Norris, PhD, RN, Associate Nursing Professor at the University of Alberta, Canada. Updated in December 2001, this easily navigated site provides access to individual authors via e-mail addresses found under "About this group project." Feedback and contributions by site visitors are encouraged.

6.   Watson's Theory of Human Caring

http://www.uchsc.edu/ctrsinst/chc/index.htm

The purpose of this Web site is to educate nurses and other caregivers about Watson's Theory of Human Caring. The three pages of the Web site are written by Jean Watson, PhD, RN, professor of nursing at the University of Colorado and director of the Center for Human Caring, in a style that is easy for any reader to comprehend. The site is well maintained by the Center for Human Caring executive director Karen Holland. The telephone number, e-mail, and fax for Watson and Holland are listed on the site. Information provided on this easily navigated Web site is current and accurate. It is available only in English. The theory of caring, its assumptions, and definitions are clearly explained. A lengthy list of publications is provided to assist interested parties in studying Watson's theory. The one weakness of the Web site is that the reference list has not been updated to include publications after 1996.

_____ Chapter **15**

Nursing Classification Systems

Erin V. Messett

Today's health care continuum challenges us to communicate health care information through many venues. The language of nursing diagnosis and classification is an important way to communicate about patients. Computerized information systems in health care document and manage clinical practice. The American Nurses Association (ANA) recognized the need for professional standards in this area and established the Nursing information and Data Set Evaluation Center (NIDSEC). For a fee, the ANA Committee for Nursing Practice reviews and recognizes nursing data and information systems voluntarily submitted against NIDSEC standards. NIDSEC and eight recognized languages for nursing are reviewed.

The Health Insurance Portability Act (HIPAA) of 1996 required national electronic standards for processing health care claims. Nurses need to understand and utilize electronic standards for coded nursing terms to convey billable information. Alternative Link and Health Level 7 (HL 7) are two other Web sites pertinent to nursing practice included in this review. All of these evolving sites provide unlimited opportunity for nursing education and research.

1. Alternative Link

http://www.alternativelink.com

Alternative Link licenses state specific Complementary and Alternative Medicine (CAM) health care and nursing databases. The strategic partners that support this Web site include Delmar Publishers, a division of Thomson Learning. A short history about Alternative Link is available on the Web site. They provide products that include coding manuals to assist with nursing terms that must be coded to convey billable information. Other products are scope of practice reports, relative values for CAM and nursing, state legal guides, ASCII data files, and database leasing. Some of the consulting and services available include teaching staff and outside PPO contractors, electronic decisions support, clarification of utilization concerns, and information that can be added to current software programs. Information on the coding system includes regulations that cover sixteen disciplines and are updated annually. E-mail addresses are provided for marketing, tech support, ordering products, job and career opportunities, questions, and a toll free access number. "Downloads," and "Press Releases and Articles" are two more easily accessed links with interesting information and links for other Web sites. This Web site was easy to use, clear, concise, and provides simple to high-level information in English. One feature to note, as stated on the site, is "Alternative Link maintains a national database to track which practitioners are allowed to offer 4000 coded services according to the laws of each state." Each year this database is updated.

2. Center for Nursing Classification

http://www.nursing.uiowa.edu/cnc

"The Center for Nursing Classification was established in 1995 to facilitate the ongoing research of the Nursing Interventions Classification (NIC) and the Nursing Outcomes Classification (NOC)." NIC and NOC were developed at the University of Iowa and assisted by a grant from the National Institutes of Health (NIH). The center's identified purposes also include updating the classifications, producing and disseminating educational materials, providing office support to assist investigators, and offering opportunities in education and research. Each NIC intervention has an associated number that can be linked to NANDA nursing diagnosis, NOC, assessment terminology in long-term care (RAPS), and OASIS outcome measures used in home health care. NIC pages include 486 intervention labels and definitions. The NOC pages include 260 outcome labels and definitions, outcome examples, student project section, dissertations, and publications. The center maintains a Web page and newsletter. The Web listserv has subscribing information and allows discussion about any standardized nursing language. A review of products with detailed description and cost is catalogued. One unique offering includes speakers and consultants identifying at least twelve topics with fees available by phone or fax. This site has multiple varied teaching opportunities with excellent clear examples and definitions. The site is colorful and easy to navigate. The Web site is up-to-date.

3. Health Level 7 (HL 7)

http://www.students.tut.fi/~viigipuu/HL7/about.html

Health Level 7 is one of the accredited Standards Maintenance Organizations (DSMOs) identified by the Department of Health and Human Services to develop specifications (sometimes called standards or protocols) in the health care domain of clinical and administrative data. Its focal point is the interface requirements of the entire health care organization. HL7 identifies its mission as "To provide standards for the exchange, management and integration of data that support clinical patient care and the management, delivery and evaluation of health care services. Specifically, to create flexible, cost effective approaches, standards, guidelines, methodologies, and related services for interoperability between healthcare information systems." It is a nonprofit organization managed by a board of directors. Its members include providers, vendors, payers, consultants, government groups, and others. This Web site contains descriptions about HL7, history and mission, the structure of various standard versions, achievements, and meetings. It has information in English and Finnish with vibrant graphics, which are easy to navigate and informative. ANA represents nursing interests as a member of HL7. One interesting aspect is that this site offers a tutorial on educational offerings and courses, meetings, library resources, news, and membership benefits. Job postings are also available.

4. Home Health Care Classification System (HHCC)

http://www.sabacare.com

This ANA recognized language Web site consists of two interrelated vocabularies: the HHCC of Nursing Diagnosis and the HHCC of Nursing Interventions that document and classify home health and ambulatory care. "These two vocabularies use a framework of 20 Care Components that represent the Functional, Health, Behavioral, Physiological, and Psychological Patterns of patient care." Virginia K. Saba developed HHCC from a federally funded research study at Georgetown University. The project was developed as a way to assess and classify patients to identify resources for Medicare home health patients. The Web offers a description of the research at the background link. The nursing diagnosis link includes a nursing diagnosis definition, coding scheme, interventions, care components, sample care plans and forms, and vocabulary lists with definitions. The versions are available in English, Portuguese, Dutch, German, and Spanish. A Web bibliography is included. The architecture of the links is very clear and concise. The design is colorful with music available on the homepage. Contact information includes phone, fax, Web and e-mail addresses.

5. International Classification of Nursing Practice (ICNP)

http://www.icn.ch/icnp.htm

ICNP was developed by the International Council of Nurses (ICN) to establish a standardized nursing classification language for describing nursing practice. The development of ICNP is a long-term project that will allow nursing data to be integrated into multidisciplinary health information systems. Three key program areas include professional practice, regulation, and socioeconomic welfare. The Web site for ICNP includes a description of its mission, objectives, goals, values, and position statements. Three elements of ICNP include nursing phenomena, nursing outcomes, and nursing actions. This is an interactive Web site with links to listings, definitions, and codes of terms in the classification, related Web sites, and publications. Some of the publications and nursing networks identified at this site are available in several languages including English, Spanish, and French. Requests for information and questions can be sent to ICN. This site is easy to use, up-to-date, and offers simple to high-level information.

6. North American Nursing Diagnosis Association (NANDA)

http://www.nanda.org/

In 1982 NANDA was created with members from the United States and Canada's National Task Force. The site includes a concise historical timetable of its history. It was the first nursing classification system recognized by ANA. The purpose of this site is to increase "the visibility of nursing's contribution to patient care by continuing to develop, refine and classify phenomena of concern to nurses." NANDA reports four key elements that are a part of nursing diagnosis and the naming and classification of its language. The elements are critical thinking, analysis, creativity, and accuracy. A site map outlines and links the user to the contents of this Web site including a strategic plan, mission and vision, programs and resources, products and publications, membership, news and events, and a resource for information and questions. NLINKS is an evolving interactive Web site for nursing language development and research. The project was identified at the 2000 NANDA Conference as an online center of communications. It depends on members for its enhancement and maintenance. The project goal is to strengthen existing relationships and advance future collaborative efforts. This site is clear and concise, easy to navigate, and continually evolving.

7. Nursing Information and Data Set Evaluation Center (NIDSC)

http://www.nursingworld.org/nidsec

NIDSEC was established and continues to be funded by the American Nurses Association (ANA). NIDSEC's stated mission is the "develop and disseminate standards pertaining to information systems that support the documentation of nursing practice, and evaluate voluntarily submitted information systems against these standards." This site provides a short background on the development of NIDSEC and then reviews the probam. Standards have been developed that model Joint Commission on Accreditation to evaluate four dimensions of nursing data sets and the systems that support them. The four dimensions include standardized nomenclature, linkages among terms in clinical content, clinical data repository, and general system characteristics. The Web gives directions for vender application and identifies and e-mail address for questions. The site discusses the voluntary review process and identifies that the review panel convenes twice a year submitting recommendations to the NIDSEC Committee. ANA recognition is given for three years. The Web site provides an example of an ANA Press Release defining recognition for the applicant's achievement.

The ANA recognized classification systems are listed. The hyperliks to each Web site provide access to their location, phone and fax numbers, and Web and e-mail addresses. Most also include the name of the developer. Several systems do not list a Web site; these include the patient Care Data Set (PCDS), the Nursing Management Minimum Data Set (NMMDS), and the Nursing Minimum Data Sets (NMDS). Each of these does list an e-mail address. These twelve sites are designed to track clinical care across the continuum for patients in acute, home, or ambulatory care settings. The site was last revised November 29, 2000. This is an excellent resource for standardized terminology in nursing and related work conducted by ANA with clearly identified hyperlinks. This site is limited to English.

8. Omaha System

http://www.omahasystem.org

FITNE, a creator of interactive training software, and the University of Florida with Karen Martin created this Web site to share information about the Omaha System (a standardized nursing vocabulary used for nursing practice and documentation) and its use in practice, education, documentation, case studies, and outcome measurement. There are four detailed case studies, which include practice cues, terminology, and documentation. The case studies also include clear examples of information application to the Omaha System. The application includes a problem classification scheme, intervention scheme, and rating scale for outcomes. A listserv and subscribing information are available to facilitate networking with frequent users of the Omaha System. The site also offers an opportunity to search the archives of the listserv. E-mail and phone numbers are provided to contact the project director, Karen Martin, for further information. The case studies are an excellent teaching tool to document patient interactions. System application examples are simple, clear, and easy to follow. Agencies, schools, and colleges using the Omaha System are identified. References with user input in mind are identified. The opportunity to review the *Journal of Nursing Informatics* is provided. A description of the portable communication system the Nightingale Tracker is available on this site. This site is up-to-date.

9. SNOMED

http://www.snomed.org

The College of American Pathologists (CAP) directs a comprehensive database known as SNOMED, Systematized Nomenclature of Medicine, to index the medical record. This system allows detailed clinical information and assessment terms from various specialties, researchers, and patients to be shared across the continuum of care and across computer systems in over forty countries. SNOMED has a Convergent Terminology Group for Nursing that links direct information on international authority, editorial board, design team, and working groups. Organizational milestones such as specific recognitions, awards, meetings, collaborations, and significant calendar events from 1965 to 2000 are included in narrative and graphic format. Links are included to press releases, programs and services, latest developments, related sites, and a customer service telephone hotline. The site includes an expansive bibliography of published articles about the SNOMED system. An e-mail address connects to the SNOMED Webmaster and further information. In May of 2000 SNOMED instituted a new clinical reference terminology, which is designated as an ANA recognized nomenclature. This Web site is in English and does not contain listings of the codes or definitions. Information is provided for purchasing the SNOMED System. This site is up-to-date

Chapter 16

Careers in Nursing

Jeanne M. Novotny

When it comes to Internet resources, nothing has changed quite like the job market search. In order to secure a place in 21st century health care, each nurse must focus on clinical and professional competencies, career development, and stress management to optimize and maintain professional satisfaction and relevance. The job market and career opportunities fluctuate so think of your career as a business: A business that is yours and one that will give you a lifetime of gainful employment and personal satisfaction. Listed below are Web sites that feature nursing career opportunities and job listings. The following sites were chosen for their comprehensive and current information for nurses.

1. American Nurses Association (ANA)

http://www.ana.org

This Internet site provides comprehensive information about nursing that is a must for all nurses and students of nursing. The information is accurate and current. Links include affiliate organizations, workplace advocacy, government affairs, ANA/AJN columns, bookstores, and continuing education online. As the Web site of the professional organization for nurses, it is so important and valuable that even though its purpose is not solely devoted to career development and job opportunities, it should not be overlooked. The site is robust in issues such as safety, standards, position statements, press releases, and current issues. The audience is across the profession and is a high-volume site that is extremely easy to use. This site is highly recommended.

2. *The Chronicle of Higher Education* Career Network

http://www.chronicle.com

This site lists available positions by job title, university, and location. Jobs listed on this Web page are academic and include faculty and research positions. A link to the advertising university site is also provided. General academic career advice may also be accessed via this site. There is an e-mail service for new positions that is sorted according to discipline and rank. The help section provides very good information on how to search for the information needed. This Web site is easy to use and the information is current, accurate, and reliable.

3. Erickson and Associates, Inc.

http://www.nursesearch.com

Erickson and Associates, Inc. is a valuable nursing resource site for nurses seeking to improve their careers as nurse managers, department heads, clinical nurse specialists, as well as matching nursing administration positions to personal goals and objectives. Based in Kansas City, MO, this site is an excellent one for nurses who are seeking opportunities in hospital settings. The site offers a comprehensive job database. The nationwide network of health care contacts provides comprehensive search services to both hiring officials and candidates. The site is well organized and easy to use. The information is up to date and the personal attention to individual career planning and placement makes it a site worth investigating, especially for nurses in hospital administration. This site is important because of its health care contacts and computerized and in-depth understanding of nursing at all levels that provides important information about trends in health care.

4. Kaplan Educational Centers

http://www.kaplan.com

This is the Internet site of Kaplan Educational Centers, which provides NCLEX review courses as well as information related to nursing careers and job opportunities. The intended audience is broad and diverse, and ranges from students in basic and graduate nursing programs to nurses with established careers who are looking for new experiences. The site provides links to educational and testing materials for the GMAT, MCAT, and GRE for nurses considering graduate education. The information is current and accurate. Books and software are available and links to a variety of services are readily available. The site is easy to access and is user-friendly. This site is exceptional for educational materials and career information. It is a dynamic and interactive site that has valuable information related to nursing careers and opportunities.

5. Johnson & Johnson's Discover Nursing

http://www.discovernursing.com

This is a general Web site about the nursing profession with information on how to become a nurse. The site is sponsored by Johnson and Johnson and is part of their multimillion dollar campaign to promote nursing. The site is intended for those considering a career in nursing. The site is also useful to those who wish to know more about the nursing profession and the options available to nurses (e.g., a nurse returning to school, media). Information on the site is current and accurate.

The best feature of this site is the searchable database of nursing programs. One can search by school name, region of the country, specific state, school type (public or private), enrollment size, or degree offered. Because the focus of the site is those wishing to enter the nursing profession, only schools with entry-level programs (diploma, associate degree, BS/BSN degree) are featured. However, schools that also have graduate programs are included in the database. School listings feature a Web address, so graduate information is easily located if that is the information desired. The site also provides basic information on nursing, searching for scholarships, profiles of nurses that are culturally and gender diverse, and information on the nursing market, benefits and salary, and a few nursing specialties. A glossary and contact information are also provided.

The only weakness of this site is in the specialty areas section. This is really just a list of links to specialty organizations and not all specialties are included. It may be that only certain organizations gave permission to have their link placed on this site. Text on the site is available in English at a simple to average level. The site is easy to navigate and the text is clear.

6. Nurseweek

http://www.nurseweek.com

This Internet site provides a forum for nurses to exchange ideas and information related to local, regional, and national issues; health care news; resources; and employment opportunities. This is a good site for nurses looking for employment. The organization of the site is divided into two main sections with specific information listed underneath each section. This organization assists in easily locating information. The homepage is somewhat cluttered and, in addition, the site contains several advertisements that are distracting. This site provides information that is useful primarily for looking at career opportunities by state and region.

7. Nursing Center

http://www.nursingcenter.com

This is an excellent Internet site that is produced and sponsored by Lippincott Publishers. Lippincott is a well-known publishing house for nursing books and journals and includes the *American Journal of Nursing*. The site provides career and clinical information, including a career center, online networking, and continuing education. There is a theme for each month, forum discussions, and a virtual university. The Nursing Center does product evaluations and explores opportunities for undergraduate and graduate education that are affordable and nontraditional. The information is current, accurate, and reliable. It is a site that is easy to use and is suitable for all nurses and those interested in a nursing career. This site is a source of general to specific information about nursing careers and is sponsored by a very respected organization. It is highly recommended.

8. Nursing Network Forum

http://www.nursingnet.org

This is the nursing Internet site of the Microsoft Network, which provides comprehensive and worldwide networking and information about all aspects of nursing practice. The site is especially interesting because of its availability on an international level in Spanish and several other languages. The homepage is dynamic and easy to use. There are vignettes about the history of nursing and other topics. The site has great pictures and easy to use links to many topics. It is useful to all nurses and students because of its NCLEX review, mentoring, career planning, and discussion groups. This site is highly recommended because it is so interesting and extremely easy to use for all levels of computer expertise. The high volume of Internet traffic is one measure of its usefulness and the information is current and accurate.

9. Nursing Spectrum: Career Fitness On Line

http://www.nursingspectrum.com

Nursing Spectrum is an online resource that is well-known and highly regarded for useful employment and career information. If you are interested in beginning or advancing a career in nursing, this site helps you navigate the intricacies of the profession. It provides a detailed look at various nursing positions, as well as leads to additional information about certification, associations, and journals. The site provides chat rooms, a bookstore, employment listings, including instant applications and resume submission, self-study modules for continuing education credit, employer profiles, and a weekly online guest lecture. It is a very useful site and the information is current and accurate. The best features of the site are the easy to use format and the variety of information that is easy to retrieve. It is an attractive, dynamic, and very useful Internet resource for all nurses and those contemplating a career in nursing.

10. Sigma Theta Tau

http://www.nursingsociety.org

This is the Internet site of the national nursing honor society. It is a valuable and important resource for career development. Sigma Theta Tau can help find answers to questions about education and career planning. In addition, there are discussions related to the following: What is a nurse? How do I become a nurse? and Where should I work? There is an online employment search that will customize the information specifically to individual needs. The important feature of this site is that it focuses on the professional aspect of nursing as a lifelong career not simply a job. An extensive online library is available. Once registered at this site, periodic updates will be automatically sent to keep you informed and updated with new and interesting aspects of career development.

11. SpringNet

http://www.springnet.com

This site is for nurses, nurse practitioners, nursing managers, students, and health care providers and is maintained by the Springhouse Corporation, which is now owned by Lippincott, Williams, & Wilkins. Springhouse publishes the following well-known journals and books: *Nursing '02, Nursing Management, The Nurse Practitioner, Advances in Skin and Wound Care, Dimensions of Critical Care Nursing*, and *Nursing Drug Handbook*. In addition to information about and from these publications, the site provides a reference library, employment opportunities, online networking events, continuing education, and conference listings. It is considered the Web site of choice among many nurses for the latest and most accurate clinical information. There are full-text articles from top nursing journals and online videos. If you are interested in writing for a nursing journal, there are lessons that will increase your chances of getting published. This site is easy to use, dynamic, interesting and very highly recommended.

Nursing Job Sites

Dara B. Walls

This section presents a variety of employment resources on the Web for nursing professionals. These resources include specific sites for registered nurses, nurse practitioners, nurse educators, certified nurse-midwives, and certified registered nurse anesthetists (CRNA). General nursing and health care employment sites that include career opportunities for certified nursing assistants, licensed practical nurses, registered nurses, and advanced practice nurses are also included. The following Web resources were chosen not only because they represent all nursing specialties, but also because they are the most comprehensive and easiest to navigate of the health care career sites.

1. The American Academy of Nurse Practitioners

http://www.aanp.org

The American Academy of Nurse Practitioners (AANP) is a professional organization that represents nurse practitioners of all specialties across the country. The AANP Career Link, a member of the HEALTHCAR-EERS Network, is an interactive service that provides an electronic forum for the exchange of career information. Visitors can perform a quick search for nurse practitioner positions for free via the 'recruitment' icon on the homepage. Several employment listings are presented, with the most recent openings appearing first. Individuals can view the job title, a one-sentence description of the position, the company name, and location. If the visitor is interested in the position, he or she may click on the job title in order to ascertain more information on date of advertisement, job description, and contact person. Visitors can apply to the posting online. Job candidates can also choose to post their resumes and to receive new job alerts for free after entering some personal information. Overall, this site is very good. It is organized, easy to navigate and the information is presented in an average level of English. However, the AANPCareerLinks.com site is new and therefore does not yet have a plethora of career opportunities listed.

2. American Nurses Association (ANA)

http://www.ana.org

The American Nurses Association (ANA) is a professional organization that represents the country's 2.6 million registered nurses. By clicking on either the 'jobs' or 'employment' icons on the left side of their homepage, visitors can search job openings that are listed alphabetically by company name. The advertisements are current and include information about job description, qualifications, and contact information. There may also be links to the company's homepage. The employment listings span a variety of nursing specialties. However, visitors and members cannot submit a resume online and one must view all of the employment listings in order to discover each company's location. Overall, this is a good site to search for job openings. It is easy to navigate and the information is clear and concise. It is written in an average level of English.

3. Hot Nurse Jobs

http://www.hotnursejobs.com

The Hot Nurse Jobs Web page is a simple site that allows nurses to post resumes and/or search job listings for free. Potential employers may advertise and/or access the resume database for a cost. Visitors must fill out a brief application in order to submit their resumes. Job search categories include certified nursing assistants, licensed practical nurses, registered nurses, nurse practitioners, certified registered nurse anesthetists, nurse educators, nurse analysts, and nurse managers. Additional categories include traveling nurses, camp nurses, paramedic and emergency medical technicians, Canadian jobs, medical jobs online, and certified home health assistant jobs. Once a category is chosen, the employment listings are presented alphabetically by state. Job title, name of company, contact information, job description and qualifications are also given. This site also contains links to other career sites and to continuing education courses presented by *Nursing Spectrum*, the print and online newspaper for nursing. Overall, this is a good site that is quite simple and easy to navigate. The job postings are current and the text is written in English at an average level.

4. Med Bulletin

http://www.medbulletin.com

Med Bulletin is a health care career site that offers a variety of tools for job seekers. Over 12,000 potential employment opportunities from more than 2,000 facilities can be searched by specialty, organization, or recruiter. Job listings with company name and location are presented, and interested visitors can click on the name of the company in order to see its bulletin. The bulletin includes information on job title, job description and requirements, location, salary, and contact person. This bulletin may also include links to Web pages about the geographic area, real estate, and the company itself. Job seekers can choose to submit their resumes at the bottom of each bulletin. A relocation salary calculator, recruiter directory, and moving services are also available. Employers and recruiters can access a searchable database of curriculum vitae and resumes, and job seekers can choose to subscribe to a free job update service that e-mails individuals about job openings in their fields. Overall, this site is very good. The career opportunities span all nursing specialties and the information is clear and presented at an average level in English. However, some of the job bulletins are quite dated and the site can be somewhat confusing to navigate for first-time users.

5. MedHunters

http://www.medhunters.com

MedHunters is an online job board for health care professionals and employers. Currently, there are over 8,000 employment listings from more than 300 hospitals and employers. Individuals may search jobs by title, location, or employer. Visitors who are interested in a job title and location can view more details regarding the position. There are nursing positions in all specialties; these include nurse practitioners and specialists, nurse educators, nurse administrators, registered nurses in clinical practice, licensed practical nurses, and nursing assistants. Interested individuals will find a link that will let them apply to the job online. This site also provides information on licensing information for registered nurses and licensed practical nurses who may be relocating, and relocation tools such as salary and relocation calculators, and city and school reports.

   It is possible to sign up for a free MedHunter account, which allows individuals to post their resumes. The MedHunter system can also match the information that the individual provides with all suitable jobs, which will continuously appear on his or her "My MedHunter" page. New jobs will be e-mailed to the individual periodically. Overall, this is a very good site. It is reasonably easy to navigate and all jobs are updated within sixty days. The information is organized, concise, and in an average level of English.

6. Midwifejobs.com

http://www.midwifejobs.com

Midwifejobs.com is an Internet career center that provides tools and services for job-seeking certified nurse-midwives as well as employers. This Web page is sponsored by the American College of Nurse-Midwives (ACNM) and can be easily accessed via a link on their homepage (*www.acnm.com*). This site allows visitors to search for jobs by location and category of employment interest (clinical midwifery, midwifery education, practice administration, practice director, research, etc.). Employment listings consist of job title, location, and date posted. Interested visitors can click on the job title to learn more about the company, job description, eligibility requirements, salary, and contact person. Individuals can also post their resumes after creating an account at no cost. Overall, this site is excellent. It is very easy to navigate and current information is presented clearly and concisely. It is written in an average level of English.

7. Monster.com

http://www.monster.com

Monster.com is a global online career network designed for individuals and employers in a variety of fields. Job seekers can post their resumes for free after filling out a membership application. Nonmembers can search jobs by entering location, job category, and a keyword. Job listings arranged according to date of advertisement are then presented along with city and company name. The health care site offers positions for certified nursing assistants, licensed practical nurses, registered nurses, nurse educators, nurse managers, nurse administrators, clinical specialists, nurse practitioners, and other advanced practice nurses. A visitor can click on the job title to obtain the job description, eligibility requirements, and contact information. It is also possible to apply online. The career center of Monster.com offers resume help, salary data, career newsletters, and information on various industries and featured employers. Overall, this is an excellent site. The site contains over 1,000,000 job postings and it is easy to follow even though the homepage contains a lot of information. The text is average level English.

8. RNWanted.com

http://www.rnwanted.com

RNWanted.com is an employment resource for registered nurses and other health care professionals. This site caters mainly to registered nurses and the employment listings are generally those of other staffing and recruiting companies. Visitors can search for employment listings by state or employer. The listings contain job descriptions, contact information, and other general details. However, many of the career opportunities do not have dates of advertisement or may not be recent postings. An advantage of this site, however, is that it allows individuals to build and post resumes for free. Additionally, there are links to most major hospitals and health centers in every state. There is a bulletin board for discussion of employment-related issues, but it does not seem to be very active. Overall, this site is good. The information is presented clearly and is written in an average level of English.

9. United Anesthesia Associates, Inc.

http://www.unitedanesthesia.com

United Anesthesia Associates in an organization that specializes in staffing services for certified registered nurse anesthetists. The site is very easy to navigate. Visitors can search for jobs by entering information on desired hospital size, location, and whether they are looking for permanent or temporary positions. Job listings include information regarding location, job status, job description, salary range, start date, hospital size, hours, primary skills, case workload, number of CRNAs, number of MDs, and number of cases per year. Interested job seekers need to contact this agency via the appropriate Web page. CRNAs may also post their resumes and employers may post their advertisements after registering online. Overall, this is an excellent site for certified registered nurse anesthetists. The information presented is current, clear and concise, and the text is in an average level of English.

Chapter 18

Writing Resources

Kristen S. Montgomery

Writing is one of the essential tools for communication among human beings. Nurses write for a variety of reasons, including documentation of patient care and progress, and as authors, to communicate new research, innovative practice techniques, or personal or professional opinions. Nurses as a group vary in their writing abilities and enthusiasm for writing. The resources listed below represent the best online writing resources for nurses. One is a general writing site, one is nursing-specific, and two offer resources for writing.

1. 11 Rules of Writing

http://www.junketstudies.com/rulesofw/

11 Rules of Writing is a concise guide to the most commonly violated rules of writing, grammar, and punctuation. The 11 rules are listed; clicking on one of the rules provides further information and examples of correct and incorrect use. The site is intended for all audiences to aid in learning and refining writing skills. The Web site is sponsored

by Junket Studies Tutoring, a private tutoring company for elementary to college level, located in Northern New Jersey. Examples, references to find information, and explanations are offered on the site. There is also a glossary to look up grammatical terms. A frequently asked questions section and word of the day are other key features of this site. There is also a teacher's section that some individuals might find helpful. An e-mail address is provided for questions. Content is provided at an average to high level in English.

2.   Indispensable Writing Resources

http://www.quintcareers.com/writing

Indispensable Writing Resources is a general writing Web site, sponsored by Quintcareers.com. Main sections of content include reference materials (a list of quality print resources), writing style guides (a list of general and subject-specific), and links to writing resources available on the Internet. There is also information on the importance of good writing skills. While the site is geared toward college students, it is useful to nurses as a general writing reference. Content is presented in English at an average level.

3.   10 Lessons on Writing for Publication

http://www.springnet.com/jrdescr/wlesson.htm

This is a one page Web site that is part of the SpringNet Nursing Communities, which is sponsored by Springhouse Publishing. Ten tips are provided on beginning as a nurse author. Each tip is followed by a discussion of the content. Tips are useful and provide clear guidance, though not all tips will work for everyone. The site is presented in English at a simple level and is easy to navigate.

4.   University of Washington Writer Toolkit

http://www.healthlinks.washington.edu/toolkits/writer.html

This Web site is a very comprehensive resource site for writing. It is sponsored by the University of Washington and is intended for college level audiences (including faculty and students). The site includes directories (e.g., journal abbreviation sources), copyright and fair use information, dictionaries, information and programs on managing references, style guides, online publishing, and Web authoring. Each of these sections provides a variety of resources for writers. While this is a very thorough site, some resources are only applicable to the University of Washington community and a few of the resources are restricted. Content is presented at an average to high level in English. The site is easy to navigate and presented in a clear and concise format.

Chapter 19

Fundraising

Joyce J. Fitzpatrick

Fundraising used to be an activity reserved for only corporate executives or college or university presidents. Now, fundraising for various programmatic initiatives is becoming part of the expected behavior of all professionals, including those in clinician and educator roles. In addition, there are professional fundraisers. As nurses become more involved in fundraising (also often referred to as development activities), they will find the following Web sites useful as both an orientation to the business of fundraising and as informative regarding sources of support. The Web sites selected for inclusion here are those that provide the broadest range of information to both the novice and the professional fundraiser.

1. Association of Fundraising Professionals

http://www.afpnet.org

This site is the official Web site for the Association of Fundraising Professionals (formerly known as the National Society of Fund Raising

Executives (NSFRE). The site provides information about fundraising primarily to its members. Access to the library is a major positive component of this site; resources are catalogued according to interest area, e.g., giving among women or among the elderly. The major weakness is the fact that membership in the organization is required in order to access many of the site components. The site will be useful to nurses who spend some part of their time in developing proposals for project funding even though the primary audience is the fundraiser within the organization. The site appears accurate and current, and is easy to read and navigate. Material on the site is available only in English.

2. Association of Healthcare Philanthropy (AHP)

http://www.go-ahp.org

This is the organization Web site for the Association for Healthcare Philanthropy (AHP), the only association dedicated exclusively to advancing and promoting the fundraising profession within North America's health care systems. AHP is a nonprofit organization with over 3,000 members. The Web site is sponsored by the AHP, and some aspects of the site are available to members only. Because of its targeted focus, even though the primary audience includes those who raise money for health care, nurses are increasingly involved in philanthropy, and, therefore, have a growing interest in this content. The information provided to nonmembers is current and accurate; there are no major weaknesses. Particularly good features of the site are the inclusion of the upcoming conferences, the bookstore, and the latest news reports about fund-raising in health care. The site is easy to use and the information available appears to be high level in the fundraising content. The site is in English only.

3. *Chronicle of Philanthropy*

http://www.philanthropy.com

This site is sponsored by the *Chronicle of Philanthropy,* the newspaper of the nonprofit world. It has many services available to subscribers;

subscription cost is $67.50 per year. This provides access to a Guide to Grants, which is an electronic database of all foundation and corporate grants listed in *The Chronicle* since 1995. Even without a subscription, this Web site provides some basic information and a number of links to products and services provided by other organizations. Daily updates of newsworthy stories are provided on the Web site. Overall, the site is easy to maneuver and is very timely and accurate. Information is available only in English.

4. Council for Aid to Education (CAE)

http://www.cae.org

The Council for Aid to Education (CAE) is a national nonprofit organization that is a part of the RAND Corporation. CAE was established in 1952 to advance corporate support of education. The Web site is sponsored by the organization, and many of the components of the site are for members only. One particularly important resource available on the site is the tracking of Voluntary Support of Education (VSE). While users must have an ID to log on and use the VSE tables, it is not difficult to get access whether as an individual user or through one's institution. Annual reports track support to educational institutions at all levels (from elementary schools to colleges and universities). The data provided is very comprehensive and detailed, and appears accurate and timely. The site is in English only.

5. Council for the Advancement and Support of Education (CASE)

http://www.case.org

This Web site is a product of the Council for Advancement and Support of Education (CASE), one of the most well-known organizations in support of development for higher education. The CASE mission is to advance and support education worldwide. Through the large network of institutions in the U.S. and Europe, CASE serves more than 38,000 members from the 3,000 participating institutions. While there are a number of site components available only to members, there are other

Web site features that are available to any user. Most striking among the features is the CASE bibliography, which includes many key fundraising references. This Web site is in English only.

6. The Council on Foundations

http://www.cof.org

This is the Web site of the Council on Foundations (COF), a nonprofit membership association of grantmaking foundations and organizations. The mission of the COF is to serve the public good by promoting and enhancing responsible and effective philanthropy. Several aspects of the Web site are of interest to nurses and health professionals who wish to access private grant funds for their projects and programs. There is a very interesting history of the COF that mirrors the growth of philanthropy in the U.S. from 2,000 foundations in 1950 to more than 46,000 foundations by 2,000. Key links are provided to other Web sites of interest in fundraising, and an extensive list of other fundraising resources is included within this site. Overall, this is a very sophisticated Web site; it is easy to use and contains much material of interest. It is only in English.

7. The Foundation Center

http://www.fdncenter.org

This Foundation Center (FC) Web site offers a wide range of information about fundraising from foundation sources. The Foundation Center is an independent nonprofit information clearinghouse established in 1956. Currently, the Center maintains a database of over 57,000 grantmakers and 243,000 grants. This Web site is very rich in resources, and links to many other resources. The FC provides free access to their publications in five professionally staffed Center-run libraries across the U.S. There also is an online version of the library that can be accessed. Individuals can purchase a subscription to the foundation directory online. This site is easy to navigate and very helpful, even to the novice Web user or fundraiser. Two features are of keen interest. First, there is an extensive "Frequently Asked Questions" section with more questions than one can imagine, and of course, the answers to the questions are provided. Second, there is an online orientation to the grantseeking process, a very easy-to-follow map for novice and experienced fundraisers or seekers. This site is available in English only.

8.   Indiana University-Purdue University Indianapolis (IUPUI) Center on Philanthropy

http://www.philanthropy.iupui.edu

This site is sponsored by the Indiana University-Purdue University Indianapolis (IUPUI) Center on Philanthropy. Basic components of the site include the description of the programs offered through IUPUI. What is most useful, however, are the links between this site and other key sites for fundraising information and programs. Links are provided to a wide range of Center on Philanthropy Affiliates. Many of these affiliates will provide basic and advanced information to the fundraiser. This site is in English only.

Chapter **20**

Economics and Financing of Health Care

Patricia W. Stone and Christine R. Curran

Although total U.S. health care costs are rising at a slower rate than in the past, national health care spending still accounts for approximately 13.5% of the U.S. gross domestic product (GDP), or $1.1 trillion, and the growth rate is expected to rise (Heffler et al., 2001). In addition, in the presence of a slowing economy we can expect increased interest in the cost and financing of health services. Changes are likely to occur regarding financial practices as a result of effort by the payers to decrease costs and providers to maximize reimbursement. This chapter includes a review of the best Internet sites currently available that address health care economics and finance issues.

1. Agency for Healthcare Research and Quality (AHRQ)

http://www.ahrq.gov

This is the Web site of the primary federal agency that funds health care research and quality initiatives in the U.S. The Web site highlights initiatives and databases available to assess the quality of health care services. Researchers, health policymakers, and consumers interested in health services research are the target audience. What will be reviewed here are the aspects of the Web site that are useful to nurses interested in the economics and financing of health care. AHRQ funds the medical expenditure panel survey (MEPS). MEPS is a nationally representative survey that collects detailed information on the health status, health services use and costs, and health insurance coverage of individuals and families in the U.S., including nursing home residents. A complete description and listing of publications using this database may be found at the following address (*http://www.ahrq.gov/data/mepsix.htm*).

The Healthcare Cost and Utilization Project (HCUP) is another database maintained by AHRQ (*http://www.ahrq.gov/data/hcup/*). The HCUP family of administrative longitudinal databases currently provides data from 1988–99. HCUP databases contain patient-level information compiled in a uniform format with privacy protections in place. The Nationwide Inpatient Sample (NIS) includes inpatient data from a national sample of over 1,000 hospitals. The State Inpatient Databases (SID) cover inpatient care in community hospitals in participating states that represent more than half of all U.S. hospital discharges. The State Ambulatory Surgery Databases (SASD) contain data from ambulatory care encounters. The project's newest restricted access public release is the Kids' Inpatient Database (KID), which contains hospital inpatient stays for children 18 years of age and younger. Many statistics come from these databases, such as the top five most expensive medical diagnoses, the top five most expensive hospital procedures, and the top five reasons for hospital admission (*http://www.ahrq.gov/data/hcup/hcupstat.htm*). The AHRQ national databases are the most comprehensive available. However, access to the databases to gain new knowledge (not already researched and published) may prove to be cumbersome and require a full research protocol. Additionally, published findings are not always available through links and often only the citation is given.

2.   American Hospital Association (AHA)

http://www.ahacentraloffice.org/

The American Hospital Association (AHA) central office Web site provides products, services, news, and reference links on coding information. This Web site is useful for information on medical diagnosis codes and procedure codes used in medical transcription and billing, e.g., International Classification of Diseases, Ninth Revision, Clinical Modification, (ICD-9-CM). Additionally, coding advice, guidelines, references and updates for the HCFA (Health Care Financing Administration) Common Procedure Coding System (HCPCS), ICD-10-CM, and the ICD-10-Procedure Coding System (ICD-10-PCS) are available. Links to multiple governmental sites on coding are especially useful. However, one cannot easily enter a diagnosis and obtain a potential list of applicable billing codes. The layout is clear, however, no site map is available. There is a current copyright date for the page displayed. English is the only language available. The level of information is average.

3.   Bureau of Labor Statistics (BLS)

http://www.bls.gov/

The Bureau of Labor Statistics is the principal Web site of the federal government for labor economics and statistics. This Web site, produced by the United States Department of Labor, Bureau of Labor Statistics (BLS), is used to disseminate essential statistical data to the American public, the U.S. Congress, other federal agencies, state and local governments, businesses, and labor leaders. The BLS is the principal fact-finding agency for the federal government in the broad field of labor economics and statistics. This Web site is an excellent source for U.S. aggregate labor statistics. Under the Wages, Earnings and Benefits category (*http://www.bls.gov/bls/wages.htm*) there is a large amount of information on the wages, earnings, and benefits of various types of workers. Generally, this information is categorized in one or more of the following ways: geographic area (national, regional, state, metropolitan area, or county data); occupation (such as nurse); and industry (such as health care). Additional categories, such as age, gender, or union membership, may be found in some cases. It also contains many health care provider salaries (*http://www.bls.gov/oes/2000/oes29 1111.htm*). For example, in 2000, the mean annual wage of a registered nurse in the United States was $46,410 and of a licensed vocational or practical nurse was $30,470. In the primary metropolitan statistical area of New York, the mean annual wage was $57,310. The data are also given by mean hourly wage and median hourly wage, which may be more useful when salary data are skewed. A limitation to the data is that advanced practice nurses are consolidated with all registered nurses. Another very useful section of the BLS Web page is the Inflation and Consumer Spending category (*http://www.bls.gov/bls/inflation.htm*). It has consumer price indices (CPI) and an easy-to-use inflation calculator that is linked to these indices. Because one hundred dollars in 1985 does not have the same buying power as one hundred dollars in 2002, to compare or aggregate these dollar figures they must be standardized into a common currency. The inflation calculator allows the user to convert U.S. dollars from a previous year into another year's currency value for such applications. In general, the BLS Web page provides high-level data. The site has dense screen, which can be challenging for novice users to navigate. However, the site selection map is helpful and eases navigation. Additionally, other useful links to economic data are available. The data are in English only.

4.   Centers for Medicare and Medicaid Services

http://cms.hhs.gov

The Centers for Medicare and Medicaid Services (CMS), formerly known as HCFA, maintains this Web site, which contains general information about these governmental insurance programs. The site is the prime federal government source for information on Medicare and Medicaid. Specifically, consumer and provider information, required forms, coding and payment system information, fee schedules, and data and statistics for researchers and health policymakers are some of the types of information available. Information is targeted to health care professionals, contractors, states, tribal governments, partners and others. This site is useful to all nurses to assist clients in obtaining information about governmental insurance coverage. Nurses (such as nurse administrators and advanced practice nurses) interested in reimbursement issues may find this site especially useful.

Up-to-date data are available. Weekly update information can be sent to your own e-mail account if requested. Links to key information are useful, e.g., HIPAA (Health Insurance Portability and Accountability Act), state Medicaid Web sites, and SCHIP (State Children's Health Insurance Program). No date is given as to the last time the site was updated. However, the data seem to be current. English is the only available language. The level of information is average to high. In general, the site presentation and usability are good. The site is user-friendly, easy to navigate, and contains a site map to facilitate information searching. Contact information is available on the site.

5. The Cost Utility Analysis (CUA) Database

http://www.hsph.harvard.edu/organizations/hcra/cuadatabase.intro.html

This Web site provides access to a database intended to help public and private policy-makers better understand the relative benefits and costs of diverse health care interventions and to aid in resource allocation decisions and evidence-based practice decisions. This Web site provides a convenient single source for clinicians seeking "benchmark" information by which to compare findings in cost-utility analyses with citations. The Harvard School of Public Health, Center for Risk Analysis, produces the site.

The intended audience includes nurses and other public and private health policymakers. Users can access the cost-effectiveness in dollars per quality adjusted life year of different interventions. The database is comprehensive up to the 1997 literature. The most important features of this site are the PDF files of study results; all data have been standardized to 1998 dollars, making results more comparable that what is usually found in the literature. Although there is a statement that the database will be updated periodically, currently the cost-utility analyses are only up to 1997 and all dollar figures are in 1998 currency. Information is available at an average level in English. Navigation is easy; however, limited links are available to other sites.

6. The Federal Reserve Bank of St. Louis

http://www.stls.frb.org/index.html

The Federal Reserve Bank of St. Louis is 1 of 12 regional reserve banks across the U.S. that together with the Board of Governors in Washington, D.C. serves as the nation's central bank. This Web site has a variety of information about the nation's central bank and economic research. Consumers, economists, and nurses will find this site useful to obtain foreign exchange rates by either monthly or daily rate information. Specific exchange rates may be found using the link to the Federal

Reserve Exchange Data (FRED) at the following address (*http:// www.stls.frb.org/fred/data/exchange.html*). In addition, historical data back to 1970 and a link to current exchange rates (within 2 days) are also available (*http://www.federalreserve.gov/releases/H10/hist/*).

A strength of the site is the average to high level of information with helpful links to other sites. Files are available for downloading, and the data are accurate and up to date. However, a calculator is not available on this Web site to aide in the conversion of currencies and the site is only available in English. Accessing the FRED (Federal Reserve Exchange Data) is suboptimal and access is through a link at the bottom of the page.

7. Healthcare Financial Management Association

http://www.hfma.org/index.html

This is the official Web site for the Healthcare Financial Management Association (HFMA). HFMA is the largest professional association for health care financial managers. The Web site contains information for visitors and members of the association, publications, jobs, and seminars. Additionally, HFMA has created a storehouse of technical information, data, and knowledge, called the HFMA Knowledge Network®. This service produces technical summaries, staff analysis, and position statements. This site targets health care management professionals and is useful to nurses who are interested in accessing a network of individuals connected with health care financial administration. It is also helpful for any nurse thinking about a career in the financial aspects of care and career services that are available. Information is organized by user focus. There is public information for visitors available as well as restricted information for members only. While the public information seems useful and up to date, accuracy of "members only" data could not be assessed. Overall, the site is easy to navigate and the level of information is average. The date of last revisions is posted and at the time of this review, current. The site is available in English only.

REFERENCE

Heffler, S., Levit, K., Smith, S., Smith, C., Cowan, C., Lazenby, H., & Freeland, M. (2001). Health spending growth up in 1999; faster growth expected in the future. *Health Affairs, (Millwood.), 20,* 193–203.

Chapter 21

International Nursing Resources

Kristen S. Montgomery

The international arena presents many opportunities for nurses in research, practice, education, and administration. Global work and communication between nurses and other health care providers is occurring at a rapidly increasing rate. International collaboration and communication can greatly benefit current nursing practice and health for the world's people. International collaboration has many benefits. Programs and innovative ideas can be shared, and nurses and other health care providers have opportunities to work in and learn firsthand about different cultures and health care practices.

1. All Nurses: International

http://allnurses.com/Boards_of_Nursing/International

A service provided by All Nurses, the site provides links to nursing in 29 countries. This site includes information on Boards of Nursing in the United States and abroad. This site was started in 1996 by Brian Short, RN, owner and operator of this independent enterprise that generates revenue through advertising. While this is a basic site, the simplicity contributes to the relative ease of use and information retrieval regarding international nursing practice. There is a simple list of board sites with a brief description of each board. Also provided is the date in which the listed site was last updated. All links are current, having been updated in the last month. One negative about this site is the use of advertisements, some of which are distracting.

2. Global Health Council

http://www.globalhealth.org

The Global Health Council is the world's largest membership alliance dedicated to improving health worldwide. The purpose of the Global Health Council Web site is to provide information on the organization and their initiatives to improve health worldwide. The Web site includes annual conference information, the women's reproductive health initiative, and the Global HIV/AIDS program. In addition, an "Updates" section features calls for abstracts, recent events, and awards. The homepage for the Global Health Council lists the above features with brief descriptions of each section. This organization makes navigation easy. All sections contain clear and concise information, though they are brief and not very detailed. Many of the features contain bulleted lists, which facilitates skimming.

3. International Network for Doctoral Education in Nursing (INDEN)

http://www.umich.edu/~inden/

INDEN is a group of nurse educators from around the world who are interested in improving the health of all people through research and doctoral education. Highlights of the Web site include news and events, conference information, papers presented at past conferences, a list of international scholarly journals, a directory of international doctoral programs, and nontraditional or summer doctoral programs. Information on membership is also available on the Web site. Overall, this is a simple site. It is easy to navigate and text is available in English at an average level.

RESEARCH/EDUCATION/ADVOCACY RESOURCES

4. International Nursing Center, American Nurses Foundation (ANF)

http://www.ana.org/anf/inc/index.htm

The International Nursing Center is sponsored by the American Nurses Foundation (ANF), a subsidiary corporation of the American Nurses Association. The Center was founded in 1991 as a result of a white paper prepared by the American Academy of Nursing (AAN), which called attention to the need for involvement in global nursing issues. The site presents information on the International Council for Nursing (ICN) and the ICN annual conference. Included is a list of related links and international conferences. International job opportunities are provided through a link to the World Health Organization (WHO) site. There are detailed sections on the history of the International Nursing Center, the mission of the center, and the related links. Donations may also be contributed to the International Nursing Center via this Web site. The ANF International Nursing Center Web site is easy to use, colorful, and pleasing to look at. It is not a complex site, a minimum of information is provided. One might expect that the site will grow as more programs are developed.

5. The International Society for Quality in Health Care (ISQHC)

http://www.isqua.org.au

ISQHC is a membership organization, including individual and institutional members, focused on quality practice and performance improvement in health care. It is funded by the Australian government. In the U.S. it is supported by the Joint Commission on Accreditation of Health Care Organizations (JCAHO), which accredits hospitals and other institutions. With today's health care focus on quality, this is an important source of worldwide information. This Web site contains information on the society, current news, international conferences, management within the organization, the advisory council, membership, accreditation, and publications. The site itself is very basic. The homepage contains membership; the *International Journal for Quality in Health Care*, a journal published by the organization through Oxford University Press; conferences; accreditation; performance indicators; noticeboard; and links. The journal section provides detailed information about the journal with links to the table of contents and author guidelines. Free online access to full-text is only available to members. A few full-text articles are available for review. Journal editors and the editorial board are also listed. This Web site is much improved both in volume of content and design since the previous edition.

6. Pan American Health Organization (PAHO)

http://www.paho.org

Originated in 1902, PAHO is the regional office of the World Health Organization (WHO) for the Americas (North, Central, and South). The Web site includes information about the organization, country health profiles, publications, databases, and a list of international conferences. PAHO materials are available in English and Spanish. A virtual disaster library, online bookstore, and press releases related to international health are available. Overall this is an excellent site. The homepage provides a list of topic areas of manageable size and scope. The site is well organized, colorful, and aesthetically pleasing. There are no advertisements to distract from the content.

7. Portfolio of British Nursing Web Sites

http://www.british-nursing.com

This site provides direct links to practice-related British Web sites. The homepage consists of a list of these Web sites, making it easy to use. The site is colorful and attractive to the eye; however, there are some blinking advertisements that are distracting. The site is supported by these commercial advertisements. There is a description of each site provided, simplifying the search process. While there is a large variety of sites contained on this page, nowhere is it indicated how these sites were chosen to appear. One wonders if these are the top sites, all the sites, or simply the ones the site creators found interesting. Information is provided in English at a simple level.

8. United Nations (UN)

http://www.un.org

The UN focuses its efforts on solving world problems that challenge humanity. Of particular interest to nursing are its programs focused on fighting disease, e.g., through improving the water supply and other public health initiatives, reducing poverty, and protecting human rights. The UN Web page includes information about the organization, conferences and events, publications, databases, human rights, UN news, documents, and maps, UN member states, peace and security, international law, humanitarian affairs, and economic and social development. In addition, there is a "Cyber School Bus" that provides international information that is appropriate for children and classroom use. The site is easy to navigate and presents information at an average level. Text is available in Arabic, Chinese, French, Russian, and Spanish.

9. World Health Organization (WHO)

http://www.who.org

The World Health Organization's primary objective is the attainment by all people of the highest possible level of health, defined as a state of complete physical, mental, and social well-being and not merely the absence of disease or infirmity. WHO has six regional offices; the Pan American Health Organization is the office for the Americas. The purpose of the WHO site is to provide information about WHO and the current initiatives. It includes past speeches given at WHO events, press reports, and fact sheets. An information services section contains WHO policy documents, the *Bulletin of the WHO,* computer-assisted translation services, health-related World Wide Web servers, and WHO library, statistical information, and *World Health Reports.*

The WHO site is easy to navigate and appealing to the eye. Information is sorted and presented in a logical manner, which facilitates finding needed information and services. Overall, it is an excellent site. Information is presented at an average level in English, Spanish, and French.

_____ Chapter **22**

Online Journals

Jean W. Lange

_____

E lectronic access to nursing knowledge is growing rapidly. New electronic journals are appearing, and many print journals are now accessible online to subscribers. Even to those without subscriptions, a visit to publisher or journal Web sites often reveals searchable databases yielding related titles and abstracts. For a fee, many publishers will send the full text of selected nursing articles. Several nursing organizations also make their journals available to members online, such as the Southern Nursing Research Society, the UK Neonatal Nurses Association, and the Gerontological Nurses Association. A listing of hundreds of journals available online, sorted alphabetically by title or publisher is available from the National Library of Medicine at *http://www.ncbi.nlm.nih.gov/entrez/journals/loftext_noprov.html*.

The following criteria guided the selection of online journals for inclusion here: currently published refereed journals originating in an electronic format that do not require membership in an organization. Ten journals met these criteria. The features of these journals are described below. All are published in English only. Some of the journals require a paid subscription or fee for access to the full text of documents; others provide full text for free. All, however, offer free access to archived titles and abstracts. Most of the journals are indexed in CINAHL.

1. *Australian Electronic Journal of Nursing Education*

http://www.scu.edu.au/schools/nhcp/aejne/

The *Australian Electronic Journal of Nursing Education* (*AEJNE*), first published in December 1995, is committed to enhancing the teaching learning experience through shared findings, insights, experiences, and advice to colleagues involved in all aspects of the educational process. Although the School of Nursing and Health Care Practices at Southern Cross University in Australia sponsors the site, authors with diverse affiliations have contributed. While the journal allows commentary specific to nursing education in Australia, most of what has been published is widely applicable.

The journal provides a forum for both refereed and nonrefereed papers, and a portion of each issue is dedicated to students' work. To date, the majority of the articles are reviewed. *AEJNE* is published one or two times per year and indexed in CINAHL. The journal is free, and full text is available through searchable archives. The table of contents can be scanned for 11 issues. A click on any title quickly brings up the full text. The site also contains a few useful links such as the Nursing Theory Page. Two of the five links were outdated, however. Although not a research journal, *AEJNE* may be useful to nurse educators in academic and health care settings and provides an opportunity for novice writers to publish their work.

2. *Graduate Research in Nursing* and *Research for Nursing Practice*

http://www.graduateresearch.com/index.shtml

Two journals indexed in CINAHL are found at this Web address, *Graduate Research in Nursing* (*GRN*) and *Research for Nursing Practice* (*RNP*). Inaugural issues appeared in summer, 1999. Five issues of each periodical have been published to date. Both journals are published by Graduate Research, LLC and maintained by faculty at the

University of Arizona College of Nursing. The site is part of the MedBan-ner Network, a community of Web site owners who exchange Web banner advertisements. Advertisements are somewhat distracting; however, one somewhat useful display offers direct links to purchase books related to journal article topics.

The purpose of *GRN* is to facilitate the sharing of graduate students' work and to encourage graduate students to submit their work for publication. Scholarly papers related to theory, practice issues, and research are sought. Research studies emphasize the findings and applications to practice rather than methodology. Unlike *GRN,* which targets nurses pursuing an advanced degree, *RNP* is dedicated to nurses in general practice. Its goal is to publish original research, case studies, protocols, or other practice-based work in language that is understandable to nurses with an entry-to-practice level of education.

The full text of both journals is free and articles are archived, how-ever, the search feature was not operational at the time of this writing, purportedly because Web site owners are seeking a new host. Both journals have links to references cited within the text and author infor-mation. This well-maintained site also offers an excellent resource page with links to research funding, instruments, methodological and statistical references, nursing issues, theorists, literature databases, writing manuals, and nursing organizations. Articles range in sophisti-cation and represent the varied interests of both generic and advanced nurse practitioners.

3. *The Internet Journal of Advanced Nursing Practice*; Internet Scientific Publications, LLC

http://www.ispub.com/journals/ijanp.htm

The Internet Journal of Advanced Nursing Practice (IJAPN) is one of 35 free, full-text periodicals published by Internet Scientific Publications (ISB), LLC in Texas. The editorial board reviews manuscripts. Although this is the only journal dedicated to nursing, ISB publishes other journals that may be of interest to nurses, including: *Internet Journal of Health-care Administration*; *Internet Journal of Emergency and Intensive Care Medicine*; *Internet Journal of Law, Healthcare and Ethics*; *Internet Jour-nal of Mental Health*; *Internet Journal of Pain, Symptom Control and Palliative Care*; *Internet Journal of Pediatrics and Neonatology*; and

Internet Journal of Rescue and Disaster Medicine. Each journal solicits case studies, original research, and reviews.

The first bi-annual issue of *IJAPN* appeared in 1997. *IJAPN* is indexed in CINAHL. Although this journal targets nurses in advanced practice, much of the content would interest nurse clinicians, researchers, and educators. All issue titles are archived with direct links to full text. Citations in the text are linked to the corresponding reference. The *Internet Journal of Advanced Nursing Practice* received the 1999 Sigma Theta Tau International Information Technology Award for Knowledge Advancement in Electronic Publishing and has been listed by Lycos, HotBot, and DirectHit as the most popular advanced nursing-related Web site on the Internet, based on user selection traffic. The ISB homepage contains an online option to subscribe to any or all of their journals. Subscribers are notified when new issues of the selected journals appear. Subscribers may also elect to receive notification of FDA alerts. There are no distracting advertisements on the site.

5. *Journal of Undergraduate Nursing Scholarship*

http://juns.nursing.arizona.edu/Default.htm

The first annual issue of the *Journal of Undergraduate Nursing Scholarship (JUNS)* was published in fall, 1999. To date, this journal is not indexed in CINAHL. Faculty at the University of Arizona College of Nursing maintain the site. Each issue contains three to four articles written by baccalaureate nursing students. Students are encouraged to submit case studies, original research, and position or policy papers addressing current issues in health care or in the nursing profession. Recent submissions expand the journal's scope to the aesthetic and artistic nature of nursing. Manuscripts are sent to external reviewers after they are deemed appropriate for the journal by the editorial board. While helping students to value publishing their work, the journal allows its authors to retain manuscript copyrights so that authors have the option to publish their work elsewhere at a later date.

This professionally designed site is uncluttered by advertisements and related links. Visitors can readily access table of contents and quickly link to the full text of any title. Authors come from varied universities in the southwestern United States. Articles are well written, and would be of interest to student or novice nurses. Because *JUNS* offers a forum for undergraduate students to embark upon the publication process, educators may wish to encourage their students to submit exemplary papers for possible publication.

6. *Online Journal of Clinical Innovations*

http://www.cinahl.com/cexpress/ojcionline3/index.html

The *Online Journal of Clinical Innovations* (*OJCI*), published by CINAHL Information Systems, contains systematic reviews of the literature regarding broadly applicable clinically based problems. The intent of the journal's founders is to facilitate the integration of research into practice by preparing reviews that provide a foundation for practice innovation. Review topics to date include such common problems as education of patients with chronic disease, pain assessment and intervention, and newborn care. The latest issue is devoted to end-of-life concerns. Each review is very thorough, ranging from 22 to 67 pages in length, and contains the latest research, practice recommendations, and a summary including tabular references to seminal work in the field. Links to each summary in the CINAHL database and to key Web-based resources are helpful.

The first issue of this fee-based journal (individual subscriptions cost $40 annually) appeared in June 1998. Since that time, approximately one to three issues have been published each year, with one to three reviews included in each issue. To date, most of the submissions are authored by three of the journal's editors; however, the board intends to gradually expand its contributor base. Nonsubscribers may view the full text of editorials, access the Internet resources, and review the titles and abstracts in each issue. Articles are also indexed in the CINHAL. Selected articles may also be ordered for a flat fee. One nice feature of this site is that it offers technical support via telephone and electronic mail.

7. *Online Journal of Issues in Nursing*

http://www.nursingworld.org/ojin/

The *Online Journal of Issues in Nursing* (*OJIN*), published by Kent State University College of Nursing in partnership with the American

Nurses Association (ANA), is a refereed publication for nurses and others with an interest in health care. Since its inception in June 1996, this thriving journal is published quarterly. The editorial board selects the topics of upcoming issues, and solicits a collection of manuscripts from national and international experts. Each manuscript receives three outside reviews. Typically, the topic is introduced with a historical review, followed by several articles that discuss its various aspects and suggest future directions.

In addition to the journal articles, latest issues include columns on information resources (particularly Web-based), legislation, ethics, and keynotes of note. The latter is a new feature that will publish topic-related speeches from major nursing conferences. The Legislative column provides legislative background on *OJIN* topics, prints opinion pieces that stimulate discussion about political issues, informs readers about newly introduced legislation or updates, and provides an international forum where readers may submit legislative information from around the world. The purpose of the Ethics column is to raise awareness of ethical issues for nurses across settings, specialties, and nationalities; inform readers about critical issues in ethics; encourage ethical thoughtfulness about ethical dilemmas that nurses face; and initiate commentary and responses from a variety of nurses globally. Clinicians, educators, administrators, policymakers, theorists, or researchers are invited to submit commentary and/or examples of ethical dilemmas they have faced.

Visitors may also access the entire listing of the 16 topics covered to date, including such timely issues as managed care, mandatory continuing education, the nursing shortage, complementary therapies, electronic publishing, the genetic revolution, and telehealth. A click on any topic quickly produces a list of all related submissions with hyperlinks to full text. The site offers online continuing education for a fee. An impressive listing of authors provides links to their publications in *OJIN*.

8. *Online Journal of Knowledge Synthesis for Nursing*

http://www.stti.iupui.edu/library/ojksn/

Online Journal of Knowledge Synthesis for Nursing (*OJKSN*) is dedicated to the scientific advancement of evidence-based practice in health care. Sigma Theta Tau International (STTI) has published the OJKSN on an irregular basis since its inception in 1993. *OJKSN* presents current scientific evidence to inform clinical decisions and ongoing discussions on issues, methods, clinical practice, and teaching strategies for evidence-based practice (EBP). Similar in mission to the *Online Journal of Clinical Innovations, OJKSN* has a much wider contributor base and produces six to twelve new reviews each year. External clinical specialist-researcher teams review manuscripts.

Each synthesis begins with an abstract summarizing the purpose, conclusions, and implications. A detailed discussion of pertinent research follows, with the citation, sample, and key findings of each study presented in tabular format. The review concludes with practice implications, needed research, and a description of the searching strategies used. References indexed in Medline have direct links to the citation in the database. Articles are also indexed in CINAHL. Users of the excellent search tool, available only to subscribers, may selectively include the journal only or the entire STTI Web site or Internet. Results are sorted by relevancy, and contain direct links to the full text.

On the homepage are links to free, full-text articles on disaster care and evidence-based practice methods, implementation guidelines, and teaching strategies. Editorials are also available to nonsubscribers. Article titles and abstracts, arranged alphabetically by title, author, or volume may be viewed from the journal's homepage. Document delivery is available for nonsubscribers. Individual subscriptions are $90 for STTI members, $105 for nonmembers. This is an excellent, high-quality journal of interest to nurses from all educational backgrounds and settings.

9. *Online Journal of Nursing Informatics*

http://www.hhdev.psu.edu/nurs/ojni/index.htm

Online Journal of Nursing Informatics (*OJNI*), first published in December 1996, produces two issues each year. Its aim is to publish original, high-quality scientific papers, review articles, practice-based articles, and databases related to nursing informatics to enhance knowledge related to nursing informatics.

All issues are indexed in CINAHL and archived. Titles are linked to full text and there are links within each article to the abstract, references, and author biography including his or her e-mail address. Ideas, comments, or questions can be forwarded to the Editor for inclusion in an interactive E-Chat. Featured in each issue are Event Monitoring, Technology Talk, a student section, and links to other nursing informatics organizations.

10. *Topics In Advanced Practice Nursing*; Medscape e-Journals

http://nursing.medscape.com/Medscape/nurses/journal/public/ nursin g.journal.html

Topics In Advanced Practice Nursing (*TAPN*) is a new journal published by Medscape. There are three issues to date; the first issue appeared in Spring 2001. At present, TAPN is not indexed in Medline or CINAHL. The purpose of this journal is to provide a free online forum for practice issues of particular interest to nurse practitioners, educators, clinical specialists, midwives, and nurse anesthetists. Each issue contains three to four articles centered on a theme. Articles are concise (less than 2,500 words) and may discuss innovative health care programs, case scenarios, novel research applications, or comprehensive reviews with practice recommendations. The articles are written by experts in the field and reviewed internally and externally. Abstract collections, featured in each issue, summarize the latest abstracts appearing in Medline about a particular topic, e.g., cardiac resynchronization therapy, depression and heart disease, and management of urinary incontinence.

Readers may register with Medscape to receive notices of new journal postings. The journal is free and issues are archived with direct links to full text. Registrants may elect a homepage that will subsequently appear on future site visits. A page has been designed for nursing that includes a smorgasbord of information and links including clinical software for PDAs; medical news headlines; monthly summaries of nursing research from the National Institute for Nursing Research; a resource center with news on major medical conditions such as bioterrorism, disaster, and trauma; conference summaries and schedules; case reviews; a searchable medical dictionary; and a link to the Medline database.

Two other notable features include free online course offerings accredited by the American Nurses Credentialing Center and "Journal

Scan." After passing a brief posttest, a free personalized certificate awarding continuing education units may be printed. A "tracker" maintains a record of registrants' completed programs. Journal Scan summarizes the latest clinical and research findings in key scholarly journals with articles of value to advanced practice nurses, and provides links to article abstracts or full text when available.

Chapter 23

Nursing Publishing Companies

Eileen R. O'Shea

D uring this age of electronic information and media, traditional nursing publishing companies have had to make great advances in order to remain abreast of exploding technology. Today's publishers offer a great deal of information, along with expanded services. One now has access to printed materials, software packages, audiovisual materials, professional resources, online shopping, interactive forums, convention and exhibit management, and advertising. To date, the amount of information offered on the Internet can be overwhelming. The following Web sites will information on nursing publishing companies.

1. Anthony J. Jannetti, Inc.—Association Management and Publishing

http://www.ajj.com

Jannetti offers complete publication management for health care professionals and specialty nursing industries. Services include: specialty journals, books, and newsletter publications; convention and exhibit management; association management; national advertising and representation; and Web site design and hosting. This Web site includes the ability to preview some content of current specialty journals, such as Nephrology Nursing or Pediatric Nursing. Regular features of the journal are listed as well as the choice to receive a complimentary issue. Under core curriculum, information of the most current texts may be previewed and ordered. There are online links for nursing practice information or association information. In the near future, AJJ will offer online continuing education courses. An attribute for this family owned company is that AJJ has made caring and personal service its motto. The company describes itself as nurturing both individuals and associations like family. This site is easy to use. It is concise and a good resource for nursing specialties and associations.

2.   Aspen Publishers, Inc.

http://www.aspenpublishers.com

Aspen Publishers services diverse professions with books, periodicals, and information services. It is a member of the worldwide Wolters Kluwer Group. When selecting the "Healthcare and Related Texts" section from the homepage, the topic of health care is divided into allied health, health administration, patient care, public health, and sports management. The homepage has a search option, which can use title or author searching. An important feature of this Web site is the ability to preview a text or manual. Listed is the product description, table of contents, price, published date, and the ability to purchase. This Web site may appear vast initially because it serves 18 different professions. Once health care is selected, the site is easy to use. It conveys clear and concise information on its publications. "Aspen Headlines," a section on the homepage, provides up-to-date information on the company itself. In general, this site offers information specific to its printed material with the ability to shop online.

3.   Delmar Nursing

http://www.delmarnursing.com/

The Delmar Nursing Web site provides nursing books and software products for instructors, professionals, and students. Nursing topics include fundamentals, community health, psychiatric mental health, dosage calculations, care plans, LPN/LVN, and health services administration. Delmar offers a variety of products for learning. These products include print, video, CD-ROM, power point slides, and online services. This publishing company is a division of Thomson Learning and has recently acquired Skidmore-Roth. The homepage displays information to access products, resources, support, company history, and a site map. Each month their most current product is featured on this page for preview or order. Information for the National Student Nurses Association can also be accessed from this page. A great benefit of this site is the availability of Nursing CE courses. Once highlighted, a brief description and the amount of credit hours are provided. Delmar Nursing Web is a colorful site that is easy to use. It offers up-to-date resources to supplement printed materials and provides the ability to shop online.

4. Harcourt Health Sciences

http://www.harcourthealth.com/

Harcourt Health Sciences consists of a team of leading publishers including Churchill Livingstone, Mosby, and W. B. Saunders. This publishing company is a division of Elsevier Science. The targeted audience is health science professionals. From the homepage one can access each of the above-mentioned publishers. Each site is organized similarly. The Mosby Web site includes a search screen; a menu for featured products and services; and an information center site. Of particular benefit is the availability of "MERLIN and SIMON" listed under featured services. Merlin stands for *M*osby's *E*lectronic *R*esource *L*inks and *I*nformation *N*etwork. Merlin provides a Web site for each Mosby published text. Characteristics of the book sites include content updates, answers to frequently asked questions, author contact information, and opportunities for feedback. Merlin sites also contain Web links to explore the most up-to-date information on a subject. Simon stands for *S*aunders' *I*nformation *M*anagement *O*nline *N*etwork. The Simon sites provide the same information as described above, but for all Saunders' published texts. Another featured product listed on the Mosby homepage is an online computer adaptive test for NCLEX-RN. This is a unique testing product that provides a realistic simulation of the exam and gives instant results and analysis of performance. This Web site provides a high level of current information to the user. It is colorful and easy to access.

5.   Lippincott, Williams & Wilkins

http://www.lippincott.com
http://www.wwilkins.com

LWW is a leading international publisher of books, journals, and new media for medical professionals and students. It is a unit of the Wolters Kluwer Company. This publisher provides information in print and electronic formats including textbooks, CD-ROM, and the Internet. The homepage states LWW offers the widest variety available in specialty journals for nurses. An important feature to this Web site is the ability to access CONNECTION. To access, one must select nursing under "specialty" on the homepage. CONNECTION offers supplemental teaching and learning tools for the classroom. It consists of sites dedicated to specific LWW textbooks. Registration is required to access protected sites. Products and services provided include sample chapters, power point slides, review and test questions, cases studies, related Web links, and chat rooms. Some areas of this Web site are still being developed. Overall, it is a useful and high-level site for referencing LWW's journals, texts, and related educational materials. A more extensive nursing Web site by LWW can be accessed at Nursing Center.com (see next entry).

6.   NursingCenter

http://www.nursingcenter.com

This Web site is owned and operated by Lippincott, Williams & Wilkins, Inc., a member of the worldwide Wolters Kluwer Group. It is an interactive Web community created by nurses for nurses. The site states it is a one-stop source for information, products, and services for nurses and health care professionals. Services and products include journals (all with abstracts and contents, some with full text articles), continuing education, forum discussions, career opportunities, nursing resources, association links, health care news, interactive presentations and features, and search engines. A benefit to this Web site is that it is free. There is not a membership fee or charges required to access its tools or resources. Also, one may subscribe to a free monthly newsletter. NursingCenter.com offers extensive nursing resources that are comprehensive and up-to-date. This Web site is easy to navigate and well organized.

7. ONLINE Nursing Editors'™

http://members.aol.com/suzannehj/naed.htm

This On-line Nursing Editors' Web page provides direct e-mail links to over 170 nursing journal editors and 9 book editors. The ease of a one-click system can link the researcher directly to author guideline pages. *Nurse Author and Editor*, a newsletter publication for nurse authors and editors, sponsors the Web site. An important feature of this site is accessing the homepage for Hall Johnson Consulting. This consulting agency offers special services, such as nursing writing, editing, and graphic services for authors, editors, and leaders. This Web site was awarded the Oncology Nursing Society Editor's Choice award and the Medical Resource Reviews Database Commended Site award. The homepage was up to date. It is a phenomenal and extensive nursing resource that is also easy to use.

8. Slack, Inc.

http://www.slackinc.com/

Slack incorporated is a leading provider of information, educational programs, and event management services for health care professionals. Products and services include journals, texts, software, online products, program development, exhibit sales and management, conventions, marketing and promotion, and sponsorship opportunities. This Web site is for medical, nursing, and allied health professionals. The best feature of this site is that information is grouped under specialty areas. A sample of specialties for the nursing profession includes critical care, gerontology, and nurse anesthesia. Each specialty area houses the most current information available, including printed materials, Internet resources, specialty products, conference schedules, and symposia on the Web. One can access the latest journal in print or browse through back issues. Full-text content is provided. This Web site has extensive resources and is presented in a businesslike and streamline format. It is certainly a high-caliber site.

9. Springer Publishing Company

http://www.springerpub.com

Springer Publishing Company publishes books and journals for health professionals in nursing, aging, mental health, social work, and medical education. The Web site contains a new releases section for all published disciplines, including nursing. This link leads to brief summaries of new publications. The site also includes an order form and a separate journals section, where detailed information regarding Springer journals can be found. The homepage for Springer Publishing Company is well organized and easy to navigate. The content provided is clear and easy to access. While these features have been present for some time, the Web site has recently been revised and now features bright colors. Some of the newer features include a list of links to authors' homepages and information for individuals who are interested in publishing a book. The manuscript questionnaire for book proposals and the authorization-to-publish form for journals and book chapters may also be downloaded online. General contact information and contact information for Springer's nursing editors is also available. A final new feature worthy of mention is online ordering capabilities. In addition, detailed information is provided on discounts for purchasing multiple books from a series.

10. Springhouse Corporation

http://www.springnet.com

This Web site states that nurses choose this company for the latest and most accurate clinical information. Springhouse Corporation is now part of Lippincott, Williams, & Wilkins Publishing. It is a member of the Wolters Kluwer Group, a worldwide publisher and information provider. Springhouse publishes nursing journals, text and reference books, licensing exam reviews, card decks, software, videos, and audiotapes. Other educational resources include continuing education programs and products, and national conferences. This Web site is eye catching. A part of the homepage displays live action video for a CE course. An important feature to this site is the continuing education course availability. The site states it possesses the largest selection of online CE offerings with new additions each month. Other features on the homepage include the section "What's New" to display SpringNet's most current products, programs, or services. The menu includes topics such as nursing library with Web site links, nursing communities, career track, nursing student center, professional services, conference calendar, journals, and products. SpringNet is easy to use. It displays accurate and current information for both students and clinicians.

_____ Part **II**

Clinical Topics

Chapter 24

General Health Care Resources

Joan Fleitas

N ever before has the concept of health been so popular. Type the word in any search engine and over five million "hits" will appear. The sites selected were chosen because of their breadth, depth, and excellence. Many of them are portals to other more specific pages.

*1. The Agency for Healthcare Research and Quality

http://www.ahrq.gov/

The Agency for Healthcare Research and Quality (AHRQ) Web site offers a plethora of information for nursing practitioners. AHRQ provides evidence-based information on health care outcomes, quality, cost, use, and access. The goals of AHRQ are to support improvements in health outcomes, strengthen quality measurements, and identify strategies that improve access, foster appropriate use, and reduce

---

*Sites suitable for consumer use.

unnecessary expenditures. The site is organized around such directories as news and information, clinical information (includes evidence-based and clinical practice guidelines), consumer health, funding opportunities, surveys and other data, research findings, and quality assessment. The pages are current, with dates listed, and authored by experts in the health professions. Contact information is included. The evidence-based practice guidelines are one of the most significant aspects of the site for nursing, reflecting the state of the knowledge on effective and appropriate care. One of the key issues on the research agenda is "Nurse Staffing and Quality of Care in Health Care Organizations."

2. Centers for Disease Control and Prevention (CDC)

http://www.cdc.gov

The Centers for Disease Control and Prevention (CDC) of the Department of Health and Human Services is recognized as the lead United States federal agency for protecting the health and safety of people, providing credible information to enhance health decisions, and promoting health through strong partnerships. The Web site offers comprehensive timely information and links to aid in the development and application of disease prevention and control, environmental health, and health promotion and education activities. Because it is a governmental site, pamphlets and other publications can be downloaded or requested without fee. The site is available in English and Spanish. Site organization is good, with consistent templates, search engines, contact information, and dated "in the news" sections on the various pages. Unique features of the site include "WONDER," which provides a single point of access to a variety of CDC reports, guidelines, and public health data; and *Healthy People 2010,* the prevention agenda for the nation. The site is current and credible.

3. Martindale's "Virtual" Nursing Center

http://sun2.lib.uci.edu/~martindale/Nursing.html

Martindale's "Virtual" Nursing Center is a very large portal to a wide range of resources, including 131,700 medical cases, 61,700 teaching files, 1,235 courses and textbooks, 1,625 tutorials, 420 journals, and 4,160 databases. The site is designed for nurses and other health professionals, and includes date of last update. Resources include interactive cases, medical dictionaries (offered in 7 languages), and anatomy and physiology resources. Links to credible, usually non-commercial Web sites are provided. The site was produced, designed and maintained by Jim Martindale who holds an MBA in finance and is employed by Paine Weber, though his primary interest is in theoretical, experimental, and applied physics. The site is endorsed by the University of California, Irvine, and has received numerous awards. It is included in this listing because of its robust and plentiful linkages to resources for nurses. The major advantage of the site is its breadth and currency, with, for example, a nursing theory page offering multimedia tutorials. The major disadvantage is the need for significant scrolling through areas that might not be immediately relevant.

4. Medscape for Nurses

http://www.medscape.com/Home/network/nursing/nursing.html

Medscape for Nursing is a site that offers robust and integrated medical information and education tools. The purpose of the site is to offer a forum for the online publication of peer-reviewed, continuing education offerings as well as summaries and highlights of material targeted to advanced practice nurses. Medscape for Nurses is built around practice-oriented content, with each specialty site filtering and delivering continually updated content from thousands of professional journals and surveys. The site's intended audience is the specialist nurse who practices in an expanded role to improve clinical practice and enhance patient care. Although particularly designed to meet the needs of nurse practitioners, clinical nurse specialists, nurse midwives, and nurse anesthetists, the breadth of content, accessibility of professional health material, and extensive resources for growth in nursing practice make this site a must for all nurses. Web MD sponsors the site, and although it is a commercial site, with advertisements for health-related products and services on the pages, the articles are generally peer-reviewed and written by acknowledged health care experts. Thus, the material is accurate and seemingly unbiased. The most important features of this site are the conference postings, the headlines and treatment of the latest health issues, and the free Continuing Education activities—planned and written in accordance with the American Nurses Credentialing Center's Commission on Accreditation, and that have been produced in collaboration with nursing-accredited CE providers. The major weakness of the site is its marketing exclusivity for advanced practice nurses when the material offered is robust and certainly of great interest to all professional nurses.

There is no accommodation for individuals who do not read English from the homepage, though the Medscape homepage itself contains Spanish and Italian portals. The site's overall appearance is busied by advertisements but enhanced by a template on the top of the pages and a search option at the bottom. Navigation is clear, with links back to the homepage from the various channels accessed on the site.

*5. National Institutes of Health (NIH)

http://www.nih.gov

The government sponsors the National Institutes of Health Web site. It is a good starting point for accessible and reliable health information. The site's purpose is to give health care providers and consumers information about health conditions, research, drugs, health organizations, publications, special programs (e.g., rare diseases, minority health), health related toll-free numbers, and links to related governmental organizations. The information is current, although since the NIH Web site is actually a large collection of sites—over 150 servers, it is difficult to give a summative answer about currency. Some are updated daily, while others are updated less frequently. The content is accurate, with authorship of the publications noted to be the Offices directly involved with the health condition of interest. The most important features of this site are its scope, accessibility to the public, provision of essential contact sources, and nonbiased information. A "what's new" section was recently added, providing visitors with up-to-date information about innovations. In addition, one of its offerings, Medline Plus, has introduced interactive health education tutorials from the Patient Education Institute that engages readers with a graphical interface to health information. The major weakness of the site is also its strength. The scope is so large that visitors might well get sidetracked and leave with their initial goal sidestepped in their excitement over the

Web site's offerings. Some sections of the NIH Web site are available in Spanish. The level of information on the site is average in terms of comprehensibility. The site's overall appearance is clean and well-organized, with intuitive navigation. A template on the bottom of the pages provides essential contact information, questions and answers about NIH, employment opportunities, visitor information, recent changes to the site, information for employees, searching, and accessibility information.

6. Pubmed

http://www.ncbi.nlm.nih.gov/PubMed/

PubMed is a governmental site offering a database developed in conjunction with publishers of biomedical literature. The site facilitates the access of literature citations and linkages to full-text journal articles. Through this portal, MEDLINE (NLM's database of 4,500 journals published in the United States and more than 70 other countries) and other citations are made available. MEDLINE is the most robust offering on PubMed's database. It includes those areas of the sciences and bioengineering needed by nurses and other health professionals engaged in research, clinical care, public health, health policy development, and educational activities. Most publications covered in MEDLINE are scholarly journals, although some newspapers, magazines, and newsletters useful to nurses are also included.

Pubmed is current and accurate, with the National Library of Medicine the umbrella agency responsible for its services. The Web site offers several unique features including a journal browser, LinkOut (links to a wide variety of relevant Web-accessible online resources, including full-text publications, biological databases, consumer health information, and research tools), and Cubby (a stored search feature that facilitates ongoing searches and updates). The site may be daunting for those without orientation to terms like MESH indexing, but is well designed with good navigational aids, a clear and consistent template, and intuitive structure.

Chapter 25

Consumer Health Resources

*Carol A. Romano, Patricia G. Hinegardner, and
Cynthia R. Phyillaier*

With the increased use of the Internet by consumers, nurse and physician health care providers face several challenges. First, they need to keep abreast of the information to which their patients have access. Second, they need to be informed about reliable consumer information resources on the Web to reference in their educational interactions with patients and family members. Finally, they need to know how and where to direct consumers who use the Internet to locate quality health care information Web sites (Jadad & Gagliardi, 1998). The difficulty of this challenge, however, rests with the principal dilemma of the Internet. The uncontrolled, open nature of the Internet fosters open debate without censorship, but it also raises concern about the quality of information available. Consumer health information on the Internet differs from printed information in two ways. First, there is complete lack of quality control, which leads to lack of reliability and the possibility of harm. Second, information may have no context; that is, it does not need to be false to be harmful. For example, consumers may misinterpret information intended for providers thus leading to false expectations about treatment options. It is also possible for consumers to miss disclaimers or warnings noted on "cover" pages (Eysenbach & Diepgen, 1998). Given this vast supply of readily available health information, and the risk of harm to consumers if the quality of information is poor, the need to identify quality consumer health resources on the Internet is vital. For a more detailed description of health Web sites appropriate to consumers, see *The Nurses' Guide to Consumer Health Web Sites* by Fitzpatrick, Romano, and Chasek.

*1. Centers for Disease Control and Prevention (CDC)

http://www.cdc.gov

The Centers for Disease Control and Prevention (CDC), an agency of the Department of Health and Human Services, is comprised of twelve centers, institutes and offices. The "CDC serves as the national focus for developing and applying disease prevention and control, environmental health, and health promotion and education activities designed to improve the health of the people of the United States." Its Web site provides access to health information, and statistics produced by the various entities within the organization. The Web site provides information for both the health professional and consumer.

Of special interest to consumers are the resources about disease and health topics that are gleaned from the general CDC Web site. These resources are arranged alphabetically under "Health Topics A–Z." New topics are continuously being added, and update information or review dates appear on many of the resources. The Web site also includes a section on "Hoaxes and Rumors" that describes bogus information that may be prevalent on the Internet or from other sources of communication. The "Travelers' Health" section contains worldwide health recommendations for travelers by destination. It also has sections with information about outbreaks, diseases, vaccinations, safe food and water, traveling with children, special needs travelers, and cruise ships and air travel.

Navigating the site is easy. The content list provides access to the major sections of the Web site, and keyword searching is also available. Since the twelve branches of the CDC design their own sites, there is variability in the format and content of the subject matter covered. A

---

*Sites suitable for consumer use.

Spanish language section provides CDC information and links to other health sites. There is also a "Contact Us" link that provides a Web-based form to send an e-mail message and toll-free number for public inquires and feedback.

*2. Healthfinder®

http://www.healthfinder.gov

Developed by the U.S. Department of Health and Human Services in collaboration with other Federal agencies, healthfinder® is a gateway to consumer health information. It provides access to selected online publications, clearinghouses, databases, Web sites, support and self-help groups, and government agencies and nonprofit organizations that produce reliable information for the public. The site provides an easy-to-use, searchable index of reviewed health information. The target audience is the general public, but health professionals will also find the site useful. A steering committee of representatives of federal agencies, nonfederal consumer health information specialists, and librarians provide guidance for development, maintenance, and improvement of the site. Information from over 1,800 government agencies, nonprofit organizations, and universities is linked using selected guidelines that are identified on the site. The currency of information varies depending on the organization.

The site has eight major sections. The "health library" contains links to health information from the various organizations. "Just for you" provides information on special health concerns based on age, gender, race, ethnic origin, or role in helping others care for their health. Links to information about health care providers, prescription drugs, hospitals, long-term care, health insurance, and medical privacy are located in "health care." The "directory of healthfinder® organizations" has information about organizations. Included in each organization's entry is its URL (Uniform Resource Locator) and other contact information, description, online and print resources, other related topics, and the date it was reviewed. "Help" offers an overview of the site for first-time visitors, search tips, a site map, and additional information about the site. "About healthfinder®" provides information about the site including accessibility, awards, information about contributing agencies, a disclaimer, feedback options, privacy policy and selection policy. Selected health care resources in Spanish are located in "Espanol." "Kids" provides links to health information designed for kids including games. Other features on the main page include "health news" and "today's online checkup," which provides a link to an interactive health assessment tool. The tools change periodically but there is an archive for accessing previous tools.

A useful feature, once a list of resources is accessed, is the "more" link. It provides detailed information about the site including its URL, sponsoring agency, description, related topics, and the date it was reviewed. Healthfinder® is easy to navigate. Searching may be done by either entering search terms in a text box or by selecting a link from within one of the major sections. Both navigation methods provide ways to tailor a search.

*3. HealthWeb

http://www.healthweb.org/

Librarians and information professionals from major academic medical institutions in the Midwest established HealthWeb. It is a collaborative project of the health sciences libraries of the Greater Midwest Region (GMR) of the National Network of Libraries of Medicine (NN/LM) and those of the Committee for Institutional Cooperation. The HealthWeb project was conceived in 1994 with the goal of developing "an interface which will provide organized access to evaluated noncommercial, health-related, Internet-accessible resources" (Redman et al., 1997). HealthWeb is a tool to facilitate access to quality health-related resources on the Internet. Information specialists collect, evaluate, and organize health information and education resources. The target audiences are health care professionals and consumers. Each library participating in the project is responsible for maintaining and updating its selected area(s).

HealthWeb is easy to navigate. An alphabetical list of diseases and health-related topics is displayed on the main page of the site. Resources within a topic are organized into categories. For example, under "Oncology" the categories include "Statistics," "Meta Sites," "Clinical Resources," "Clinical Trials," "Research Grants and Funding," "Organizations and Communication." Categories vary depending on the topic. After choosing a category, there is an option to choose a "Long

Display" that includes brief descriptions of the sites listed. A keyword search feature allows for searching within the specific topic area or the entire HealthWeb site.

Other features of the site include "User Guides" providing links to guides that will help health care professionals and consumers use Internet resources more effectively, a "FeedBack" link that gives people the opportunity to provide general feedback about the site, report a dead link or suggest a site to add, and a "Search" link that provides a text box to enter search terms and provides tips for more effective searching.

*4. HIV InSite

http://www.hivinsite.ucsf.edu/InSite

This site is a project of the University of California San Francisco AIDS Program at San Francisco General Hospital and the UCSF Center for AIDS Prevention Studies, both programs of the UCSF AIDS Research Institute. UCSF faculty and staff select the information found on the site. The editorial policy states that, "Materials posted to the site are reviewed for credibility, reliability and accuracy." Information about the advisory and editorial boards is provided, and although the site has some commercial sponsors, they are not involved in editorial decisions.

Designed as a gateway to in-depth information about particular aspects of HIV/AIDS, HIV InSite provides numerous links to many authoritative sites. Information provided usually contains a date of "publication." Its major categories include: "Knowledge Base," which is a comprehensive textbook on HIV/AIDS; "Medical," which contains treatment resources, medical literature, and listings of clinical trials; "Prevention," which includes information on what works and what does not for prevention of HIV infection; "Policy Analysis," which covers information on policy and legislation, resource allocation and ethical dimensions; "Basics," which contains a list of answers to commonly asked questions; "Countries and Regions," which provides worldwide information; and "Links," an extensive categorized list of major HIV/AIDS sites.

A useful feature at this site is HIV ForeSite, an e-mail-based newsletter produced by the staff. It provides brief updates about new information available on HIV InSite and elsewhere concerning HIV/AIDS. Other features include direct links to major medical databases (PubMed, National Library of Medicine Gateway, The Cochrane Collaborative Review Group on HIV Infection and AIDS, AIDS Clinical Trials Information Service), "Ask HIV InSite," where questions may be asked or a list of answers to previously submitted questions can be browsed, and a collection of "Patient Fact Sheets," which provide information for clients in English, Spanish, and French.

The site is well-organized and provides a variety of access points. Buttons across the top of the site permit quick access to the major categories. A text box for searching allows a specific topic to be entered and searched from any page. An e-mail address and survey form are provided for feedback and "whenever possible and relevant, the author or creator and date of creation of last review are identified." This site has extensive information; however, a disclaimer clearly states that, "it cannot substitute for the advice of a doctor or lawyer or other relevant professional."

*5. MayoClinic.com

http://www.mayoclinic.com

Although MayoClinic.com (formerly the Mayo Clinic Health Oasis) has changed its name and format since the previous edition of *Internet Resources for Nurses,* it continues to maintain its reputation as an excellent source for consumer health information. It is compiled by over 2,000 people who are physicians, nurses, scientists, and educators at the Mayo Clinic, a nonprofit institution. The site is an extension of the Mayo Clinic commitment to provide health education to patients and the general public, and a disclaimer states that it is not intended to replace health care by a professional. The newer format places more emphasis on wellness.

The authoritative source of the site is clearly identified as the Mayo Foundation for Medical Education and Research. Editors and their credentials are defined and the opportunity to contact the staff for feedback is available. The editorial board identifies important and timely health topics and selects specialists as expert sources for articles. The purpose of the site is defined as educational; however, there is some advertising by commercial sponsors. Ads are kept to a minimum and must meet strict guidelines. The editorial policy states that Mayo does not endorse any company or product.

The site's original format has been expanded considerably with its new name. In addition to the major centers of health information that existed previously (e.g., Allergy & Asthma, Arthritis, and Cancer), interactive applications and tools to assist consumers in managing their health have made the site more comprehensive. In addition to the "Find Information" section on the old site, a new "Take Charge of Your Health" section has been added. "Take Charge of Your Health" includes a "Personal Health Scorecard," "Healthy Lifestyle Planners," "Disease Self-Managers," and "Health Decision Guides." They present a series of multiple-choice questions with results that are tailored based on the responses entered. A free, weekly e-mail newsletter, "Housecall," which includes new health and fitness information, is available to anyone who wishes to subscribe.

Another significant new feature of the site is "My Mayo." This allows an individual to choose preferences in a "My Mayo Profile," which is then used to select and display articles on subjects of interest to that individual. The feature also allows saving of specific articles and pages to a "My Mayo Bookshelf" area for easy retrieval. A "Drug Name" search box continues to be available on the homepage for searching by generic or brand name drugs in the *USP (United States Pharmacopeia) Drug Guide for Consumers*.

The site is well designed and user-friendly but more cluttered than was noted in the previous review. It is easy to navigate, and those few advertisements that appear do not interfere with the content of the site. As might be expected with a site that permits individual health profiling and interactivity, MayoClinic.com requires registration for security reasons. There is no fee to register, and the user must agree to an extensive online agreement and privacy policy. Information at MayoClinic.com is timely and accurate. The site is updated every weekday, all material is dated, and everything is reviewed at least on an annual basis.

*6.   Medem™

http://www.medem.com

Founded by leading medical societies in the United States including the American Academy of Ophthalmology; the American Academy of Pediatrics; the American College of Allergy, Asthma and Immunology;

the American College of Obstetricians and Gynecologists; the American Medical Association; the American Psychiatric Association; and the American Society of Plastic Surgeons; Medem™ was created "to become the most comprehensive and trusted source of healthcare content on the Internet." The four main sections on the site are "Medial Library," "For Physicians," "Find a Physician," and "Corporate Information."

Consumers will find the "Medical Library" and the "Find a Physician" sections of most interest. The "Medical Library" is divided into four major categories: "Life Stages," "Diseases and Conditions," "Therapies and Health Strategies," and "Health and Society." These categories are further subdivided. For example, "Therapies and Health Strategies" includes the sections "Complementary and Alternative Medicine," "Fitness and Nutrition," "Medical Tests and Medications," "Pain Management," "Physical Medicine and Rehabilitation," "Plastic Surgery/ Cosmetic and Reconstructive Procedures," and "Preventive Medicine." A list of document titles displays under a specific topic. Next to each title is an icon that indicates whether the information provided is introductory, general, advanced or at the professional/research level. Following the document title is the acronym of the organization supplying the information. The information in Medem™ is provided and approved by the nation's leading medical societies making it an excellent source of information for consumers. Documents may be read on the screen or printed using the printer-friendly format option. Resources range from peer-reviewed journal articles to medical news. There is a section in "Diseases and Conditions" that provides articles in Spanish.

"Find a Physician" is another useful section for consumers. It provides links to physician finders from several of Medem™'s founding societies including the American Medical Association. Physicians can be located by specialty or name within a specific geographic area. The "For Physicians" section provides secure communications and integrated Web-based services for a physician practice. Physicians can create a practice Web site and set up a secure messaging mailbox. "Corporate Information" provides information about the participating societies and also provides information for organizations that want to become partners. Overall the site is well organized and easy to use. One can browse through the site using the category links or search the site using the text box provided. A "Search Tips" link offers suggestions for searching. Search results within the "Medical Library" are ranked by relevancy.

*7. MEDLINEplus

http://medlineplus.gov/

MEDLINEplus is a consumer-oriented Web site established in 1998 by the National Library of Medicine (NLM), the world's largest biomedical library. The NLM expert staff select and revise the content from governmental and nongovernmental publications, brochures, databases and Web sites. The NLM is part of the National Institutes of Health (NIH), an agency of the Department of Health and Human Services. The site's purpose is to provide accurate and current medical information to anyone with a medical question. Although targeting consumers, both consumers and health care professionals will find useful information here.

Information can be obtained by selecting from an alphabetical list of hundreds of Health Topics on specific diseases, conditions, and wellness issues. Individual topics are covered with reliable resources that are unrivaled in subject comprehensiveness (O'Leary, 2000). Each health topic page contains links to authoritative information on that subject, and an optional link to a preformulated MEDLINE database search with results on that subject. MEDLINE consists of citations with abstracts to eleven million research articles published in 4,300 biomedical journals and is considered the "gold standard" of medical databases. By having the search results preformulated, the consumer does not have to know special searching techniques in order to retrieve useful information from the database. An alternate method for locating information on a particular subject is a search box in which a word or phrase may be entered.

MEDLINEplus is much more than results from the MEDLINE database since it provides a number of additional resources. There are many useful directories that include locations and credentials of hospitals, doctors, and other health care providers. A list of links to several online medical dictionaries provides access to definitions of unfamiliar medical terms. Drug information for consumers is available from the United States Pharmacopeia (USP) in easily understood terms and can be searched either by generic or brand name. A number of resources listed at the site include links to full-text publications available from the NIH and other governmental and nongovernmental organizations.

MEDLINEplus is easy to navigate. There are no advertisements or cluttered graphics obscuring the information. The homepage and major sections of the site can be quickly accessed without having to go through multiple "back" buttons. Each health topic page displays the release date for that topic and all sections of the site are continuously updated. New health topics are added frequently; "Anthrax" was a recent addition. A new feature added in the last year is a series of interactive tutorials on approximately seventy topics. Although it requires downloading a plug-in application, the software loads quickly and provides the consumer with self-paced audio/video information. An automatic link checker is in place and broken links are corrected on a daily basis in order to assure currency of information. A Spanish language format is also available.

*8. National Women's Health Information Center (NWHIC)

http://www.4woman.gov

This population specialty site is a gateway to selected women's health information resources. Its purpose is to provide a single site on the Web where women nationwide can locate reliable and timely information for themselves and their families. It is intended for a variety of audiences, which includes consumers and health care professionals. NWHIC is a service of the Office on Women's Health in the U.S. Department of Health and Human Services. It consists primarily of federal resources and selected nongovernmental sources that are approved by NWHIC's editorial advisory board.

The site may be searched by entering keywords, or by selecting from an extensive alphabetical directory of "Health Topics." An A to Z search under "Health Topics" yields results divided into publications and organizations. A unique feature for consumer searching is the menu of "Frequently Asked Questions About Women's Health" (FAQs). The FAQs section is arranged alphabetically by health topics with links to numerous questions and answers. Some of the subject links have "Easy to Read" counterparts (e.g., Breast Cancer, Latina Women's Health, Heart Disease), for basic readers of English. NWHIC contains a number of special features. One feature is a menu selection on every page to "Contact Us" for feedback. The NWHIC toll free telephone number and e-mail address are provided. Another feature is monthly guest editors who provide articles on issues of relevance to women's health. Several links on the homepage are helpful: a "Women's Health News Today" section which is updated daily; "Hot Topics in Congress," which includes links to women's health-related legislation in the U.S. Congress; and links to resources for "Minority Health Information" and for "Women with Disabilities." The homepage also contains a link "En Espanol," which provides access to a Spanish version for many of the resources available at NWHIC. The site is easy to navigate. There are no advertisements, but there are public service graphics that look like ads. The homepage has more graphics and links than previously, but for clarity, a "Text Only Homepage" may be selected. Web pages are current and production/revision dates are posted.

*9.   NOAH: New York Online Access to Health

http://www.noah-health.org/

NOAH: The New York Online Access to Health is one of the oldest established consumer health sites on the Web. Launched in 1995, it is comprised of a collection of state, local, and federal resources selected by volunteer librarian editors with the assistance of a scientific advisory board consisting of interdisciplinary health professionals (Vogue, 1998). The mission of NOAH, "to provide high quality full-text information for consumers that is accurate, timely, relevant and unbiased" is clearly accomplished with the current site. The original four site sponsors (The City University of New York, The New York Academy of Medicine, The New York Public Library, and The Metropolitan New York Library Council) have been joined in recent years by additional sponsors, the majority of whom are libraries. NOAH is unique in that it is completely bilingual. Consumers can access all menus and resources beginning from the site's homepage in either English or Spanish. Content includes a number of broad "Health Topics" which are arranged alphabetically and then broken down into numerous subcategories to include definitions, care and treatment, and lists of information resources. Sources are linked to content. For example, the content on the basics of diabetes is linked to full-text items by the American Diabetes Association, the Joslin Diabetes Center, and *The Merck Manual.* The quality and depth of the sites chosen provide consumers with much needed information in terms that they can comprehend. A disclaimer is also provided that identifies NOAH as an information guide that should not be interpreted as professional or medical advice.

NOAH is designed with the easy navigability required by the novice user. A directory format allows selection of broad health categories, which lead to more specific subcategories. "Word Search" provides the option of entering a word or phrase into a text box. The "Word Search" at NOAH uses the Excite search engine; however, it only searches documents located at the NOAH site. Information throughout the site is presented in a clear and logical manner and there are no advertisements. The currency of the information is noted with the posted month of update in a "What's New on NOAH" section by subject area.

*10. Oncolink

http://www.oncolink.com/

Oncolink is an excellent example of a disease specialty Web site. Cancer specialists at the University of Pennsylvania established the site with the mission "to help cancer patients, families, health care professionals and the general public get accurate cancer-related information at no charge." The editorial board for the site includes both physicians and nurses. The site is updated daily and provides introductory to in-depth information.

Major categories on the site include "Types of Cancer," "Treatment Options," "Coping with Cancer," "Clinical Trials," "Cancer Resources," "Ask the Expert," "Oncolink Library," and "Sponsors." User-friendly menus within many of the categories provide easy access to valuable information. "Cancer Resources" includes links to many interesting sections including "Oncolink TV," a multimedia service that provides access to videos on conferences, news, and supportive care. This category also includes "Financial Information for Patients," "Global Resources," and "Causes and Prevention." Other features of the site include "Cancer News," "What's new this week," "Oncotip of the Day," and "OncoLink Art Gallery," which features artwork produced by people who have been impacted by cancer.

The site is easy to navigate. Information may be located using the user-friendly menus or by using "Quick Search" or "Advanced Search." From the homepage, a word or phrase may be entered in the "Quick Search" text box and all of Oncolink is searched. From within a category,

"Quick Search" gives the option of searching all of Oncolink or only that specific category. "Advanced Search" provides the option of using AND and OR to create a search. It also provides the option of choosing a specific category, type of article, and years.

REFERENCES

Eysenbach, G., & Diepgen, T. (1998). Towards quality management of medical information on the Internet: Evaluation, labeling, and filtering of information. *British Medical Journal, 317,* 1496–1500.

Fitzpatrick, J. J., Romano, C., & Chasek, R. (2001). *The nurses' guide to consumer health Web sites.* New York: Springer.

Jadad, A., & Gagliardi, A. (1998). Rating health information on the Internet: Navigating to knowledge or babel? *Journal of the American Medical Association, 279,* 611–614.

O'Leary, M. (2000). MEDLINEplus: MEDLINE for the masses. *Information Today, 17,* 20–21.

Redman, P. M., Kelly, J. A., Albright, E. D., Anderson, P. F., Mulder, C., & Schnell, E. H. (1997). Common ground: The HealthWeb project as a model for Internet collaboration. *Bulletin of the Medical Library Association, 85,* 325–330.

Vogue, S. (1998). NOAH-New York Online Access to Health: Library collaboration for bilingual consumer health information on the Internet. *Bulletin of the Medical Library Association, 86,* 326–334.

Chapter 26

Pharmaceutical Resources

Doris Troth Lippman

A ccess to pharmaceutical information via the Internet has provided consumers and health care practitioners alike with unlimited opportunities to expand their knowledge. While this has
been advantageous in some ways, it also has presented many challenges for those who provide care to consumers. The challenges include helping clients to understand the information they have obtained,
directing them to reliable resources, and staying current in the ever-
evolving field of health care practice.

*1. Center Watch

http://www.centerwatch.com

Center Watch is a clinical trials listing service. It aims to be an information source for both the clinical trials industry and research professionals and patients interested in clinical trial participation. The site is useful

---

*Sites suitable for consumer use.

because it divides the material into 2 categories: "Patient and General Information" and "Professional Resources." Each category is further divided into sections that cover topics ranging from drug trials, dosages, and an online bookstore. Industry resources are also extensive and include information such as research center profiles, career opportunities, and publications. Overall, this site is well-organized, comprehensive and up to date. It is also visually appealing and easy to navigate.

*2.   HSLS Health Resources

http://www.hsls.pitt.edu/intre/health/pharm.html

This Web site is an online version of the University of Pittsburgh Health Sciences Library. The site is quite extensive, providing information for both health care providers and consumers. Professionals who use this site will have access to Internet guides such as "The 'Virtual' Pharmacy Center," "A Pharmacist's Guide to Internet Health Care Resources," and links to professional organizations, associations, and electronic newsletters and journals. The section on databases includes information on new medicines under development. The health care consumer can find information on medications such as those used to treat mental health conditions. The HSLS Health Resources Web page is quite extensive. Information is current and easy for the user to follow.

*3.   Mayo Clinic

http://www.mayoclinic.com

This site is produced by the Mayo Clinic in Minnesota. The purpose of the site is to provide educational material to both the public and professional health care provider. The site provides a section titled "Drug information" where the browser can find information on more than 8,000 prescription and over-the-counter drugs. The material is easily accessed since it is listed alphabetically and can be browsed by name or category. Information is also provided on avoiding drug interactions and how to use medications correctly. Overall, this site produced by the world renowned Mayo Clinic is visually attractive and provides information in a very user-friendly manner. The material is current, well-organized, and concise.

*4.   MedExplorer

http://www.medexplorer.com

This is the site of a commercial company that was created by Marlin Glaspey in 1996. The site is free to users and is supported by advertisements and sponsors. This site provides information for both health professionals and consumers. The information for health professionals related to pharmaceuticals is provided through a list designating such categories as an online pharmacy, patient guides, drug management, resources, products, and software. Overall, this is a good site providing extensive search capability for nurses and other health care providers. It is simple to use although somewhat bulky. It does not provide information about when it was last updated although it does provide a disclaimer related to liability.

5.   Medical World Search (MWS)

http://www.mwsearch.com

Medical World Search (MWS) is the first search engine on the World Wide Web developed especially for the medical field. It aims to provide access to health care information for health care providers and consumers. It is a private company headed by Theresa L. Chang, BS; Ifay F. Chang, PhD, and Humbert H. Suarez MD, PhD. The site requires that users register before accessing the services provided. Among the services included are an acronym dictionary for pharmaceutical terms, a medical vocabulary spell check, and access to a MWS staff as needed. The site developers have responded to users' requests by selecting a number of health-related listservs. Additionally, the developers of this site are experimenting with providing wireless Internet users with a wireless interface. The site is clear, concise, and easy to use. It is well-organized and an excellent resource for nurses and other health care providers.

*6.   *The Merck Manual*

http://www.merck.com/pubs/mmanual

This site is produced by Merck and Co., Inc., a leading research-driven pharmaceutical products and services company. This site provides free online access to the classic resource for drug information, *The Merck Manual of Diagnosis and Therapy* (17th Edition, 1999). *The Merck Manual of Medical Information—Home Edition* is available now in a new interactive version. Pharmaceutical information can be accessed by using the Table of Contents or by asking specific questions in the search box. This site is comprehensive and easy to use. The online nature of its format allows updating on a regular basis and thus ensures that the information is current.

*7. RxList

http://www.rxlist.com

RxList.com was developed by Neil Sandow, PharmD. It is free to the Internet community and is a Health Central Network site. This site provides information in both English and Spanish. It also includes access to over 53,000 medical definitions found in Taber's Medical Dictionary. Users of this site will also find information on alternative medicines such as Ginkgo, Ginseng, St. John's Wort, and many other Western herbs and Chinese herbal remedies. A unique feature of this site is a section titled RxBoard, the first drug-specific discussion board on the Web. An example of the type of content in this section includes a discussion about the most searched drugs on the RxList. This site also provides a medical abbreviation finder and a helpful guide to links through RxList. Overall, this site is very comprehensive and easy to use.

*8. RxMed

http://www.rxmed.com

RxMed decribes itself as a site for physicians, patients, and their families. Its purpose, according to the mission statement, is to provide valuable and thorough illness and medication information, as well as access to various medical products and services. All of the material found on the site is authored or critiqued by RxMed's ten-member Medical Advisory Board. The site includes a section on pharmaceutical information that contains documented, authoritative, and detailed information on over 3,000 prescription medications. The listings cover general pharmacology, indications, warnings, dosage, and adverse effects information for each pharmaceutical monograph. Extensive material on herbal and dietary supplements, travel health, and illness is provided. The site is comprehensive and peer-reviewed. Ongoing announcements about nonpharmacy or health-related products that are for sale is distracting. Overall, though, this is a current and user-friendly site.

*9.   United States Food and Drug Administration (FDA) Center for Drug Evaluation and Research (CDER)

http://www.fda.gov/cder

This site provides access to the Federal Drug Administration's Center for Drug Evaluation and Research (CDER). The homepage for CDER provides consumers and health care providers with many categories of information from which to choose. These selections include drug information, regulatory guidance, and new consumer information related to buying and using drug products. The section on drugs includes CDER regulation in the areas of new prescription drug approvals, drug safety, and clinical trials information. Health care providers are able to access new drug information from an interim page that provides timely information on new drug products while a more comprehensive page is being developed. Other features of this site include a CDER Handbook on how the Center for Drug Evaluation and Research works, a MedWatch section on safety alerts for FDA-regulated products, and current "Highlights in the News." This site is very extensive, well-organized, current, and easy to use.

_____ Chapter **27**

Physical Assessment

Suzanne Hetzel Campbell

_____

This section provides information about resources on the Web aimed at nursing students and practicing nurses in the area of physical assessment. Various features allow for online practice of auscultation techniques as well as case studies specific to age groups or disease processes. Accurate physical assessment skills are important in all areas of nursing. This chapter provides insight into maintenance and enhancement of those skills.

1. Advanced Physical Assessment: Breast

http://nsweb.nursingspectrum.com/ce/ce85.htm

This site is a Continuing Education Module offered by Nursing Spectrum. CEUs are available for a fee. A case study approach is used to demonstrate a comprehensive breast history beginning with a description of the structure and development of the breast. Key issues related to family and social history are reviewed and specific details are provided in technique for breast palpation. Documentation is described and various breast abnormalities are reviewed (including male conditions). Content was written by an advanced practice nurse and is current. The site is available at an average level in English only.

2. Assessment of Abnormal Growth Curves

http://www.aafp.org/afp/980700ap/legler.html

This site is a 1998 journal article from *American Family Physician* written by Drs. James Legler and Lewis Rose, Associate Professors in the Department of Family Practice at the University of Texas Health Science Center at San Antonio, Texas. The article can be printed out and it provides a wealth of information to evaluate assessment findings with hints on performing assessments according to growth and development guidelines. This site is an excellent reference source for advanced practice nurses working with children in primary care settings and for registered nurses who work with children in a variety of contexts.

3. Assessment Tips and Techniques

http://www.nursing.about.com/cs/assessmentskills/index.htm

This site contains links to ten valuable assessment sites that are easy to access and which are described below: Advanced Physical Assessment of the Breasts; Assessment of Abnormal Growth Curves; Auscultation Assistant (see above); Cardiovascular Examination (see PE study guides above); Identifying Structural Hip and Knee Problems; LEAP (Lower Extremity Amputation Prevention) Program; McGill University Virtual Stethoscope; Pediatric Assessment in the Home; Physical Assessment of the Well Woman; and Prenatal Screening and Assessment Tool. The site provides a few sentences describing each link and a hyperlink. It has consolidated a group of worthwhile assessment sites with different foci that appeal to a variety of practitioners at different levels. The site itself is busy with advertisements and has a subject listing ranging from bioethics to transcultural issues in nursing. There are links for articles and a search capability. Disclaimers and information about the site developers is provided. Specific sections are discussed below.

4. The Auscultation Assistant

http://www.wilkes.med.ucla.edu/index.htm

For practitioners learning or seeking to review heart and lung sounds, this is the site for superb education and assistance. Easy to navigate with section tabs including physiology, systolic murmurs, diastolic murmurs, rubs, gallops, and lungs, this site allows for auditory cues in conjunction with written explanations of the various conditions, underlying pathology, and relationship to physiology of the heart. Each section differentiates the sounds in a list on the left, and direct links in the text allow one to compare similar or differentiating conditions. For example, early versus late peaking murmurs in aortic stenosis can be compared with one link. Michael Wilkes, MD, a University of California at Los Angeles Medical School Professor, developed and maintains the site. The last update was December 2000 with information that he had acquired an electronic stethoscope to enhance recordings. The site is aimed at residents, student nurses and practitioners, and has an educational focus. Contact through e-mail is available. The cardiovascular examination is the strong point, but basic lung sounds are provided at this site as well. Attractive, user-friendly, good for review and to enhance skills.

5. Cardiovascular Exam

http://www.medinfo.ufl.edu/year1/bcs/clist/index.html

See #3, Assessment Tips and Techniques, this exam is only one small part of this site, click on cardiovascular exam or use the direct link from the Assessment Tips and Techniques site.

6. Geriatric Assessment

http://www.vhct.org/case1199/index.shtml

This site is a collection of interdisciplinary cases, appropriate for medical students and other health professionals with a focus on education. Using a case presentation approach, a patient is presented with an illness, past medical history is described as well as current physical status (physical exam report, lab tests, diagnostic tests). The extent of assessment, description of pathophysiology, diagnostic and treatment options provide an excellent learning scenario. Current (revised 12/24/01), well-organized, and with excellent hyperlinks throughout the text to sites such as the family doctor, DAVID (atlas of anatomy), and Heart and Diabetes Associations, this site provides excellent resources. Overseen by School of Health Professions and School of Medicine Missouri-Columbia, the assessments are written by physicians and nurses. Beyond this specific site, cases are available on a variety of diseases and populations. This site is highly relevant to this chapter on physical assessment.

7.   Identifying Structural Hip and Knee Problems

http://www.postgradmed.com/issues/1999/12_99/skinner.htm
http://www.postgradmed.com/pearls.htm

This site is a 1999 journal article from *Postgraduate Medicine*. It is written by Harry Skinner, MD, PhD, Professor and Chair of the Department of Orthopedic Surgery and Joseph Scherger, MD, MPH, Professor and Chair of the Department of Family Medicine, both at the University of California in Irvine. Developed for advanced practitioners, this site reviews history and exam techniques for hips and knees across the life span. References and contact information are provided, and the full-text article can be printed. A nice addition is a separate link to each of three other symposiums including topics on musculoskeletal problems in primary care, painful shoulders, and back pain. Finally, tabs at the top of the first page allow the user access to "PEARLS" (or go straight to the second Web site listed above). This is a great resource for advanced practitioners (especially students) as experienced practitioners write in helpful hints.

8.   LEAP Program (listed on this site as "Best of the Net")

http://www.bphc.hrsa.gov/leap/default.htm

This site is well maintained by the Bureau of Primary Health Care. It is a program developed to provide practitioners with a system of sequential assessments and tools for patient education with the goal of reducing lower extremity amputations in diabetics and others suffering from circulation problems. The Self-Testing Instructions, available in English and Spanish, can be printed and the monofilaments used for screening may be ordered for free. The site includes access to a 12-minute video demonstrating the assessment and has many links to orthopedic and diabetic care sites. This site is definitely appropriate for all levels of practicing nurses and student nurses, colorful, easily navigated, and a worthwhile site.

9. McGill University Virtual Stethoscope

http://sprojects.mmi.mcgill.ca/mvs/mvsteth.htm

This incredible site is sponsored by McGill University and provides a "virtual stethoscope" to listen to both respiratory and cardiovascular assessments. There are colored images, an extensive written description of the conditions, excellent diagrams, and it is easy to follow and learn from. Quizzes allow students to test their knowledge at the end of the lesson. The homepage offers a directory of sites on everything from embryology to gastroenterology with laparoscope images and extensive information. Directed at medical students, beginning physiology information is appropriate for nursing students and definitely for advanced practitioners. Updated regularly, overseen by a reputable university, this site is sure to enhance assessment skills and techniques. RealPlayer 3.0 is necessary to use the virtual stethoscope, and although touted with "easy free downloading," this was not the case. The most up-to-date computer equipment should be recommended for full access to the site.

10. Pediatric Assessment in the Home

A direct link to this site is not easily accessible, but it can be bookmarked from the original Assessment Tips and Techniques site. This site includes a continuing education article from Nursing Center.com written by Janice Thompson, Professor at Quinnipiac University School of Nursing. It is from December 2000, includes a test, and for a fee can award continuing education credits. Specific to assessment of pediatric patients in the home, it includes the role of the nurse and home risk assessment tools that help to focus on evaluation of the child's physical and psychosocial needs. The article is concise, contains easily referenced tables with information such as guidelines for communication, and common defense mechanisms used by children. Only a portion of the article is printable and no hyperlinks from the site were available. However, as a specific learning tool the site is very useful.

11. Physical Assessment of the Well Woman

http://www.umanitoba.ca/womens_health/nephys.htm

This site is specifically designated for nursing education and listed as a "guide for nurses." It includes information on the interview; examination approach, technique, criteria, and method; and reviews each major body system from head to toe. Similar to the physical exam study guides mentioned above, this is a more concise format, and appropriate for beginning level nursing students. Nothing flashy, but relevant, accurate, and a good starting point. References are supplied, updated last May 1998, supervised by the Department of Obstetrics, Gynecology and Reproductive Sciences at the University of Manitoba and the Health Sciences Centre. The site is available in English at an average level.

12. Prenatal Screening and Assessment Tool

A direct link to this site is not easily accessible, but it can be bookmarked from the original Assessment Tips and Techniques site. This site provides a flowchart that can be downloaded and printed. It is useful to assess for prenatal use of drugs and alcohol and provides some basic important information for beginning nurses and advanced practitioners working with pregnant women. The site is produced by Santa Clara County in California and has links to many other sites from parenting to child abuse reporting. Telephone number, address, and e-mail are available for contact persons.

13. Physical Exam Study Guides

http://www.medinfo.ufl.edu/year1/bcs/clist/index.html

This site, produced by the University of Florida, provides study guides for a comprehensive head to toe physical exam. The site was developed for medical students by Dr. Richard Rathe, MD (Professor, School of Medicine, University of Florida). The lists of equipment, general information, inspection and palpation techniques with notes that give helpful hints at the end of each section, provide accurate information that is relevant for beginning nurses as well as advanced practitioners. Lecture slides are available with some pictures and drawings. However, these slides were developed in August of 1998 and have not been modified since December 2000. The cardiovascular exam is especially well-presented and has a table of vital sign averages for children at different ages. There is a link to a mini-mental exam and "The Heart in Action," which can be downloaded. The download can take a bit of time, but it is well worth the wait. Easy to navigate and well-organized, this site provides basic information that is concise and to the point. One key aspect of the organization is the layout of each part of the exam separately. The site is appropriate for learning beginning assessment techniques and more advanced procedures (e.g., varieties of murmurs). Weaknesses include the lack of links to other sites and not being updated recently. The site is available in English at an average level.

14. RALE (Respiration Acoustic Laboratory Equipment) Repository

http://www.RALE.ca/Recordings.htm

This site was developed by Chris Carson at PixSoft, Inc. in Canada. Its purpose is described as follows: "This computer aided instruction on respiratory sounds is designed for students, educators, doctors, nurses, allied health professionals, and anyone who uses a stethoscope." Like the Auscultation Assistant site, it provides digital recordings of lung sounds, including normal, bronchovesicular, bronchial, tracheal, wheezing, crackles, squawk, stridor, and grunting. In addition, there is text describing what is being heard, a respirosonogram in color, and an electrocardiogram (ECG) tracing with explanations. The digital recordings play well on newer and older versions of "Real Player," and the clear sounds are easily recognizable and distinguishable. The site lists its current updates, as well as phone, fax, address, and e-mail for contact persons. It is a well-organized and stable site focused on respiratory sounds. There is minimal advertising for stethoscopes and versions of this Repository for purchase on CD ROM. Case presentations and quiz files are included with purchase. The site is available in English at an average level.

Chapter 28

Clinical Decision Making

Tener Goodwin Veenema

M edical care is often said to be the art of making decisions without adequate information. Health care providers must frequently choose treatment modalities long before they know which disease process is present. Even when the illness is known, they must frequently select from among several treatment options, and the consequences of each cannot be predicted with certainty. Indeed, uncertainty is intrinsic to the practice of medicine and nursing. The domain of clinical decision making is concerned with two questions: "How do clinicians (and patients) make important clinical decisions?" and "What can be done to improve the overall quality of clinical decision making (how can we reduce uncertainty)?" The following alphabetical list of Web sites attempts to answer both of these questions by providing nurses with description analyses of the components of clinical decision making and access to prescriptive measures of various kinds, including clinical practice guidelines, computerized decision support, and decision analysis.

*1. Agency for Healthcare Research and Quality Clinical Practice Guidelines

http://www.ahrq.gov/clinic/epcix.htm

One of the most clinically useful resources is the Agency for Healthcare Research and Quality (AHRQ) evidence-based practice Web site containing Clinical Practice Guidelines. These guidelines are available for both health professionals and consumers in English and Spanish and cover a broad array of clinical scenarios. A summary and evidence report is provided for each clinical topic and many are in files that can be easily downloaded from the Web. A powerful search engine allows information to be retrieved by keyword. The site also contains a list of Evidence-based Practice Centers, technical reviews, and some conference summaries.

*2. CenterWatch

http://www.centerwatch.com

CenterWatch is a publishing and information services company that provides information services used by patients; pharmaceutical, biotechnology, and medical device companies; investigators; and research centers involved in clinical research around the world. Founded in 1994, CenterWatch publishes a wide range of newsletters, books, and custom research reports. This Web site represents a clinical trials listing service, and provides an extensive list of Institutional Review Board (IRB)-approved clinical trials being conducted internationally as well as profiles of approximately 600 clinical research centers. The site contains several drug directories, and includes lists of promising therapies newly approved by the FDA (Food and Drug Administration), drugs currently in clinical research, and a drug trials results database. CenterWatch contains a search engine based on detailed keywords that allows the user to search for either patient (consumer) or professional resources. The professional bookstore gives health care providers book reviews and access to the most current publications on conducting clinical research. Users need to keep in mind that this is a

---

*Sites suitable for consumer use.

commercial (for-profit) Web site; however, it remains a great source of information for anyone interested in the clinical trials industry.

3. Centre for Evidence-Based Medicine

http://cebm.jr2.ox.ac.uk

This is a great Web site sponsored by the Centre for Evidence Based Medicine located in Oxford, United Kingdom. The site provides nurses and physicians with an overview of the concept of evidence-based medicine, explains how levels of evidence are assigned, and provides a vast array of accurate, up to date information for clinical decision making. It contains teaching activities and teaching materials that are easily accessible and access to eight evidence-based journals including the *Journal of Evidence-Based Medicine, Evidence-Based Nursing,* and the *Journal of Evidence-Based Mental Health.* Also contained within the site is the EBM 'toolbox' of useful analytic tools for using evidence in clinical decision making and the CATbank, a creation, storage, and retrieval facility for CATs (Critically Appraised Topics), including the CATmaker. The site is well-maintained and extremely easy to use. Nurses who are new to the concepts of evidence-based practice will find this site particularly valuable.

4. Cochrane Clinical Reviews

http://www.cochrane.org/cochrane/revabstr/mainindex.htm

Cochrane Reviews, sponsored by the National Library of Medicine and Milbank Memorial Fund, are summary reviews of the evidence for a particular clinical topic. Cochrane has assembled international experts into 50 collaborative review groups such as the Cochrane Breast Cancer Group, Stroke Group, Neonatal Group, and the Cochrane Musculoskeletal Group. These groups make the results of research assessing the effects of health care more easily available to those who want to make better decisions. The site stresses to providers that well-informed decisions require information, and judgments about needs, resources, and values, as well as judgments about the quality and applicability of evidence. This Web site contains a wealth of clinical information that is both valid and reliable.

5. Medical Matrix: Decision Making and Tools

http://www.medmatrix.org/_spages/Decision_Making_and_Tools.asp

The Medical Matrix Project is devoted to posting, annotating, and continuously updating "full content, unrestricted access, Internet clinical medicine resources." The target audience for this Web site is primarily physicians and health care providers who are on the front line in prescribing treatment for disease conditions. It is a "supersearch" engine that constructs ranked, peer-reviewed, annotated, clinical medical resources on the Web. Medical Matrix assigns ranks to Internet resources based on their utility for point-of-care clinical application. Quality, peer review, full content, multimedia features, and unrestricted access are emphasized in the rankings. The homepage for the site contains a search engine that allows the user to keyword search topics in medical specialties, diseases, clinical practice, current literature and educational modalities, and medical computing, imaging and technology. This Web site links the user directly to the Decision Making and Tools page that contains a broad list of links to clinical decision making sites. The user must register to first access this site; however, it is free of charge and the registration takes less than a minute. This Web site is attractively designed, fun to visit, and easy to use.

6. National Guideline Clearinghouse

http://www.guideline.gov/index.asp

This Web site is the home of the National Guideline Clearinghouse™ (NGC), a public resource for evidence-based clinical practice guidelines. NGC is sponsored by the Agency for Healthcare Research and Quality (formerly the Agency for Health Care Policy and Research) in partnership with the American Medical Association and the American Association of Health Plans. This site contains a number of valuable features including detailed key word searching, a browser function based on Disease or Condition; Treatment, Intervention, or Organization categories; and guideline comparison capabilities. The site also provides direct links to other guideline sites including the AHRQ guidelines listed previously and the current CDC guidelines. NGC, as part of their normal site maintenance, requires all guideline developers to provide evidence that their guideline was developed, reviewed, or revised within the past 5 years and not superceded by a more recent version. Guidelines not meeting these criteria are removed and listed in the HGC Guideline Summary archive. This process makes this site one of the best in terms of validity and reliability of information provided.

*7. National Library of Medicine (U.S.)

http://www.nlm.nih.gov

The ultimate medical knowledgebase is found in the National Library of Medicine (NLM) site. This site is home to the world's largest medical library and links to all of the NLM databases including Medline, PubMed, AIDSline, CancerLit, Toxline, CINAHL, and MeSH. Note that some of these databases require an account and are fee-based. Also available is access to Computational Molecular Biology, Medical Informatics, and the Visible Human Project, with downloadable high-resolution CT and MRI sections of both male and female bodies. The site is vast and includes numerous other high-quality medical resources. Nurses can link to *http://clinicaltrials.gov* to provide their patients with information and recruitment criteria for current clinical research studies and to *http://gateway.nlm.nih.gov*, a "supersearch" engine contained within the National Library of Medicine. The target audience for the Gateway is the Internet user who comes to the National Library of Medicine not knowing exactly what is here or how best to search for it. The NLM Gateway presents a single interface that lets users search in *multiple* retrieval systems. The user enters one query that is sent automatically to multiple retrieval systems having different characteristics but potentially useful results. Results from the target systems are presented in categories (journal article citations; books, serials, and audiovisuals; consumer health information; meeting abstracts; other collections) rather than by database. In some categories, multiple collections are searched. Nurses can go to Gateway for an overview scan of NLM's resources. Some will find what they need immediately. Others may find that one resource, such as PubMed® or MEDLINEplus, has information they would like to know more about. They may then choose to go straight to that resource for a more focused search. This is the quickest and easiest way to navigate the National Library of Medicine.

8. Ottawa Health Decision Center

*http://www.ohri.ca/programs/clinical_epidemiology/OHDEC/decision.
asp*

The Ottawa Health Decision Center (OHDeC) was established in November 1995 as part of the Clinical Epidemiology Unit of the Loeb
Health Research Institute at the Ottawa Hospital. The OHDeC consists
of a team of investigators who are conducting clinical research projects
and are interested in clinical decision-making analysis. This site is of
particular interest to research nurses working in aging, clinical epidemiology, cancer, endocrinology, molecular medicine and vision, and clinical nurses from a broad array of settings. The Web site contains access
to clinical decision rules (e.g., Ottawa Ankle Rules, Ottawa Knee Rules,
CT Head Rule, Cervical Spine Rule), clinical practice tools, education
modules and evaluation measures, and to its Decision Support Framework. This decision support framework was developed for practitioners
and patients considering health care decisions that are stimulated by
a new circumstance, diagnosis, or developmental transition; require
careful deliberation because of the uncertain and/or value-sensitive
nature of the benefits and risks; and need relatively more effort during
the deliberation phase than the implementation phase. The Center is
funded by the Canadian Institute of Health Research and seems to be
well-maintained.

*9. PharmInfoNet

http://pharminfo.com

The Pharmaceutical Information Network, or PharmInfoNet, is a Web
site specializing in new drug information. PharmInfoNet contains information of relevance to both health care professionals seeking technical
information and to consumers wanting to know more about health care.
The site is extremely well-organized, easy to navigate, and attractively
designed. The major areas of content are Drug Information, Publications, Disease Centers, Glossary, Medical Meeting Highlights, Discussion Groups, PharmMall, Pharmacy Corner, PharmLinks, and even a
Gallery. One of the most useful areas in PharmInfoNet is the DrugDB
(drug database). While the number of drugs listed does not compare

in number to what one would find in works such as the *Physician's Desk Reference* or the *Merck Index,* much more recent information is available on drugs such as Viagra and Propecia (a new hair loss remedy). There are even entries for common medications such as ibuprofen and acetaminophen. A typical drug entry lists trade name, generic name, manufacturer, use, and links to full-text online health and medical journals. The Web site provides access to full-text articles from clinical publications, economic data, symposium information from scientific meetings, and links to other relevant drug information and pharmaceutical sites. It is important to note that all of PharmInfoNet's online publications are either produced by them or their affiliates. None of these journals is peer reviewed. However, their articles often contain references to standard professional journals like the *New England Journal of Medicine* and *Lancet.* PharmInfoNet is produced by VirSci Corporation, a high-tech company that applies virtual technologies to medical communications, medical and pharmaceutical marketing, and pharmaceutical sales training. They are adamant, however, about not being affiliated with any specific pharmaceutical company; however, users should remember that this is a commercial site.

10. Society for Medical Decision-Making

http://www.smdm.org

This is the homepage for the Society for Medical Decision-Making. Founded in 1979, the Society for Medical Decision-Making is an international, interdisciplinary organization dedicated to the study and improvement of all aspects of medical decision making. The Society's diverse membership includes trainees to senior researchers as well as educators, clinicians, managers, and policymakers. Members come from a variety of backgrounds and academic disciplines and are dedicated to promoting rational and systematic approaches to decision making that will improve the health and clinical care of individuals and assist health policy formation. This Web site is designed primarily for researchers and academicians interested in medical decision making, but may be of interest to nurses working in this arena as well. Segments of the Web site are password protected and restricted to society members, such as the discussion board and some of the educational modules, but most of the site is not restricted. The site has its own search capability and includes links to other professional societies, related journals, and medical decision making-related academic departments nationwide.

Chapter 29

Infants, Children, and Adolescents

Kristen S. Montgomery

A though there are many challenges to caring for infants, children, and adolescents, childhood and adolescence typically are healthy periods of time. Health care appropriately focuses on prevention, primary care, building healthy attitudes, and life skills. The Web sites below are intended to offer information on appropriately caring for infants, children, and adolescents.

*1. American Academy of Pediatrics (AAP)

http://www.aap.org

The American Academy of Pediatrics Web site provides general information related to the health care of children and adolescents. The Web site includes current news for the AAP, AAP policy statements, bookstore, continuing medical education (CME), and contact information. Information on advocacy, research, membership, professional

---

*Sites suitable for consumer use.

education, and publications is available. A new section on children, bioterrorism, and disasters has recently been added. Overall, this is a very good site. The American Academy of Pediatrics is the leading authority on children's health care, and this commitment to high quality is also evident in the Web site. The site is comprehensive and easy to use. Content is presented in English at an average level.

*2.　Bright Futures

http://www.brightfutures.org

The goal of the Bright Futures Initiative is "promoting and improving the health, education, and well-being of children and adolescents age 0–21 and their families." A nationally recognized panel of experts has developed guidelines in specific focus areas to help achieve this goal. Guidelines are available for use online or a hard copy may be purchased. The online guidelines are very user-friendly. The user can choose a general topic area of interest or a specific age group to obtain information. These files are in PDF format and may be downloaded and printed. The special topic guides include nutrition, oral health, mental health, physical activity, and families. Also available is *Guidelines for Health Supervision*. A 2001 update is available for the pocket guide. The site and initiative are sponsored by the Maternal Child Health Bureau, HRSA, the National Center for Education in Maternal Child Health at Georgetown University, and Pfizer Pediatric Health. In addition, the entire Web site is available in Spanish. The site is very user-friendly and presents information at a simple to average level.

3.　Centers for Disease Control Adolescent and School Health

http://www.cdc.gov/nccdphp/dash/

The homepage of the CDC Adolescent and School Health Web site is intended for health care providers, researchers, and policymakers. Some of the key features of this site are the national school health strategies, research and evaluation content, risk behaviors, guidelines for school programs (includes AIDS, healthy eating, violence, physical activity, and tobacco), resources and tools, and project partners. The site is easy to navigate and interesting to browse. The text is presented in English at an average level. There are no distracting advertisements.

*4. Children's Intensive Caring

http://www.intensivecaring.com

Children's Intensive Caring is a comprehensive medical resource regarding caring for children. The site was developed and is managed by a pediatrician. The Web site is divided into professional and consumer sections. The professionals section includes "Intensive Thinking: Pediatric Critical" which is a question and answer review book and CD-ROM regarding caring for ill children. The "Cool Baby Hall of Fame" features a topic with test questions. Teaching tools are included for asthma, bronchiolitis, coarctation, Guillain-Barre Syndrome, Henoch-Schonlein Purpura, and Kawasaki Syndrome. There are also sections on interpreting blood gases, urinary analysis (UA), drug dosages, poisons and antidotes, and diabetes guidelines. The site also features continuing medical education (CME) and a section just for nurses. The site is presented in English at an average level. Navigation is easy.

*5. Health Resources and Services Administration (HRSA) Focus on Child Health

http://www.hrsa.dhhs.gov/childhealth

HRSA's Focus on Child Health Web site provides information about its various programs. Content is appropriate for a wide audience including health care providers, policymakers, consumers, and other concerned persons. The site is sponsored by the U.S. Department of Health and Human Services (DHHS). The main categories of this site include outreach models, HRSA child health programs, state resources, model programs, and insurance/HCFA. A key feature of this site is the *Report to the President by the Interagency Task Force on Children's Health Insurance Outreach,* which can be downloaded and printed from the site. The site is clear, concise, and easy to use. The language level is simple and there are no distracting advertisements. The site is available in English only.

*6.   Institute for Child Health Policy

http://www.ichp.edu

The Institute for Child Health Policy Web site is a comprehensive resource for governmental and political information related to child health that is located at the University of Florida at Gainesville. The Institute was established in 1986 and is funded by HRSA and the Maternal Child Health Bureau (MCHB). The site's intended audience is health care providers, policymakers, and other interested persons. Content is presented in a simple way that is useable for consumers as well. The homepage is divided into several main categories including organization and financing of care for children, youth with special health care needs, and research. Highlights of the site include the section on children in managed care, the various state child health insurance programs, supplemental security income (SSI), and the section on access and quality care for low-income adolescents. The text is available in English at an average level.

*7.   MSNBC Children's Health Headlines

http://www.msnbc.com/news/CHILDRENSHEALTH_front.asp

This Web site is sponsored by the MSNBC Television Network. It is designed for the general public, but is also useful for nurses who wish to remain current on news related to pediatric health care. Several interactive sections are available on the site, including fast facts, immunization schedules, and an interactive check-up. The site provides a very detailed list of the latest news related to children's health care. There is a link to the MSN homepage. The text is presented in an average level in English. The site is easy to navigate and contains only a few advertisements.

*8.   National Center for Youth Law

http://www.youthlaw.org

The National Center for Youth Law is a private nonprofit law office serving the legal needs of children. The Web site includes articles and analyses, general publications, and information on recent bills passed regarding child support and the rights of children in foster care. It links to California's Welfare and Health Programs—A Guide for Teens, Childhood Lead Poison Training, Requests for Cases: Familial Status Housing Discrimination, and Foster Care. Information on employment, fellowships, and internship opportunities; development and support; and contact information are included. Overall, this is a good resource for legal information. The site is well-organized, easy to use, and presented at a simple level in English.

*9. National Institute of Child Health and Human Development

http://156.40.88.3/default.htm

This is the homepage for the National Institute of Child Health and Human Development at the National Institutes of Health (NIH). The purpose of the site is to provide a variety of information about children to researchers, clinicians, administrators, policymakers, and the general public. The information provided on the site is current and accurate. The following sections are included: news and events, health information and media, funding, research, epidemiology, statistics, prevention, employment, fellowships, and research resources. In addition to this professional information, there is information on national child health initiatives including the Back to Sleep Campaign to prevent Sudden Infant Death Syndrome (SIDS), and Milk Matters to encourage the consumption of milk among children and youth. Information on clinical trials and the institute's strategic plan is also included. The site is only available in English and is presented at an average level. The site is easy to navigate.

10. World Health Organization (WHO) Child and Adolescent Health and Development

http://www.who.int/child-adolescent-health/

This department of the WHO is responsible for interventions concerning health, growth, and development outcomes for the age group 0–19 years. Main areas of the site include news, integrated management of childhood illness, rights, adolescent sex and reproductive health, neonatal health, prevention and care, nutrition, development, resources, collaborators, and HIV/AIDS. Each of these sections contains a wealth of information. The site is mainly geared toward health care providers. The site is well-organized, easy to navigate, and presented in English and French at an average level.

Chapter 30

Women's Health

Kristen S. Montgomery

W omen are the primary seekers of health care in the United States, and often oversee the health care needs of the entire family. Women's health encompasses the range of adolescence through older adulthood. Resources related to pregnancy and childbirth, while part of women's health, are included in a separate section of this book, titled *Maternity*. The Web sites below represent clinical resources related to the care of women and range from clinical information resources to organizations that support clinical work and research to advance the science regarding women's health care.

1. American Medical Women's Association

http://www.amwa.doc.org/

The American Medical Women's Association is an organization of 10,000 women physicians and medical students dedicated to serving the unique needs of women. The organization was founded in 1915. Their vision statement is to empower women to lead in improving health for all within a model that reflects the unique perspective of women. They are an organization that functions at local, national, and international levels to advance women in medicine and improve women's health. Although this organization is mainly geared toward physicians, there are some pearls of wisdom for nurses as well. For example, the organization provides and develops leadership, advocacy, education, expertise, mentoring, and strategic alliances to advance their mission. The Web site also highlights recent news in women's health. In the "Health Topics" section, a range of full-text articles appears with author name, credentials, and source. Information is provided on upcoming meetings and there is a section that addresses priority educational initiatives for both consumers and health care providers (e.g., breast cancer education for primary care providers and women). Finally, information is provided on the *Journal of the Medical Women's Association,* the official journal of the organization. Several recent supplements are available free online including tobacco and women's health, medical abortion, and emergency contraception. Full-text back issues are available online for free (includes 1997 and 1998). The current table of contents, editorials, and abstracts are available free online as well. Interested persons may also sign up to receive free e-mail updates for upcoming chats, issues, and forum sessions. At this time, information is only available in English. The Web site is easy to navigate and information is current and accurate.

2. Jacobs Institute of Women's Health

http://www.jiwh.org

The Jacobs Institute of Women's Health was founded in 1990 by the American College of Obstetricians and Gynecologists to promote the study and reporting of women's health issues. It is particularly concerned with the interface of medicine and the social sciences. The Web site includes information on publications of the institute, current events, the Board of Governors, awards and prizes offered by the institute, state profiles on women's health statistics, membership information, and managed care. The site also features search capabilities and a staff list; the site is intended for use by health professionals. An "Insights" section features the compilation of briefing papers from symposia sponsored by the Jacobs Institute of Women's Health. The

"State Profiles on Women's Health" section features ordering information on this publication offered by the Jacobs Institute. Overall, this is a comprehensive resource for information relating to women's health care. The site is well-organized, accurate, up to date, and easy to use.

3. *Journal of the American Medical Association (JAMA)* Women's Health Information Center

http://www.ama-assn.org/special/womh/womh.htm

This is part of the larger American Medical Association Web site. It includes free continuing education. The purpose of the site is to provide current information to health care providers who care for women. A news line features top stories and in-depth special reports. A library provides the top new literature related to women's health. There are also separate information centers on sexually transmitted diseases and contraception. These information centers include a library and best of the net (top sites selected by reviewers). The best of the net section also contains a "last update" date. Overall, this is a very helpful Web site. The site is well organized and succinct. The organizational structure facilitates information retrieval. Information presented on the site is current and accurate and presented at an average level.

*4. The National Women's Health Information Center (NWHIC)

http://www.4woman.org

The National Women's Health Information Center is a project of the U.S. Department of Health and Human Services. It is a database of women's health information. Main sections of the Web site include search by health topic, health news and current events, dictionaries and journals, health information for special groups, announcements, information in Spanish, and information on the Office on Women's Health. One can also download *Bodywise Handbook,* an eating disorders information source for middle school personnel. NWHIC's mission

---

*Sites suitable for consumer use.

is described as "a one-stop gateway for women seeking health information." The resource is free and directed toward a vast audience, including consumers, health care professionals, researchers, educators, and students. The page also features the Health and Human Services *Blueprint for Action on Breastfeeding*, that can be downloaded for free, and information on violence against women and women with disabilities. This very comprehensive Web site presents a wealth of information to the user. The site is generally easy to navigate, though the homepage is somewhat busy. Information is up to date and presented at an average level.

5. Society for Women's Health Research

http://www.womens-health.org

The Society for Women's Health Research was established in 1990 to improve the health of women through research. It was formerly called the Society for the Advancement of Women's Health Research. One important mission of the Society is to advocate for more funding for research of common women's health problems. The site is intended for researchers and health care providers. The Web site includes information about the society, research findings from the annual society meeting, publications, policy and advocacy, the Women's Health Research Coalition, gender-based biology, clinical trials, research funding, health facts, public education, and online shopping. Information is also provided on job opportunities, the *Journal of Women's Health and Gender-Based Medicine* (official journal of the Society), and upcoming events. The Web page also features a topic series on information that is of concern to women's health, e.g., women at risk for cancer. Overall, this is a good resource for information related to women's health research. The site is well organized, current, and easy to navigate.

*6. Women's Health Interactive

http://www.womens-health.com

Women's Health Interactive is a company based in Colorado that specializes in providing health information for women through the use of digital interactive technologies. This Web site features top health news, online health centers, and an option to create a "personal action plan" for health and wellness. The health centers include gynecology, headache, mental health, midlife, natural health, and assessment. The "Frequently Asked Questions" section has entries on cysts, endometriosis, fibroids, infertility, menstrual disorders, menopause, midlife sexuality, Pap tests, and vaginitis. The Women's Health Interactive site also includes a women's service directory that helps interested persons locate specialized health care services, professional associations related to women's health, and organizations. Finally, there is a section on current research topics, opportunities to participate in research online, and a women's opinion survey. General site information is also provided, including contact information, search capabilities, discussion lists, affiliates, and a section about the site. While this is an informative site for nurses, it does focus on information that is appropriate to the general public. The site is very comprehensive, covering a wide range of topics related to women's health. The Web site is cluttered in some areas and the pictures featured within the text do not add any value to the information presented.

Chapter 31

Older Adults

Meredith Wallace and Kathleen Perfetto

T he year 2030 will bring with it an estimated 20% of the population being elderly (> 65 years of age). This presents the necessity of having valid and reliable information as well as evidence-based practice to care for this population appropriately. The continuous need for education not only for health care providers but also for family and friends is a vital component to the growing needs of this population. Currently, there are an estimated 5,000 related sites. The sites presented here provide information with respect to common diseases and illnesses, commonly asked questions regarding care of the elderly, and difficult issues that may arise in this population. Information on continuing education, assessment tools, up to date research findings, support groups, booklets, and educational materials are provided in these sites.

*1.   Go60.com

http://www.go60.com/

Go60.com is a Web site produced by Robert Knechtel, a computer savvy older adult committed to harnessing the Internet to bring seniors

---

*Sites suitable for consumer use.

(and those concerned about them) vital information, products, and services to enrich and prolong quality, independent living, and when extended care is unavoidable, assist them in managing it in ways that maintain dignity and humanity. Knechtel describes the site as a no-nonsense Internet destination devoted to helping seniors improve with age and is not about dazzling readers with an eye-popping, animated Web site. The site's best features are its sections entitled: "Health News," Alzheimer's Watch," "Caregiving," and "Myths About Aging." Nurses, as well as seniors and family members, may find the most current news articles on alcoholism, depression, and fitness, as they relate to older adults, as well as on more standard topics like arthritis, cancer, and heart disease. Alzheimer's Watch contains a list of signs and symptoms, as published by the Alzheimer's Association, to aid loved ones and caregivers to spot potentially disease-related behaviors that require medical evaluation. This section also serves as an avenue for obtaining the latest news on Alzheimer's Disease. Caregiving supplies consumer tips on choosing nursing care facilities and services (written in accordance with the American Association of Homes and Services for the Aging), and is also an excellent way to find current, full-text articles on this subject. Some articles, however, are not readily accessible; others must be purchased from the source. This section also contains recommendations for additional Web sites that provide excellent information on caregiving services and organizations that support caregivers. Myths about Aging consists of a synopsis of the evidence from the MacArthur Foundation Study dispelling common myths of old age, as well as facts about the older adult population. Because this site is mostly an avenue for obtaining current news articles, readers must evaluate sources for credibility. Overall, this is an enlightening, informative, and recommended Web site.

*2. Health and Age

http://www.healthandage.com/

Health and Age is a Web site dedicated specifically to education on the aging process, and is sponsored by the Novartis Foundation for Gerontology, an independent, nonprofit organization whose mission is to make its fund of knowledge available to a wider audience, in an effort to promote human well-being. The site's editor-in-chief is Robert

Griffith, MD, an Oxford-educated general practitioner, researcher, and consultant on new drug development. The site is also supported by specialists in the fields of nutrition, psychological counseling, and complementary medicine. The information on this site has been carefully selected from major medical journals or is provided by the site's associates, which include the National Institute on Aging, Harvard Medical School, and Tufts University. Nurses, other health care professionals, and the public may use this site to access the latest health news, recent reports, and in-depth articles on a myriad of health topics and to obtain precise information on health products, and prescription drugs. Specific health questions may be answered via the site's "Ask the Doctor" service within five business days, under full confidentiality. This outstanding Web site also offers access to disease digests (which may be downloaded via additional software); information on alternative medicine, including herbs, supplements, and treatments, ranging from acupuncture to yoga; and self-assessment tools, including those used to calculate body mass index, sleep, stress levels, and more. The Health and Age Network offers two mini-sites, one containing higher-level information intended for health care professionals and medical educators, and one intended for the layperson. The site's most impressive feature is its "Primer on Aging," which offers excellent graphics and detailed information on age-related body changes in the brain and cardiovascular, respiratory, and digestive systems. This Web site is user-friendly and offers information in English. Of all the Gerontological sites offered, this one provides the most current, comprehensive, credible, and readily accessible data.

*3. Mature Connections

http://www.matureconnections.com/

Matureconnections.com is an Internet magazine created for seniors (ages 50 and up), by seniors who recognized the need for a prime Web site to present interesting and informative material for mature adults in a straightforward, easy-to-use manner. Mature Connections is published by Connections, LLC of Los Angeles, CA, a company dedicated to publishing Internet Web sites that provide products and services in user-friendly formats. Although the bulk of information, products, and services offered on this site are geared toward entertainment (e.g., food, travel, and hobbies), some sections contain valuable information for nurses and health care consumers. The most comprehensive and useful categories for nurses on this site are "Women's Health Interactive" and "Health and Fitness Archive." Women's Health Interactive is a subsection of the "Health and Fitness" category, which specializes in the development and delivery of health education for women through the use of interactive digital technologies. It contains learning centers on cardio health, gynecologic health, mental health, headaches, and more. Each center provides tools for assessing current knowledge, education on the topic, an avenue to interact with others, resources for accessing current information, and a mechanism for creating a personal action plan to promote health. The Health and Fitness Archive consists of full-text articles on subjects like joint discomfort, preventing vision loss, and improving sleep patterns. Articles are informative, current, and provided by credible resources such as the Arthritis Foundation and the National Eye Institute. The site is attractive, easy to navigate, and contains average to high-level information. Drawbacks include limited information in categories such as medical equipment and supplies, pharmacy, and vision. Information is available in English only.

*4. Senior Net

http://www.seniornet.org/

Seniornet.org is a Web site offered by Senior Net, a nonprofit organization of computer-savvy older adults whose mission is to provide seniors with education for, and access to, computer technologies to enrich their lives. Senior Net is based in San Francisco, CA, and is funded by membership dues, learning center fees, and altruistic donations. This site offers access to online computer courses for older adults and access to information and discussion on areas of interest, such as books, finances, and health matters. Nurses may use the site to obtain simple to in-depth explanations of health conditions for their clients by accessing the "Health Matters" category. This category also provides listings of credible, pertinent resources for further information and support. One may also access the "Healthy Aging Center" from the Health Matters section to obtain current articles on areas of health that are of special concern to older adults. The articles are written by Michael

Castleman, a well-known San Francisco-based health writer. Nurses may also refer clients to this site to participate in Round Table discussions on specific health matters. Although information contained in this site cannot substitute for information and advice from a health care practitioner, it may help one make more informed health care decisions and it may serve as a source of peer support for seniors who may have limited emotional supports of their own. The Healthy Aging Center also teaches seniors how to search the Web for trustworthy health information and warns them that some of the medical information available on Web sites is questionable or even dangerous. The site is easy to use and contains a tool for increasing or decreasing text size to facilitate reading for older adults. Information is available in English only. One does not have to be a member to access information or participate in discussions.

*5.   Yahoo Seniors

http://www.seniors.yahoo.com/

Seniors.yahoo.com offers access to the Yahoo search engine, which nurses, other health care providers, and consumers may use as a gateway to health information. The homepage offers a link to major geriatrics-related categories, such as Gerontology, Elder Abuse, and Elder Law. The "Health" category provides access to subcategories of special interest to geriatric nurses, including death and dying, long-term care, nursing, pharmacy, and senior health. The death and dying category offers site listings for information on advance directives, bereavement, and palliative care. The long-term–care category offers links to sites on caregiving, hospice, and nursing home care. By accessing the senior health subcategory, nurses may find sites for topics like aging, Alzheimer's, consumer products and services, long-term care, and organizations (e.g., Consumer Ombudsman Program, Heath Advocates for Older People, and Meals On Wheels). The Nursing subcategory, found under the Health section, offers information specifically designed for nurses—for example, information on conferences, education, government agencies, nursing institutes and organizations, and Web directories. From the nursing Web directories, nurses may access a nurse Web search index, which features full-text searching of major nurse topics and Internet information resources. For example, one may use the search tool to access geriatric and other nursing journals, like *Geriatric Nursing, Geri-Nurse News, Home Care Journal,* the *American Journal of Nursing,* and *Nursing Research.* Both print and online versions of journal articles may be obtained via paid subscription or pay-per-article. A nurse directory provides categorized listings of nurse-related Internet sites. The seniors.yahoo.com Web site serves as an excellent avenue for obtaining precise information of special interest to those who provide health care to older adults. Because it is part of a major search engine, research may be time-consuming and requires a fair amount of Internet savvy.

Chapter 32

Nutrition

Kristen S. Montgomery

N utrition plays a key role in health and well-being. Advances have been made in recent years to advance nutrition therapy for various age groups and to manage certain conditions. Adequate nutrition is crucial throughout the life span, from infancy to old age. The following is a list of nutrition resources for clinical nurses to use in their practices. The sites range from general nutrition sites to organizations that specialize in nutrition and food science. When evaluating information from a "nutrition" site it is imperative to carefully critique the site from which you retrieve information. Many of the sites labeled "nutrition" are actually advertisements for various types of supplements and untested weight loss plans.

*1. American Dietetic Association

http://www.eatright.org

The American Dietetic Association (ADA) is a membership organization of dietetic professionals, founded in 1917, with approximately 70,000

---

*Sites suitable for consumer use.

members who focus their work on improving the nutritional status of the public. The purpose of the site is to provide a resource to health care providers who work with the public on nutrition-related matters. The ADA Web site includes sections on nutrition resources, member services, classifieds, services to find a dietician, and government affairs. A nutrition tip of the day is also offered. There are sections on home food safety and ADA employment. Abstracts for the ADA journal are available via link. Additionally, there are sections that provide information on nutrition-related careers, including specific schools and programs, and there is a list of upcoming meetings and exhibitions related to nutrition. The "Nutrition Resources" section is divided into separate sections for consumers and professionals. Each section provides a variety of publications and information related to nutrition. Some of these publications are available in Spanish. An e-mail address is provided for questions. The Web site provides excellent, current information and is creatively organized on the site page. The site is simple to use and provides information that is clear and concise.

*2. Arbor Nutrition Guide

http://www.arborcom.com

This is an educational site providing a broad range of nutritional information. According to its editor-in-chief, Dr. Tony Helman, it is a nonprofit site operated as a public health service by volunteers. Dr. Helman is a physician-nutritionist based in Australia. The site is intended for health care providers and includes sections that are appropriate for consumers. The information presented in these pages is current and accurate. A "last updated" date is displayed centrally on the homepage. The most important feature of this site is the comprehensiveness of the content. The site contains the following broad categories: "Applied," "Clinical," "Food," "Food Science" and "Home." The "Applied" section includes dietary guidelines, journals/newsletters/books, and lay and patient information. The "Clinical" section includes nutrition-related diseases, nutritional deficiencies, nutrition assessment, special diets, and sports nutrition. The "Food" section includes information on the food industry, agriculture, cooking and dining, cultural nutrition, and ancient diets. The "Food Science" section contains information on food composition, genetic engineering, food law/labels, and food safety/additives.

Text is available in several languages and the site also has search capabilities. Finally, a free e-mail nutrition update service is available to those who wish to sign up. Information is provided in English. The site is well-organized and easy to use. The major categories of information are presented in a way that facilitates locating information efficiently.

3. Food and Agriculture Organization of the United Nations

http://www.fao.org

The purpose of this Web site is to provide global food and agriculture information. It contains information on agriculture, fisheries, forestry, nutrition and sustainable development. Additionally, access to statistical databases is provided. There are sections to help locate regional offices, employment opportunities, publications, events, the World Health Organization calendar, special programs, and a link to the World Food Summit, which provides a newsletter. The newsletter is available in English, French, and Spanish. Links to other WHO organizations and news and highlights are also provided. The entire site can be viewed in English, French, Spanish, Chinese, or Arabic. This is a very comprehensive site intended for the general public interested in issues of global health. The information is well-organized and concise. The information provided is accurate and up to date. Different sections are segregated, facilitating information retrieval. Information is average to high level.

*4. Food and Nutrition Information Center

http://www.nal.usda.gov/fnic

The Food and Nutrition Information Center is the information center of the National Agricultural Library, which is part of the U.S. Department of Agriculture's Agricultural Research Service. The Food and Nutrition Information Center Web site includes a section on healthy school meals; information on food safety, dietary supplements, food composition, and dietary guidelines [including the Recommended Daily Allowances (RDAs)]; the food guide pyramid; reports and studies; and Internet resources. "Topics A–Z" is a very comprehensive, alphabetical listing of food and nutrition topics. There are also databases for food and nutrition software and multimedia programs, nutrition education training (NET) program materials, USDA/FDA training programs, and nutrition education materials developed by WIC (Women, Infants, and Children Nutritional Supplementation programs). Overall, this is a very good site. The information is clearly organized and informative. The site has the endorsement of the USDA and is noted to be an official Agricultural Network Information Center.

5. Food Safety and Nutrition Info: International Food Information Council

http://www.ificinfo.health.org/

The International Food Information Council, a nonprofit organization founded in 1985, sponsors this site. Its mission is to communicate science-based information on food safety and nutrition to health professionals and others providing information to consumers. It is based in Washington, DC, and focuses primarily on U.S. issues. The Food Safety and Nutrition Info Web site includes information on sugars and sweeteners; food labeling; food biotechnology; adult, adolescent, and child nutrition; health and physical activity; food additives; food safety; international food issues and resources; fats and fat replacers; food allergy and asthma; and food irradiation and technologies. This site also contains searching abilities and a glossary. Nutritional literature is available for ordering from this site. The "Scientific Reporting" section includes background information, related publications, and Food *Insight* Reports. One can also customize the site to display categories of information one needs. Specifications can be remembered based on one's computer settings. This is a very useful site. The simplicity of the page adds to the ease of use and efficiency of this site. Information is current and accurate and presented at an average level.

6. Food Service and Nutrition Journals

http://www.sciencekomm.at/journals/food.html

This site provides links to major nutrition journals, many of which are available full text. Minimally, a table of contents and bibliography information are provided. The site links to 97 different journals and Barnes and Noble. Searching capabilities are provided. Searching can be done via 3 different lists: interdisciplinary (nature, science), medicine, and books on scientific writing, or via the alphabetical list of major subject areas. Clicking on one of the major subject areas leads the user to a list of homepage links for the major science journals included. The Food Service and Nutrition Journals Web site also links to online resources (writing, presenting, online dictionaries), book corner (writing guides, medical dictionaries, drug guides), and a self-help (writing) guide. This Web site is sponsored by science.komm, a Web site with almost 4,000 links to bioscience and medical journal homepages, designed and managed by Mark Brownlaw. The Food Service and Nutrition Journals Web site provides an invaluable service to health care providers seeking information regarding the latest nutrition research. All journal links are current with the latest journal issue. The site is quite simple, which contributes to its ease of use and efficiency. The language level is average.

*7.   Mayo Clinic.com Food and Nutrition Center

http://www.mayohealth.org click on Healthy Living Centers, then Food and Nutrition

This is the nutrition section of the Mayo Clinic consumer health Web site. The Mayo Clinic.com Food and Nutrition Center includes a virtual cookbook, ask the Mayo dietician, quizzes and reference articles, nutritional updates via e-mail service, and links to other nutrition related sites. The Web site also includes a database of searchable recipes. Other features of this site include a "Nutrition and Disease Management" section, nutrition basics, and weight management tools. Pages can be formatted for easy printing or e-mailed. Unfortunately, registration is required to use the interactive tools. However, the registration is short. The site provides helpful, clear, and concise information. The site is well-organized and user-friendly.

8.   Nutrition and the Pregnant Adolescent: A Practical Reference Guide

http://www.epi.umn.edu/let/nmpabook.html

This is an online textbook for clinicians caring for pregnant adolescents. It is mainly geared toward nutritionists, but is applicable to nurses and other health care providers as well. The text was produced by the Leadership, Education, and Training Program in Maternal Child Nutrition at the University of Minnesota School of Public Health, Division of Epidemiology with the financial support of the Maternal Child Health Bureau, Health Resources and Services Administration, U.S. Department of Health and Human Services. Mary Story, PhD, RD, and Jamie Stang, PhD, MPH, RD, co-edited the book. The book has a copyright date of 2000. Information is presented in brief descriptions and bullet points for easy reading. A very comprehensive list of chapters is available for free download and printing. Chapters cover basic areas such as adolescent development and nutrition basics, to more complex nutrition topics. Appendices include nutrition assessment forms, dietary guidelines, and sample menus. The book is available in English at a simple to average reading level. The separate chapters make navigating the site very efficient.

9. Tufts Nutrition Navigator

http://navigator.tufts.edu/

The Tufts Nutrition Navigator is a rating guide to nutrition Web sites sponsored by the Tufts University Center on Nutrition Communication, located at the School of Nutrition Science and Policy, in Massachusetts. This site is intended for nutrition professionals. The homepage of the site includes 9 main categories to access needed information. These categories include general nutrition, family, women, men, journalists, health professionals, educators, special dietary needs, healthy 2002, and hot topics. Selection of a topic leads to a very comprehensive list of Web sites on the given topic area. Each of the Web site listings is given a rating score (0–25) and a brief 1–2 sentence critique of the site. This format offers the user a quick way to assess the sites that are most useful to them. At the time of publication, the health care provider section contained 147 sites that were currently rated. The 25-point scale represents the sum of content and usability scores that were developed by an advisory board of distinguished nutrition experts. Names, place of employment, and a biographical sketch are available for all members of the panel. No weak points were noted for this site. The site is easy to use and information is presented at an average level.

Chapter 33

Pain

Laree J. Schoolmeesters

P ain is a complex and subjective experience, influenced by behavioral, cognitive, affective, and physiologic factors. Pain is defined by the American Pain Society (1992) as " . . . an unpleasant sensory and emotional experience associated with actual or potential tissue damage, or described in terms of such damage" (p. 2). McCaffery (1979) defines pain, as whatever and whenever a person experiencing pain says it is. Self-report of pain is the single most reliable indicator of pain (Acute Pain Management Guideline Panel, 1992). There are three classifications of pain: acute, chronic, and malignant. In addition to these Web sites, many sites exist for specific types of pain (e.g., headache, low back pain, and phantom pain). Links to these topical areas are included in selected Web sites.

*1. American Academy of Pain Management

http://www.aapainmanage.org/

The American Academy of Pain Management (AAPM) is a membership organization comprised of pain clinicians from many different disci-

---

*Sites suitable for consumer use.

plines. The site provides information about its membership, congressional record, and continuing medical education. Resources for the nurse and consumer include guides to United States pain management programs by zip code and pain management professionals from the AAPM Membership. Examine the Patients' Bill of Rights, pain management definitions, related links, and discussions regarding various pain-related topics. The site's most valuable feature is the National Pain Data Bank, which is an outcomes measurement system that provides resources for health care professionals and researchers. The Data Bank is used by over 100 pain management programs and manages a patient database of over 13,500 as of October 1999. The Research Assistant provides for researching any specific condition paired with specific treatments, modalities, disciplines, and medications in the National Pain Data Bank. This information is in English with an above-average reading level. A good foundation of pain material is provided on this site.

2. Dick Chapman's Pain Research Homepage

http://painresearch.utah.edu/crchome/

This site is the homepage of C. Richard Chapman, PhD, Professor and Director at the University of Utah. The site will be undergoing major revisions in the coming months. The site is a resource for individuals in the field of pain research and clinicians concerned with pain control. The section for researchers includes consciousness, cognitive and behavioral, multidisciplinary sciences, research funding sources, ethics, medical imaging, and anatomy. Clinicians are provided with introductory information on pain terminology, acute pain, chronic pain, and cancer pain. The pain resources section contains sites with information about pain organizations, state cancer pain initiatives, cancer pain, clinical guidelines, pain measurement resources, pain journals, homepages of pain researchers and clinicians along with commercial links. Examine the resources regarding palliative care and clinical resources. A separate link is provided for patients and their families. The topic links are general resources, general and chronic pain, specific pain syndromes and pain disorders, cancer pain and survivorship, pain-related psychological problems, and therapeutic music and art. Each heading has Web sites listed alphabetically. The information is in English at a simple to average level. The site subscribes to the HONcode principles of the Health On the Net. The site is well-organized, provides unique features, and may become a favorite site for pain researchers.

*3.   InfoMIN: Medical Information Network for Chronic Pain, CFS, FMS, and Other Medical Resources

http://www2.rpa.net/~lrandall/index.html

InfoMIN is a private, nonprofit health information resource maintained by a chronic pain sufferer that provides medical information for patients, family members, and health care providers. A magnitude of topics are covered such as chronic pain, chronic fatigue syndrome, fibromyalgia, reflex sympathetic dystrophy, myofascial pain syndrome, Crohn's disease, and depression and chronic illness. The site uses large font and provides information on how to obtain Social Security Disability. Healthcare providers and consumers will be able to use the Pain Inventory Form and Pain Diary Worksheet. Links to pain research and a large amount of pain and medical information are accessible through this site. There are also links to *The Merck Manual* and pain policy and the law. The site is a good source for information about a wide variety of chronic pain disorders. All information is in English at a simple reading level. It is an excellent resource for health care professionals, patients, and family members. Another positive is the frequent updates to the site.

*4.   NOAH: New York Online Access to Health

http://www.noah-health.org/

New York Online Access to Health (NOAH) seeks to provide high-quality full-text health information for consumers that is accurate, timely, relevant, and unbiased. NOAH currently supports English and Spanish. Nurses can use this resource and refer their clients to it as well. There are three categories: What is Pain?, Care and Treatment, and Pain in Children. What is Pain? has two subcategories: (a) the Basics and (b) Types of Pain with an A to Z topical listing. Care and Treatment has three subcategories: (a) Basic Care, (b) Body Specific Therapies (back, pelvic, and vulvar), and (c) Types of Therapy (acupuncture, biofeed-back, chiropractic, chronic pain therapy, and medications for pain). The Pain in Children subcategory provides the basics, which includes anesthesia; chest pain; colic; cramps; earaches; growing pains; heel, hip and knee pain; and teething. The site has won multiple awards and has all information in both English and Spanish. The site also includes health topics, search by word, and a list of the recently added items. The site is very simple to use and has an average reading level.

*5. North American Chronic Pain Association of Canada

http://www.chronicpaincanada.org

The North American Chronic Pain Association of Canada (NACPAC) is affiliated with the American Chronic Pain Association (ACPA) and provides links to American pain clinic directories. This nonprofit site provides self-help for those in chronic pain. It provides a listing of support/self-help groups, pain clinics, and pain specialists throughout Canada. A toll free phone number is listed to contact representatives from this organization. Other links include general and chronic pain information; related associations and resources; media; and medical; articles on pain; forums, newsgroups, chats, and online conferences; medical information references; pain research; and management resources. A one-sentence synopsis is provided with each Web site and new updates are easily noticeable. The pain clinic directories are one of the key features of this site. All information is in English and the links are good resources for patient referral and health care professional use.

*6. Pain.com

http://www.pain.com/

Pain.com is funded by the Dannemiller Memorial Educational Foundation. The site provides information for professionals and consumers and is divided as such. This comprehensive well-designed site provides subheadings for cancer pain, interventional pain management, migraine/headache pain, regional anesthesia, and perioperative pain. For the professional, programs for Continuing Medical Education (CME) and Continuing Education (CE) along with free CME and CE are provided. The *Online Pain Journal* has full-text articles. Under the Pain Expo heading one can search for pain products or medications. Scanning the extensive Virtual Library one can find articles, abstracts, case studies, and journals. *Pain News* lists pain articles by date. The Pain Resource will link to pain societies and associations, a pain glossary, a drug checker to determine any medication or food interaction, and pain program accreditation standards. Refer consumers to the 'Ask the Pain Doctor' for free service or to find a pain specialist or pain clinic in the US or Canada by zip code. The Pain Support provides access to drug assistance programs for those unable to afford medications, pain assessment tools, and political and health-related support groups. Professionals and consumers will benefit from this easy to use site. All information is in English with an average to high level of information for the professional and a simple level for the consumer. The principles of the Health On the Net Foundation are followed.

7. PainLink

http://www.edc.org/PainLink/

PainLink is a virtual community of health professionals working in institutions that are committed to alleviating pain. An initiative of *Education Development Center, Inc.*, with funding from The Mayday Fund of New York City. The fee-based membership for health care institutions include technical assistance, teaching cases, access to pain management resources, and administration of the Pain Management inventory (a clinician survey of knowledge, attitudes, institutional barriers, and pain management learning needs). The site provides a variety of resources for health professionals. A pain survey may be completed with the results graphed. The Guidelines heading contains links to guidelines, standards, position statements, and other resources developed by institutions, professional societies, and other organizations. A strength of the site is the Pain Resources database, which is divided into pain management, institutional change, clinician education, clinical pain syndromes, and pain in special populations. Once in the area of interest, the search can be limited or expanded based on key words or type of material (e.g., journal, book, Web site). The Resource heading provides an alphabetical list to related Web sites. The Archives heading provides transcripts of online discussions, such as addiction, and Mayday newsletters with various institution strategies on improved pain management. All information is in English at a high level. Although a drawback of the site is that it is mainly intended for institutions, health care providers will appreciate a well-organized, user-friendly site.

8. PainNet, Inc.

http://www.painnet.com/

Pain Net, Inc. was developed by physicians, educators, and business professionals to provide educational and support services to physicians and other health care professionals. Services include Credentialing by Procedure, Educational Programs, Managed Care, Patient and Physician Advocacy, Practice Development, and Quality Assurance. Public Information includes a patient Bill of Rights, questions to ask your caregivers, and a state-by-state listing of qualified pain care physicians. Free information is listed, for example, AHRQ guidelines and online counseling. Links to other sites are also available. Physicians have an opportunity to register their practice on the Web site or register for continuing medical education programs. Informational links and a newsletter are other areas accessible to health care professionals. The bookstore provides a variety of information for consumers and health care professionals. Look for the online educational programs, doctor-locating directory, and free brochures. All information is in English. The target audience is physicians, although it is a good site for client referral. The Public Information area provides simple and concise information.

9. Pediatric Pain

http://is.dal.ca/%7Epedpain/pedpain.html

The site is sponsored by Dalhousie University, located in Halifax, Canada, in conjunction with the IWK Health Centre Pediatric Pain Research Lab. The site provides professional and research information, a pediatric pain sourcebook of protocols, policies, and pamphlets, and self-help resources. Examine the links section for self-help, research and professional, and journal Web sites. Health professionals and researchers can explore the Child Facial Coding Scale—a behavioral coding system to estimate a child's pain and the International Forum on Pediatric Pain that is focused on cutting edge research and clinical practice. Other resources are a Pediatric Pain Letter, containing abstracts and commentaries, and a Mailing List, which is an international forum for discussion about children's pain. Investigate the listings of publications. The sourcebook section contains 19 listings from the FACES pain scale to sickle cell. To find specifics, there is a search that may limit by disease, audience, pain, drug, and others. Each listing may be downloaded. Submission guidelines are noted. The self-help section is a wonderful tool for parents and health care workers. Two online booklets are available. *Pain, Pain Go Away: Helping Children With Pain* is illustrated with suggestions for pain relief with an above average reading level. *Making Cancer Less Painful: A Handbook for Parents* discusses potential pain involved with cancer and procedures. This is an excellent well-rounded site for use by researchers, health professionals, and parents. Information is in English at an average to high level. The site gives particularly useful and research-based educational material.

REFERENCES

Acute Pain Management Guideline Panel. (1992). *Pain management: Operative or medical procedures and trauma. Clinical practice guideline.* (AHCPR Pub. No. 92-0032). Rockville, MD: Agency for Health Care Policy and Research, Public Health Services, U.S. Department of Health and Human Services.

McCaffery, M. (1979). *Nursing and pain management.* Philadelphia: Lippincott.

Chapter 34

Mental Health

Patricia A. Wilke

The incidence of mental illness is steadily increasing. The constraints imposed by the current system of managed care and limited community resources create a growing need for psychiatric mental health nurses to direct consumers and families to existing mental health care resources. With the increasing frequency of Internet use and the proliferation of mental health-related Web sites, the Web is rapidly becoming one of the most essential resources for professionals and consumers alike.

*1. Alzheimer's Association

http://www.alz.org

The primary objective of the Alzheimer's Association Web site is to provide information and support to family members and caregivers of individuals diagnosed with Alzheimer's disease (AD). This well-de-

---

*Sites suitable for consumer use.

signed site is separated into five distinct Web pages; each is targeted at a particular audience: "People with AD," "Family Caregivers and Friends," "Physicians and Healthcare Professionals," "Researchers," and "Media." The pages created for consumers and caregivers mainly focus on Alzheimer's information and support services. Information for caregivers is also available in Spanish. A unique feature of this site, geared for the nonprofessional, is a glossary of the vocabulary that is commonly used in conjunction with AD. On the page designated for physicians and health care professionals, issues related to diagnosis and treatment of AD, quality care, family and caregiver counseling, and insurance are discussed. Information on funding, grant programs, current research, and clinical trials is available on the page written for researchers. The last page focuses on media concerns. Other regular features found on this site include news and legislative updates, chapter information, upcoming events, on-line polls, weekly tips, message boards, and links to additional resources. The Alzheimer's Association Web site is accurate, well-organized, and regularly updated.

2. American Psychiatric Nurses Association

http://www.apna.org/

The American Psychiatric Nurses Association (APNA) Web site includes information on legislative, policy, and clinical news that may affect the practice of psychiatric mental health nursing. The aims of APNA are to provide professional leadership, enhance the quality of mental health care for all individuals, and assist in the development of mental health policy. APNA membership information, a calendar of events, annual conference news, and a listing of APNA publications are also included. The *Journal of the American Psychiatric Nursing Association* is accessible from this site. There are also links to individual APNA chapters, international psychiatric nursing organizations, and government resources. The homepage provides a recruitment service for nurses called "CareerLine." The APNA site is easily navigated and frequently updated, with offerings that are useful and relevant to psychiatric nurses.

*3. Internet Mental Health

http://www.mentalhealth.com

The stated intent of the Internet Mental Health Web site is to share information about the diagnosis and treatment of mental illnesses worldwide. It was created and funded by Phillip W. Long, MD, a Canadian Psychiatrist. Internet Mental Health was written for consumers, their families and friends, mental health professionals, students, and anyone with an interest in mental health. The site is very colorful, well-organized, and offers an extensive amount of mental health information in English, French, German, Portuguese, Spanish, and Italian. The homepage contains links to the following topics: "Disorders," "Discussion," "Medications," and "Magazine." In keeping with the international focus of the Web site, the "Disorders" page contains both American and European descriptions of 54 of the most frequently occurring mental disorders. There are also descriptions of 72 different psychiatric medications with indications, adverse effects, and research findings. Furthermore, an online diagnosis feature is available for 37 of the most common disorders for a modest subscription fee. Another useful feature is the "Help" page, designed to assist readers in locating information on this site and elsewhere on the Internet. In addition, an "Internet Link" page provides external links to a variety of mental health Web sites. Because of its comprehensive nature and online diagnostics, Internet Mental Health is truly a unique site that has much to offer both consumers and mental health professionals. It is accurate, informative, and updated on a regular basis.

4. Medscape Psychiatry and Mental Health

http://www.medscape.com/Home/Topics/psychiatry/psychiatry.html

The Medscape Psychiatry and Mental Health Web site is one of the Medscape "specialty" home pages. Owned and operated by WebMD, it is an excellent resource for mental health professionals. The aim of the site is to provide professionals with up to date clinical information to enhance patient care. Dr. Robert Kennedy is the Editor and Program

Director of the Psychiatry and Mental Health Web site. The homepage displays links to psychiatry news articles, continuing medical education courses, a physician directory, and medication information. The list of psychiatry resource links is listed on the lefthand side of the homepage for easy navigation. The site offers clinical updates, practice guidelines, conference information, journal articles, and a page with interactive case presentations for clinicians. There are also psychiatry links to government sites, journals, and other sources. The "Patient Resources" page contains links to information about various mental disorders and medications. In addition, there is a link to Medscape Health, the site for consumers where informative articles and news about many kinds of health conditions can be found. Articles for consumers are written at a lower level for easy comprehension. Like other Medscape Web sites, Medscape Psychiatry and Mental Health is a valuable resource for mental health professionals. The site is frequently updated, well-organized, accurate, and easy to use.

*5.   Mental Health InfoSource

http://www.mhsource.com/

Mental Health InfoSource is a large expansive Web site consisting of seven individual content areas: "What's New," "MH*Interactive*," "Continuing Education," "Healthier You," "Disorders," "Classifieds," and "Resources." There is an enormous amount of mental health information available on this site for consumers and mental health professionals. In addition to information on mental disorders, the reader can find news briefs, home study courses, and two online journals, *Psychiatric Times* and *Geriatric Times*. Journal articles are available in a variety of languages. Other useful features include links to treatment centers and managed care Web sites. Of particular interest to nurses, a Psychiatric Nursing Discussion Forum is located on the "MH*Interactive*" page, uniting psychiatric nurses with their colleagues around the world for consultation and collaboration. The "Healthier You" page contains the link to the official homepage of the National Alliance for Research on Schizophrenia and Depression (NARSAD). This organization is dedicated solely to the study of brain and behavior disorders in an effort to discover the causes of mental illness and develop effective treatments. The NARSAD Web site offers a great deal of helpful information for consumers and their families, health care providers, and the public. Nurses will find this site especially useful as a mental health teaching resource. Fact sheets, brochures, and videotapes about schizophrenia, depression, and bipolar disorder are available here as well as news of ongoing research studies. Mental Health InfoSource is produced by Continuing Medical Education, Incorporated, a division of the CMP Healthcare Group. The information provided on this site is current, research-based, and frequently updated. The organization and design of the homepage enhance its ease of use, despite the extensive amount of material available on the site.

*6.   Mental Help Net

http://mentalhelp.net

The comprehensive award-winning Web site, Mental Help Net, offers readers online mental health news, information, and numerous other resources. Directed by Mark Dombeck, PhD, the site is sponsored by CMHC Systems, an information technology company. CenterSite, LLC is responsible for the Web site's content and evaluates the quality of all recommended Web links with a four star rating system. The mission of Mental Help Net is to provide discourse and collaboration among professionals of different disciplines, provide mental health education to the public sector, improve access to mental health care, and support continuing mental health research. The homepage is well designed with a feature article at the top and news articles in the right margin; links to issues and disorders, resources, information, and professional services complete the page. Each disorder listed is linked to articles on basic information and news, support groups, treatment facilities, research, personal narratives, and other helpful consumer resources. Some of the services offered to consumers and professionals on this site are particularly noteworthy. Consumers are able to locate a psychiatrist, psychologist, social worker, or psychiatric nurse using the "Clinicians Yellow Pages." In addition, professionals can find a conference, job, or continuing education course. Other important consumer resources offered here include mental health and managed-care glossaries. Mental Help Net is easy to navigate and offers a large variety of mental health information that would be of interest to just about anyone. It is written at a level that can be understood easily by most people.

*7.   National Alliance for the Mentally Ill

http://www.nami.org

The official Web site of the National Alliance for the Mentally Ill (NAMI) is useful to professionals and consumers alike. In keeping with the stated aims of NAMI which include support, education, advocacy, and research, this site contains current information on mental illnesses and treatments, educational programs, local affiliates and support groups, publications, policy and legal issues, research news, and links to related sites. Mental health professionals can direct consumers to this site for illness-related information and support. In addition, there are fact sheets and other helpful materials available for distribution to consumers by health care providers. The information on this site is relevant, accurate, and regularly updated. Because it is written with the consumer in mind, it is easy to comprehend. In addition, many of the educational articles and brochures are available in Spanish.

*8.   National Depressive and Manic-Depressive Association

http://www.ndmda.org

Congruent with their mission, the National Depressive and Manic-Depressive Association (DMDA) Web site is designed to help educate consumers, professionals, and the public about depression and manic-depression. The aims of the National DMDA are to increase public awareness about these disorders and their treatments in order to improve access to mental health care, reduce the associated stigma, and encourage further research. The site is divided into various content areas and contains helpful information on mood disorders, support groups, publications, and many other resources. The site is easy to navigate and has proven to be useful to many. It is updated regularly and the information is reliable and research-based. The National DMDA does not, however, sanction any particular treatment method found on its site and encourages appropriate professional consultation.

*9.   National Institute of Mental Health

http://www.nimh.nih.gov

The Web site sponsored by the National Institute of Mental Health (NIMH) is well-organized and easily navigated. Information is current, accurate, and regularly updated. The homepage contains links to news and events, including reports of the Surgeon General, educational programs, research and clinical trials, and funding opportunities. In addition, there are links to pages specifically designed for practitioners, researchers, and the public. The organization of the site is an important feature and contributes to its ease of use. Included on the "For Practitioners" page are links to current research reports, NIMH-sponsored events, information on specific disorders, available clinical trials, and patient educational materials. Links to funding, employment, research, and policy can be found on the "For Researchers" page. In addition, links to information on selected mental disorders, medications, clinical trials, and fact sheets can be accessed on the "For the Public" page, some of which are available in Spanish.

*10.   National Mental Health Association

http://www.nmha.org

The National Mental Health Association (NMHA) claims to be the oldest and largest nonprofit mental health and illness organization in the United States. The NMHA Web site has much to offer mental health care providers. The homepage is expertly designed to facilitate quick and easy navigation. Timely articles and a section on "Coping Resources" tailored for specific groups of individuals are included here. In addition, the site offers information on current news and legislation, advocacy, mental illnesses, educational resources, upcoming events, and NMHA affiliates. There are informative articles written with all age groups in mind. Nurses can direct consumers and their families to this site for support and mental illness information; in fact, the NMHA strongly advocates consumer participation in their organization. Nurses can also obtain illness-related fact sheets on this site. The site is well-organized, accurate, and frequently updated.

Chapter 35

Critical Care

Laree J. Schoolmeesters

The field of critical care began to develop because of the effectiveness of the intensive care for critically ill patients such as burn patients and those afflicted with polio. Intensive care units began opening in the 1960s and 1970s, initially for postanesthesia care. Thus the need for specialized training for health care professionals also evolved. Along with this came the introduction of diagnostic (e.g., electrocardiograms) and life saving technology (e.g., mechanical ventilators). The needed education became part of curriculums and professional organizations. The field of critical care may encompass trauma, neurology, cardiology, transplantation, emergency, and more. The top 10 selected sites provide links for a large number of subspecialties. Many of these sites provide or have links to interactive educational resources.

1. Acid–Base Tutorial

http://www.acid-base.com/

This interactive Web site on acid–base was developed by A. Grogono, MD, a professor in the Department of Anesthesiology at Tulane University School of Medicine, New Orleans, LA. This is an in-depth tutorial for health care professionals at all levels of critical care. The introduction gives a simple overview of acid–base for beginners. An alphabetical index provides a quick reference to any acid–base queries. A terminology directory is also helpful to the beginner. The history section identifies individuals and dates of important events. The physiology section gets into the details of acid–base balance. Clinicians will find the following sections helpful: acid production, clinical considerations, respiratory or metabolic correction, interactive pages, and simple arithmetic. Areas for the advanced learner include computing, Henderson equation, pH playground, and acid–base diagram. A pocket acid–base card can be purchased for a nominal fee. This tutorial is a referenced, comprehensive examination of acid–base. The humor is appreciated in one topic labeled "Henderson without the Hassel." This Web site is time-intensive but worth the effort. The high-level information is in English.

2. American Association of Critical-Care Nurses (AACN)

http://www.aacn.org/

The AACN is committed to providing the highest quality resources to maximize nurses' contribution to caring and improving the health care of critically ill patients and their families. Unfortunately the site provides minimal information to the general public or nurses unless they are members of AACN. Most areas now require a password. The following areas are accessible to all. To view job postings, click on careers, then career development services. AACN certification exam blueprints, synergy questions, and tips for taking the certification are available. The General Practice section has 3 areas—Databases, General Practice Information, and Public Policy. Under Databases, General Rx provides information on the 200 most common drugs. The Clinical Practice section has AACN fact sheets on registered nurse statistics, advanced practice (what it is; reimbursement; and prescriptive privileges), AACN critical care nursing, mandatory overtime, and Patient's Bill of Rights. Pocket cards are available for a nominal fee and two are free (blood gas and cardiac monitoring). Standards for acute and critical care nursing practice are available. The site is in English with average reading level. The format of this Web site has improved and is frequently updated, though the information available to nonmembers has decreased.

3. Cardiac Trace Tutorials

http://www.healthsci.utas.edu.au/physiol/tute1/Intro.html

These tutorials were developed by faculty and employees from Royal Hobart Hospital with financial support from the University of Tasmania. The data was recorded from patients undergoing cardiac surgery. There are two tutorials, hemodynamics and rhythms. The hemodynamic tutorial begins at a basic level and provides illustrated examples of venous, atrial, and arterial pressures with interactive questions. There are 16 exercises in identifying waveforms. There are multiple choice and true/false exercises throughout both tutorials. The rhythms tutorial describes and explains common rhythms and demonstrates the effects on cardiovascular hemodynamics. The tutorial begins with the conduction system of the heart and the normal electrocardiogram. It then progresses through 10 different abnormal rhythms, such as pacing and conduction blocks, using graphics and descriptions. At the end of the tutorials are approximately 11 exercises (with answers) that can be worked through to enhance learning. The waveforms in both tutorials are clear and easily understandable. All information is in English. One drawback is the lack of updates since 1998. The Web site will enhance the knowledge of health care professionals and students.

4. The ECG Library

http://www.ecglibrary.com/ecghome.html

Stephen Gerred (medical registrar Auckland, New Zealand) and Dean Jenkins (Specialist Registrar, Llandough Hospital, Cardiff, Wales) have published a book on ECGs and developed this Web page to provide information on 12 lead ECGs. The table of contents is simple and straightforward. Sections include ischemic heart disease, hypertrophy patterns, atrioventricular blocks, bundle branch blocks, supraventricular rhythms, ventricular rhythms, pacemakers, Wolf Parkinson White Syndrome, and Miscellaneous (e.g., electrolyte imbalances, implantable cardioverter defibrillator, Lown-Ganong-Levine Syndrome, and piggy back heart transplant). In addition, there is a section that includes axis deviation, and a history of electrocardiography. There are ECG links for over 30 related Web sites. The information is in English, simple to understand, but of a high level, as a basic understanding of rhythm interpretation is needed. The 12 lead ECG graphics are of high quality and fully interpreted and explained with hypertext for further exploration.

5. Gloria's Critical Care and Nursing Pages

http://w3.one.net/~gloriamc/index.html

This site, constructed by a U.S. based coronary care nurse, is an index to critical care, nursing, and medical links. Links are organized by categories and alphabetized, usually with a short synopsis. The "What's New?" section provides dates that new links were added. The following are the categories with the number of Web sites they contain: the Critical Care Web (28); Anesthesia (5); Cardiology (20); Emergency and Trauma (50); Neurology (4); Pediatric (16); Pulmonary (9); Organ Donation (6); Nursing Resources (36); History of Nursing (30); Student Nurses (4); Online Nursing journals (23); Nursing Associations (46); Home pages of Other Nurses (19); Nursing Web Rings (2); and Web-tools (21). Some of the links appear in more than one category. Of interest may be the chemical exposures found under the Emergency category. For ease of searching, the Medical and Health categories are organized by Medical Indexes, Miscellaneous, Virtual Hospitals, Journals, and specialty or disease. Examine the Webtools category for Internet searching tools and software. All information is in English with an easy reading level. The site abides by Health On the Net Foundation. The Web page gives a holistic feel with fun links to music and gardening.

6. Narelle's NetNurse Pages

http://www-personal.usyd.edu.au/~nacolema/njc_nursing.html

Narelle is a nurse education consultant in Sydney, Australia who compiled a comprehensive search Web site for nurses. The main page contains Netlinks, LAMP Links, Citing Electronic Sources, and Net-NurseNotes. The NetLinks are divided into four topics: trailblazers (search engines and search engines specific to health), nursing (colleges, nurses' homepages, and nursing), medical (general interest A–Z, critical care nursing, and critical care and trauma), and assorted (informatics and journals). Narelle's LAMP Links are from the author's column "Nursing the Net" from *The Journal of the New South Wales Nurses Association.* Links to critical care and trauma include 28 Web sites with such topics as pediatrics, cardiology, flight, and emergency. There are 10 Web sites on critical care nursing though the majority are nursing associations. The NetLinks is user-friendly, but the LAMP Links section is a bit dated. The outstanding feature of this Web site is the referenced lecture notes from the author and her colleagues. Health care professionals and students will appreciate the logical and comprehensive nature of the topics on acid–base balance, evaluating ABG's, and shock.

7. Pediatric Critical Care Medicine (PedsCCM)

http://PedsCCM.wustl.edu

The PedsCCM is an independent Web site that provides peer-reviewed original content with integrated links about critically ill children and infants. The site is organized into Clinical Resources, Clinical Research, Organization Meetings, Opportunities, Internet Resources, Interact with PedsCCM, and Other Stuff. The following information can be found under Clinical Resources. The "picuBOOK" is a compilation of high-level media information that can be translated to different languages with a click. There is a head injury topic, a video of minimally invasive cardiac surgery, and graphics and slides of neurosurgery CT scans. The "PedsCCM File Cabinet" contains original peer-reviewed educational and practical materials that are indexed (from anatomy to systemic diseases). The "Case Reports in Pediatric Critical Care Background" are a collection of brief patient reports that are rare cases or unusual presentations of common conditions. Downloadable items for medical software and interactive programs are also available. The Clinical Pathways information can also be downloaded. A section for nurses or advanced practice nurses (APNs) contains information on roles, training programs, and examples of units with APNs. The following information can be found under the Clinical Research heading. The evidence-based journal club has an online tutorial, citations, and reviews by date and subject. Researchers will find information on clinical trials, surveys, and grants, with links to funding and articles on grant writing. Under Opportunities, pediatric critical care practitioners have the opportunity to search the fellowship and job database. Internet Resources provides information on Web sites, journals, and e-mail lists. Other Stuff has newly added information to the site and parent resources. This is a dynamic and comprehensive site for pediatric critical care practitioners. The information in some areas can be seen in English, French, Spanish, and Russian. This multidisciplinary resource has something for researchers, students, and consumers. The PedsCCM is by far one of the largest innovative and most informative sites.

8. Springnet

http://www.springnet.com/

This site provides free articles and continuing education (CE) credit for fee. It is now operated by Lippicott, Williams and Wilkins, a large commercial publisher. Click on "critical care" on the pull down menu for a custom page and then choose from drugs, general critical care, professional issues, cardiac monitoring, cardiovascular disorders, pulmonary artery pressure monitoring, pulmonary, or point-of-care testing. Each topic has two to five complete articles with references and some have CE credits. The main page has 300 plus online contact hours available with certificates sent via e-mail. CE offerings (1.5 to 3.0 credits), with corresponding cost ($8.95 to $21.95), are organized by clinical category, publication date, journal, article title, or CE with video. Links for students, nursing communities, and calendars are available. This organized database provides health care professionals, educators, and students with information and CE credits in a topical area. Other notable features include a career directory and opportunities for authorship. All information is in English and of average reading level. A major drawback is the need for up to date articles in the critical care section as some information is as old as 1996 or the CE testing date has expired.

Emergency Care

Tener Goodwin Veenema

This collection of Web sites represents a diverse collection of agencies, associations and organizations that produce, analyze or distribute information of specific interest to emergency and trauma care providers. These Web sites will guide nurses to the most current information and guidelines available for clinical practice, updates on emergency and trauma nursing research, primary and secondary injury prevention strategies, and management of patient care services. Several of these agencies are responsible for the development and implementation of national policy addressing both adult and pediatric emergency services.

1.   American Association of Critical Care Nurses

http://www.aacn.org

This is the Web site for the American Association of Critical Care Nurses (AACN). Much of the Web site is password protected and limited to AACN members. However, there are quite a few sections that are not. The site includes trauma best practices (e.g., "Family Presence During Invasive Procedures and Resuscitation"). It also features numerous critical care abstracts and continuing education articles on critical care from *AACN Clinical Issues: Advanced Practice in Acute and Critical Care, American Journal of Critical Care,* and *Critical Care Nurse.* The 'discussion' group is divided into limited access and general access sections.

2. American Trauma Society

http://www.amtrauma.org

This Web site is home to the American Trauma Society and provides comprehensive overviews and resources for all aspects of trauma management. The site includes detailed information about the society and its membership, updates on meetings, specific to trauma care, educational resources, and information about the ATS Bystander Care of the Injured Program or "Red Light Running" campaign. The trauma prevention section includes a board game for children and updates on National Trauma awareness month. The site includes a link to trauma nursing opportunities (*http://www.amtrauma.org/employ/trauma _nursing.cfm*) accompanied by a description of the requirements necessary to become employed as a trauma nurse coordinator. Portions of the Web site are password protected and restricted to members.

3. Children's Safety Network National Injury and Violence Prevention Resource Center

http://www.edc.org/HHD/csn

This center is 1 of 4 Children's Safety Network Resource Centers funded by the Maternal and Child Health Bureau of the US Department of Health and Human Services. The site includes case studies on community injury prevention interventions, such as community traffic safety programs, farm injury prevention, youth violence prevention programs, and occupational health and safety for teens.

4. Emergency Medical Services for Children

http://www.ems-c.org

Emergency Medical Services for Children (EMS-C) is a national initiative designed to reduce child and youth disability and death due to severe illness or injury. Its goals are to ensure that state-of-the-art emergency medical care is available for all ill or injured children and adolescents; that pediatric services are well integrated into an emergency medical services system; and that the entire spectrum of emergency services, including primary prevention of illness and injury, acute care, and rehabilitation, are provided to children and adolescents. There is a lot of information available at this Web site including data and research, family information, health policy, emergency medical services development, education and training resources, and information on the rehabilitation of children with special needs. Users can find out what their state and others are doing to improve pediatric emergency care. The Web site is attractively designed and very easy to use.

5. Emergency Nurses Association

http://www.ena.org

This is the Web site of the Emergency Nurses Association (ENA). It contains detailed information including the history of the organization, mission and values statements, board of directors, state councils and chapters, calendar of events, and forms and employment opportunities. The site provides information on funding and scholarship opportunities, and ENA-sponsored publications, such as the ENA newsletter and previews of the *Journal of Emergency Nursing*. The site provides an overview of the association's programs and services, patient advocacy and legislative initiatives, information on how to obtain certification in Emergency Nursing and an introduction to EN CARE—the Emergency Nurses Association Injury Prevention Institute. The site is simple to navigate and appears to be regularly maintained. The Web site is focused on recruiting and serving members, and fundraising for its foundation. Much of the site is restricted to ENA members, and there is room for improvement in providing substantive information to the general emergency nursing audience.

6. Emergency Nursing (UK)

http://www.emergency-nurse.com/resource/tutorials.htm

This site aims to provide a resource for nurses working in emergency-related fields, anywhere in the world. Billing itself as "one of the first sites on the net for Emergency nurses," this is a fun Web site to visit and contains a vast array of information, quick tips, and links to other sites of interest for emergency practice. The collection of resources includes information on triage, illustrated tutorials on cannulation and EKG interpretation, an X-ray library, emergency nursing quiz, and a guide to neurological observations. Users can find nursing humor, sign up for a mailing list, and a wide selection of free emergency clipart for downloading and incorporating into presentations.

7. Mosby

http://www.mosby.com/ijtn
http://www.mosby.com/jen

The International Journal of Trauma table of contents and abstracts from 1997 to present are available at this site. Articles and abstracts from *Journal of Emergency Nursing* are available at *www.mosby.com/jen*. Full-text articles are available starting with 2000, with table of contents and abstracts from 1997 to the present. Access to abstracts is complimentary. Access to full-text articles is via paid subscription or pay-per-article. Users can subscribe online and order bulk reprints of articles as well.

8. National Center for Injury Prevention and Control

http://www.cdc.gov/ncipc

The U.S. Centers for Disease Control and Prevention (CDC) began studying home and recreational injuries in the early 1970s and violence prevention in 1983. From these early activities grew a national program to reduce injury, disability, death, and costs associated with injuries outside the workplace. In June 1992, CDC established the National Center for Injury Prevention and Control (NCIPC). As the lead federal agency for injury prevention, NCIPC works closely with other federal agencies; national, state, and local organizations; state and local health departments; and research institutions. As part of the CDC, the NCIP works to reduce morbidity, disability, mortality, and costs associated with injuries. This is one of the best sites on the Web for emergency nurses looking for information and statistics on injury prevention. This vast Web site is well designed, easy to navigate and search, and hosts a wealth of resources. It contains the *Injury Fact Book 2001–2002*, guidelines for injury care, and comprehensive information on violence and unintentional injuries. The site provides a broad scope of information including instructions for securing research grant funding, safety tips for parents, resources for being safe at work, equipment use recommendations, and a description of the epidemiology of traumatic brain injury in the United States.

9. National Highway Traffic Safety Administration (NHTSA)

http://www.nhtsa.dot.gov/people/injury/ems/

This Web page hosts the Emergency Medical Services division of NHTSA—The National Highway Traffic Safety Administration. NHTSA's mission is to save lives, prevent injuries, and reduce traffic-related health care and other economic costs. The goal of NHTSA's EMS Division is to develop and enhance comprehensive emergency medical service systems to care for injured patients involved in motor vehicle crashes. The agency develops, promotes, and implements effective educational, engineering, and enforcement programs toward ending preventable tragedies and reducing economic costs associated with vehicle use and highway travel. The site contains access to databases, reports, public information on injury prevention programs, ongoing research and evaluation, leadership activities, and NHTSA's Intelligent Transportation Systems Program. The site is well designed and maintained, and includes a list of the agency's partner organizations.

*10. National Safekids Campaign

http://www.safekids.org

This is the Web site for the National SAFE KIDS Campaign, which describes itself as "the first and only national organization dedicated

---

*Sites suitable for consumer use.

solely to the prevention of unintentional childhood injury—the number one killer of children ages 14 and under." This site should be book-marked by all pediatric and emergency nurses as it represents a great source of information and safety tips for parents of young children. The site features a family safety checklist and fact sheets that include statistics and prevention tips on topics such as shopping cart injury, motor vehicle occupant injury, and sports injuries. It contains a media center, list of product recalls, and a teacher's desk and kids' corner with specific information targeted to these groups. The site has its own search engine that allows the user to search for child safety legislation and regulations for all 50 states.

Chapter 37

Community Health

Mary K. Bailey

Public Health/Community Health nurses are health educators; patient teachers; client advocates; home caregivers; alcohol, drug abuse, and violence counselors; case finders; resource finders; medical collaborators; and infant early interventionists. They function as hospice nurses, occupational health nurses, public health agency nurses, school nurses, community case managers, nurse practitioners, and community health nurse specialists. Because of their multiple interests, it is difficult to choose which sites to feature for community health nurses. Because of the depth and breadth of the information available from the United States Department of Health and Human Services, that Web site and the links to the divisions of the Department have been selected. Other sites have been selected in consideration of the practicing public health/community health nurse.

*1. American Academy of Pediatrics (AAP)

http://www.aap.org

The American Academy of Pediatrics is a well-respected organization established for practicing pediatricians. Its Web site has links to topics

---

*Sites suitable for consumer use.

on advocacy, research, consumer information, publications (fee-based), and professional education. The professional education site is probably the most useful for the practicing community health nurse. The online otitis media case studies section presents several short case studies followed by videos of tympanic membranes under pneumonoscopy followed by multiple-choice questions that give instant feedback. The AAP Clinical Practice Guidelines are valuable tools for nurse practitioners working in ambulatory care. There is a link to the "Pediatric Internet" that presents reviews by AAP Fellows of Internet resources and guides appropriate for use by children.

2. American Public Health Association (APHA)

http://www.apha.org

The American Public Health Association represents more than 50,000 public health professionals throughout the world. The organization publishes *The American Journal of Public Health* and the newspaper *The Nation's Health*. The Web site claims that APHA "is a quality resource for public health professionals" and offers news about the annual meeting, links to continuing education online, legislative issues and advocacy, state public health associations, the World Federation of Public Health Associations, and other Public Health links. The Public Health link opens a page with links to other national and professional organizations, Schools of Public Health, Epidemiologist, and resource locators. There is an extensive listing of jobs at the Career Mart. This site is most helpful in keeping the public health practitioner informed about National health care issues and legislation, and for career enhancement.

*3. Centers for Disease Control and Prevention

http://www.cdc.gov/

The USDHHS site that is probably the most serviceable for nurses working in the community is the Centers for Disease Control and Prevention (CDC) site. CDC is located in Atlanta, Georgia, and is the lead federal agency charged with protecting the health and safety of the nation. The agency maintains surveillance of diseases, performs detection and investigation of services related to health problems, does research, develops health care policies, facilitates strategies, and provides training for public health providers. In addition, the CDC seeks to be a resource for providing reliable information for consumers. Of the 12 *Centers, Institutes, and Offices* that make up the CDC the following would appear to be the most useful for the nurse working in the community: The National Center on Birth Defects and Developmental Disabilities (*http://www.cdc.gov/ncbddd*), National Center for Chronic Disease Prevention (*http://www.cdc.gov/nccdphp.htm*), and the National Center for Health Statistics (*http://www.cdc.gov/nchs*).

*4. KinderStart

http://www.kinderstart.com

KinderStart site claims to be the largest and most popular directory focused on children ages zero to seven. There are links for child development, bringing home baby, food and nutrition, pregnancy and birth, and society/culture/environment. The link to Health/Medical/Dental, leads to 13 pages of useful sites with information about child abuse detection, common illnesses, first aid for children, hospitals and clinics for children, major diseases such as asthma, autism, cerebral palsy, cleft lip, fetal alcohol syndrome, dental first aid, gum and tooth problems, and dental insurance. Many of the pages are also in Spanish. There is a Child Care Locator link, a "chat" room for parents, a kids' playground and a kids' classroom link. This site would be of use for health education, professional education, or as a handy referral to give to parents, caretakers, and grandparents. The site has a copyright date of 2000.

*5. National Center on Elder Abuse (NCEA)

http://www.elderabusecenter.org

The National Center on Elder Abuse (NCEA) is a group of six partners involved in the care and study of elder abuse and is funded in part by a grant from the U.S. Administration on Aging. The purpose of the

organization is to provide information about elder abuse to professionals and the public, to offer assistance and training to professionals who
work with elders, develop policy, and perform some research. A click
on the link to "The Basics" brings up a page with facts about the major
types of elder abuse including physical abuse, sexual abuse, emotional
and psychological abuse, neglect, abandonment, financial or material
exploitation, and self-neglect. Additional information is presented about
caregiver stress, the cycle of violence, law enforcement, and profiles
of the abused and the abusers. The Adult Protective Service (APS)
link provides a downloadable file "Ethical Principles and Best Practice
Guidelines" for health care providers. There is a link to "Hotline Phone
Numbers" that leads to a State-by-State directory of elder abuse agencies. The site offers a downloadable "Speaker's Kit on Elder Abuse" that
was prepared by the National Association of Adult Protective Services
Administrators. From the homepage there are links to a listserv, clearinghouse, statistics, elder abuse laws, newsletters, conferences, research, and families. This site would be helpful for orientation of new
public health nurses and nursing students.

*6. National Institutes of Health

http://www.nih.gov/health/

The National Institutes of Health (NIH), an agency within The USDHHS,
conducts its own research and also funds research in universities,
medical schools, colleges of nursing, and hospitals in this country and
abroad. In addition, the NIH Web site presents some very practical
health and illness information for consumers and health care providers.
Of particular interest is the link "Learn about Health Conditions" that
leads to the NIH Health Information Index that lists over 2,000 health
topics. The link to Healthy Vision 2010 links to the Healthy People toolkit
which furnishes information about eye examinations and prevention of
eye diseases, how to prevent eye injury and promote safety, and programs for vision rehabilitation. Many of the other sections are linked
this way as well. The link to Medline Plus presents information on
health topics, diseases, and a medical encyclopedia. There are links
to over 100 topics sorted by body location, procedure, or demographic
group. Information provided is extensive and practical. Medline Plus
also features an Interactive Health tutorial site that provides animated

slide shows with spoken and written text that are available for download and printing. There are slide shows for over 100 common diseases such as asthma, irritable bowel syndrome, congestive heart failure, and diabetes. The diabetes link has information about eye complications and foot care. There is also information about tests and diagnostics, surgery and procedures, prevention, and wellness. The slide presentations for diabetes and hypertension are available in Spanish (spoken and written) and can be downloaded in a printable format in Spanish. These presentations would be invaluable in instructing new Spanish-speaking diabetics or hypertensives or nonreading English speakers. In addition to the Interactive Health site there is a link "Look up Drug Information" that leads to information about more than 9,000 prescription and over-the-counter medications. "Read about Special Programs" leads to topics such as Complementary and Alternative Medicine, AIDS Research, rare diseases, Women's health, Minority health, behavior and social sciences, bioethics resources, and NIH clinical alerts.

7. U.S. Department of Health and Human Services

http://www.dhhs.gov

The Department of Health and Human Services (USDHHS) is the principal agency in the United States government whose mission is to protect "the health of all Americans." The programs of the Department are administered through 11 HHS operating divisions that include eight agencies in the U.S. Public Health Service which is directed by the Surgeon General (*www.surgeongeneral.gov/ophs*) and three human services agencies. As the collection site for health information, the Department maintains a vast amount of data about the Nation's health. The USDHHS divisions address problems of interest to nurses working in the community such as Medicare and Medicaid (HCFA, *www.hcfa. gov/*); health resources and services (HRSA, *www.hrsa.gov/*); food and drug safety (FDA, *www.fda.gov/*), prevention of the outbreak of infectious disease and immunizations (CDC, *www.cdc.gov/*); prevention of child abuse and domestic violence and early childhood education through the Head Start program (AFC, *www.acf.dhhs.gov/*); substance abuse treatment and prevention (SAMHSA, *www.samsha.gov/*); services for the elderly including home-delivered meals (AOA, *www.aoa.*

gov); health care for Native Americans (IHS, *www.ihs.gov/*); and research to improve and assure the quality of health care in the nation (AHRQ, *www.ahrq.gov/*). Also of special interest to public/community health nurses is the Community Health Status Indicators site (*www.communityhealth.hrsa.gov*). At the "find a county" link county statistics can be viewed online or downloaded in a pamphlet version. The format of this site is simplified making access to data quick and easy to get. There is information about life expectancy, causes of death, infant mortality, environmental health risks, infectious diseases, and health disparities. All of the data of the selected county is compared to a nationwide list of peer counties making it possible to identify problem areas in the county. The USDHHS site is updated often and is important as the source of the latest information based on reliable research.

Chapter 38

Advanced Practice

Emily E. Drake

A dvanced practice nurses need quick access to current medical and nursing information. Nurse practitioners and clinical nurse specialists will find many of the Web sites useful in everyday practice. For example, sites such as the *Merck Manual* online or MD Consult provide a wealth of disease and treatment information at your fingertips. Other Web sites may be used less frequently but are just as valuable, such as sites that list job opportunities, advertise continuing education programs, or track legislative issues. The Internet also provides an opportunity to network with other nurses in advanced practice roles around the country and around the world. There are many discussion lists, listservs, and bulletin boards specific to clinical areas and nursing roles (for example, psychiatric-nursing or school nurse lists). These lists allow nurses to receive advice or consultations from colleagues online or by e-mail. Web sites can also help APNs connect to specialty professional organizations and provide needed certification and re-certification information. This section is separated into three sections: general information Web sites, practice guidelines and clinical resources, and lists of links.

GENERAL INFORMATION WEB SITES
FOR NPS AND APNS

1. NP Central, Information For and About Nurse Practitioners

http://www.nurse.net/

The goal of NP Central is to provide useful information in a usable format to nurse practitioners, colleagues, and potential clients. This site contains general information for nurse practitioners and information about nurse practitioners for consumers. It includes a resources and issues section, information about employment, education, and shopping. It also includes information about e-mail discussion groups for NPs. This Web site was established in 1994 by two nurse practitioners, Robert T. Smithing, MSN, FNP, and Madeline D. Wiley, MSN, FNP. Sponsors include Fitzgerald Health Education Associates, 3M Littmann, and Amazon. This Web site provides valuable information for both new and experienced nurse practitioners in a variety of specialties. This site would be a good resource for NP students. The employment information includes job postings, salary data, and links to recruiters. It also contains information about continuing education offerings. This Web site is professionally maintained and provides clear contact information, disclaimers and terms of use, and frequent updates. While this site provides some useful information it is not comprehensive.

PRACTICE GUIDELINES AND CLINICAL RESOURCES

1. Cochrane Collaboration

http://www.cochrane.org/

Abstracts

http://www.update-software.com/ccweb/cochrane/revabstr/ mainindex. htm

The Cochrane Library is a major source of information about reliable evidence-based health care. It is a fee-based service that offers full-text research-based reviews and protocols (The Cochrane Library). However, on the Web the summaries or abstracts of the Cochrane Reviews are accessible for free. The Cochrane group includes over 45 health care categories or groups of reviewers that summarize the current research in areas from breast cancer, diabetes, peripheral vascular disease to wound care, and many more. Within each general topic area there are many reports and protocols. The abstracts include background and objectives, information about the meta-analysis, main results, and conclusions. Information about purchase of the entire Cochrane Library collection, for use either by CD-ROM or by Internet subscription, is available on the Web page. The Cochrane Library is based in the United Kingdom but collaborates with centers all over the world. The abstract page is straightforward and fairly easy to navigate using the "back" key and includes a search function. It is updated regularly. Unfortunately, only the reviews are offered on the Web page and not protocols. Do not expect any fancy graphics; this site is all text but easily printable. Only well-controlled, randomized research trials are included in the reviews. Although it attempts to be comprehensive, some topics areas are covered more thoroughly than others. This site lacks a disclosure or disclaimer statement.

2.   MD Consult

http://www.mdconsult.com/

This is a fee-based online medical reference site. Subscribers are allowed full-text access to nearly 40 medical reference books, 50 journals, and over 600 Clinical Practice Guidelines. It also includes GenRX, a major drug reference. There are also more than 3,000 patient education handouts, some in Spanish. It includes two frequently up-dated sections called "Today in Medicine" and "What Patients are Reading" that help health care providers stay current with media reports. There is also a Continuing Medical Education (CME) component. MD Consult was founded by three medical publishers, Mosby, W.B. Saunders, and Lippincott Williams & Wilkins. This site is well-organized, easy to navigate, and quite extensive in content. But, it is not free. Annual rates vary ($99–$199.00). Group practices and institutional special rates are available. A free 10-day pass is offered to preview the site before buying.

*3. *The Merck Manual**

http://www.merck.com/pubs/mmanual/

The seventeenth edition of the *Merck Manual* is now offered online free of charge for unlimited use. According to the Web site information, the *Merck Manual* provides research and educational information used by more medical professionals worldwide than any other general medical textbook. This "virtual" medical textbook offers 23 chapters on everything from infectious disease to hematology/oncology and ear, nose, and throat disorders. It is over 300 pages long and is formatted with hyperlinked text so that terms are cross-referenced throughout the text. This Web site also contains its own internal search engine so that any symptom, disease, medication, or other term can be searched for within the site. The *Merck Manual of Geriatrics* is also available through this site. The *Merck Manual* is a classic medical reference. The content is excellent and its online version is wonderful because it is free and easily searchable. However, there is an evident lack of pictures or graphics. All material is presented in text format. This site is well-organized and easy to navigate, although the internal search engine is not tolerant of spelling errors. There is no clearly identifiable point of contact, or disclaimer. There is definitely a potential for commercial bias; Merck is a company that sells medical products. However, they are providing a valuable service to health care providers and consumers through this site.

4. National Guideline Clearinghouse

http://www.guideline.gov/index.asp

The National Guideline Clearinghouse™ (NGC) Web page is a public resource for evidence-based clinical practice. It is essentially a government-sponsored database of evidence-based clinical practice guidelines and related documents and it contains over 1,000 clinical guideline summaries. NGC is produced by the Agency for Health Care Quality (formerly the Agency for Health Care Policy and Research), in partnership with the American Medical Association (AMA) and the American

---

*Sites suitable for consumer use.

Association of Health Plans (AAHP). Nearly 200 organizations have guidelines posted on this Web page, including the American Academy of Pediatrics, the American Heart Association, the Oncology Nursing Society, and many others. All guidelines contain summaries, recommendations, annotated bibliographies, and contact information. This site is easy to navigate. It includes a search function. The information is current and up to date. All guidelines can be easily printed from the site. All information is presented as text only.

5. Primary Care Clinical Practice Guidelines

http://medicine.ucsf.edu/resources/guidelines/

The purpose of this Web site is to provide easy access to clinical resources for primary care providers. It includes guidelines, clinical reviews, cross-cultural health, teaching, and more. All information is hyperlinked. The homepage is organized like a table of contents and includes a site map. Within the site is an impressive resource page that provides a long list of links organized as On-line Textbooks and References, Superlists of Links, Teaching Resources, Patient Resources, and Other Sites of Interest to health care providers. Most links provided also include a short description or evaluation. This site is easy to navigate and is straightforward in its layout; however, it is not particularly pretty to look at. It is primarily a list with text, little color, and no graphics. This award-winning site appears to be extremely comprehensive. It contains a search function and an alphabetical list of topics. This site is very well maintained. The site is hosted by the Department of Medicine at University of California, San Francisco and includes both disclaimer and disclosure statements. Unlike the National Guideline Clearinghouse, this site offers not only guidelines, but also journal articles, and other Web sites, for each topic.

LISTS OF LINKS

1. Internet Resources for Nurse Practitioner Students

http://nurseweb.ucsf.edu/www.arwwebpg.htm

This is a list of Web sites compiled to assist NP students; however, it is also useful for practicing NPs and other APNs. It was compiled by a nursing student at University of California, San Francisco (UCSF). She includes links organized under the following categories: health information gateways, nursing resources, clinical practice guidelines, case studies and interactive tutorials, evidence-based health care, government agencies, and pharmacology. She also includes sections for various specialties: primary care, pediatrics, adolescent health, school-based health, women's health, HIV/AIDS, and complementary and alternative health care. This site is linked to the UCSF School of Nursing. This is an extremely well developed list of links. Although the actual site contains little information and has not been updated since July 1999, it is still useful. The site is well-organized and contains applicable links. A short description of each link might make this a better site.

_____ Chapter **39**

Primary Care

Jennifer Okonsky

The following is a list of Web sites with a primary care focus. In this era of cost consciousness and health care reform, more and more emphasis is being placed on primary prevention and primary care. This comprehensive list of primary care sites is intended for the primary care practitioner who cares for a wide variety of patient populations. The sites below include a wide variety of resources, including professional organizations, clinical information resources, databases, and diagnostic tools useful in the clinical setting. The majority of these sites have a multidisciplinary or interdisciplinary focus; that is, the sites are appropriate for a variety of types and levels of practitioners. Increasingly, health care providers are being encouraged to work more collaboratively with interdisciplinary teams of health care providers. This model of health care delivery is particularly crucial to building a better primary care system for the future, enhancing health care delivery to all persons.

*1.   Agency for Healthcare Research and Quality

http://www.ahrq.gov/

The Agency for Healthcare Research and Quality is a very comprehensive site. It provides four navigational tools: search, browse, what's new, and frequently asked questions. The content is extensive and the site divides the information into six categories. The categories of Clinical Information, Consumers and Patients, and Data and Surveys (3 of the 6) would be most beneficial for primary care. Subcategories are more specific and contribute to quick and easy searches. This AHRQ site is updated regularly and provides guidelines that are used in everyday practice. The site will keep the viewer abreast of state and local policies, funding opportunities, and latest research. Information is also provided in Spanish.

2. American International Health Alliance

http://www.aiha.com/english/programs/phc/index.cfm#overview

The American International Health Alliance mission is to advance global health through volunteer-driven partnerships that mobilize communities to better address health care priorities, while improving productivity and quality of care. The intended use of this Web site is international involvement in volunteer partnerships. The AIHA has created an innovative, broad-based partnership model that enables individuals, institutions, and communities to unite their voluntary resources and energy in a global quest for improved health. Primary health care is one of the many cross-partnership programs. The primary health care page offers the Program Overview, Program Description, Program Contacts, Participating AIHA Partnerships, Conferences and Workshops, Sample Equipment List for PHC Centers, and Presentations on Model PHC Centers. This site also offers a EuroAsiaHealth Knowledge Network that supplies database links. Some of the unique links include the multilingual library and the glossary with English and Russian translations. This is an exceptional site that offers a variety of information ranging from getting involved with international primary care to simply keeping current with primary care initiatives. The text is clear and information tabs and links are sorted in a logical and structured manner.

3. The Emergency Medicine and Primary Care Home Page

http://www.embbs.com/

The purpose of this Web site is to provide information relating to primary care practice. Distinguishing features include a radiology library, CT scan, medical photograph library, Medgacode simulator, and sample electrocardiograms. Health care job listings are provided, along with in-depth clinical reviews, a toxicology corner, challenging clinical cases, medical software showcase, medical images, best picks of the medical Web link, and telemedicine connection sections. This site is written at a higher than average level. Information is also available on how to contribute an article or image to the Web site for consideration. This is an excellent site for professionals. The site is very comprehensive and extensive. The main sections are listed on the homepage for easy navigation. All information is current. There is also contact information for the physicians who maintain the site. The Emergency Medicine Bulletin Board System, created in 1994 by two physicians, sponsors the site; copyright to Triple Star Systems, Inc.

4. Medscape Primary Care

http://www.medscape.com
http://PrimaryCare.medscape.com/Home/Topics/PrimaryCare/
PrimaryCare.html

Medscape is a large commercial Web site featuring information for physicians, nurses, and other health care professionals. The homepage is broken into four segments: Primary Care Resources, Medscape Network, Your Account, and MedicalLife and Partners. The segment on Primary Care Resources includes the following sections: news, treatment updates, clinical management, practice guidelines, conference summaries and schedules, a journal room, an exam room, library, patient resources, managed care, and primary care links. The conference summaries section features next day summaries by leading authorities in the area. A wide variety of conferences are represented with links. The conference calendar allows one to select conferences based on geographic location, and to submit CME events to be included in the calendar listings. An exam room features a question of the day and interactive cases that examine a variety of conditions and age groups. The library contains reference textbooks and a dictionary. Patient resources provides a variety of information that is appropriate for patients, according to broad categories of diseases and conditions. The managed care section contains news and current legislation relating to managed care and includes news articles, editorial opinions, and tools to use in primary care settings. The Medscape Network segment features not only a specific section for nurses, which includes nurse practitioners, but links you to Medscape International that offers news in different languages. This is a very comprehensive, well-organized site with text that is clear and concise.

5. Mental Disorders in Primary Care

http://www.who.int/msa/mnh/ems/primacare/edukit/

The Mental Disorders in Primary Care site is excellent. Primary care providers are often the first line providers to observe and/or assess a mental disorder. This site is geared mainly toward providers. The site is an educational packet provided by the World Health Organization (WHO). It offers quick but comprehensive information on depression, anxiety, alcohol use disorders, sleep problems, chronic tiredness, and unexplained somatic complaints. Tabs at the top of the page sort sections into topics, flowchart assessment guides, and checklists, or the entire packet can be downloaded. Some of the documents are in PDF format so acrobat reader is needed to view them. The information provided is clear and succinct.

6. Office of Disease Prevention and Health Promotion

http://odphp.osophs.dhhs.gov/odphpfact.htm

The Office of Disease Prevention and Health Promotion (ODPHP) was created by Congress in 1976 to play a vital role in developing and coordinating a wide range of national disease prevention and health promotion strategies. Sponsored by the U.S. Department of Health and Human Resources, this page is a vehicle of links to provide information for health care providers as well as the public. The six links provided are as follows: Healthy People 2010, Leading Health Indicators (LHIs), healthfinder® (information offered in English and Spanish), National Health Information Center (NHIC), Task Force on Environmental Health and Safety Risks to Children, Dietary Guidelines for Americans, and Healthy People in Healthy Communities. The information provided in each of the six links is updated frequently. Each site offers a colorful display of prompts that make navigation of the site effortless. The sites offer a range of information that is all very useful for primary care providers. The sites encompasses the Healthy People 2010 objectives, major health issues, health referrals and resources, children's health and safety information, dietary guidelines and strategies for healthy communities.

7.   Primary Care Clinical Practice Guidelines

http://medicine.ucsf.edu/resources/guidelines/index.html

The University of California at San Francisco School of Medicine produces the Primary Care Clinical Practice Guidelines site. The homepage features 22 clinical content categories and 4 clinical resources for the primary care provider. Navigating from the homepage is simple; one can highlight the specific category or search by alphabet. The link provides comprehensive information. Guidelines that appear are not limited to one agency and article references are often used. The clinical resources provided on the homepage include links to guidelines and clinical reviews, cross-cultural health, teaching, patient information, and Users' Guides to the Medical Literature-Rational Clinical Exam. This site is complete, well-organized, and of high quality.

8.   The Quality Center of the Bureau of Primary Health Care

http://bphc.hrsa.gov/quality/

The Quality Center of the Bureau of Primary Health Care is part of the Health Resources and Service's Administration, which is sponsored by the U.S. Department of Health and Human Services. The site is provided for clinicians to assist them in reaching the goal to continuously improve the quality of patient care, service delivery, the health care workforce, and health outcomes in the delivery systems. The BPHC Web site's homepage offers plenty of information to aid health care providers in promoting resources for quality improvement. The homepage sidebar provides information about the program, staff, latest up-to-date information and resources, quality Web links, quality tools, and training opportunities. Although searching specific topics may not be simple because there is no search function, the subcategories are clear. There are multiple links to information offered in Spanish including health history forms written in English and Spanish. The quality tools section not only makes available resources and links to other sites, but also provides power point presentations from other providers. Although the site provides a lot of references and resources that may decrease the swiftness with which one can obtain information, once familiar with the site, it is an asset to the health care provider.

*9. University of Michigan Health System Primary and Preventative Health

http://www.med.umich.edu/1libr/primry/prim00.htm

The University of Michigan sponsors the University of Michigan Health System Primary and Preventative Health site; the site is developed and maintained by The Department of Public Relations and Marketing Communications. This site is aimed at consumers, however, it is an excellent site for primary care providers as well. This site provides general information about primary and preventative health. The health care provider can utilize this site as a referral page to consumers or use the information in the site for teaching and educational purposes. The homepage is precisely organized to answer your basic questions regarding primary care. To start, a link is provided that defines primary care, managed care, HMO, and family practice. The other topic links listed include how to choose a health care provider, early detection, fitness, community nutrition education programs, health education resource network, health lifestyle, immunization, nutrition, prevention, warning signs and risk factors, how to get a referral, and how to make an appointment. The site's information is simple and presented in a straightforward manner. An excellent source of information for consumers, ease of navigation is great for first-time computer users. A nice additional feature the site offers is the "tip of the week" link.

10. Virtual Hospital

http://www.vh.org/

The University of Iowa produces the virtual hospital Web site. This site provides an extensive amount of information for providers and patients.

---

*Sites suitable for consumer use.

Welcome to Virtual Hospital, For Healthcare Providers, For Patients, Common Problems, and Beyond Virtual Hospital are five key links that provide information. Each link gives subcategories. The patient information section presents excellent educational information. The Provider site allows for links to clinical practice guidelines and up-to-date research. The site not only offers information and research but also provides continuing education credits. Information for providers also consists of multimedia textbooks, simulations, diagrams, lectures, and case studies. This site can be used as a quick reference for patients, providers, and as a teaching tool. The information content provided for patients is simple and can either be a quick reference or used in an educational discussion. A nice feature is the ability to e-mail patient information pages. Although there is an enormous amount of information, the navigation is simple and easy.

Chapter **40**

Palliative Care

Joan T. Panke

P alliative care is a nursing and medical specialty that focuses on the prevention and relief of suffering through the management of symptoms and other physical needs, and psychological, social, spiritual, and practical support of the patient and family from the early through the final stages of an illness. The field of palliative care emerged in response to the continued pressure to improve care of patients and families facing serious illness. The philosophy and principles of palliative care include the consideration of both patient and family as the unit of care.

1. American Academy of Hospice and Palliative Medicine

http://www.aahpm.org

The American Academy of Hospice and Palliative Medicine (AAHPM) is an organization committed to the advancement of hospice/palliative medicine, its practice, research, and education. This Web site includes AAHPM position statements, press releases, publications, and products. Information regarding upcoming events and meetings, job listings, and related links is also available on the site. Members of AAHPM can access valuable member services that include slide presentations. One of the most valuable aspects of this site is the related links. The Web site is well-organized, easy to navigate, and filled with useful current and accurate information. Membership is NOT limited to physicians, and the information accessed from this site is useful for all professionals.

*2.   Americans for Better Care of the Dying (ABCD)

http://www.abcd-caring.org

This important Web site serves to link the nurse with critical resources related to public policy and system change. ABCD came about through a grant from the Open Society Institute's *Project Death in America* (see *www.soros.org/death.html*). ABCD is dedicated to ensuring that all Americans can receive high-quality end-of-life care. The goals of ABCD are to (1) build momentum for reform; (2) explore new methods and systems for delivering care; and (3) shape public policy through evidence-based understanding. The site's intended audience includes all individuals dedicated to improving care of the dying. One of the most important features includes access to an online version of Lynn and Harrold's (1999), *The Handbook for Mortals: Guidance for People Facing Serious Illness*, a factual, comprehensive guide for patients and families facing serious illness. Health care organizations and providers will find this an invaluable resource in planning patient and provider educational programs. Other important features of this Web site include a section on "Shaping public policy" that offers links to important policy sites related to end-of-life care; "reading room" which offers action tips and multicultural end-of-life care; and valuable resource links. Information is updated frequently, so readers can rely on its accuracy. ABCD's Web site contains high-level information, and is easy to navigate.

*3.   Approaching Death: Improving Care at the End of Life

http://www.nap.edu/readingrooms/books/approaching

From the Web site the National Academy Press, one can access the Institute of Medicine (IOM) Division of Health Care Service's Committee

---

*Sites suitable for consumer use.

Report on Care at the End of Life, *Approaching Death: Improving Care at the End of Life*, edited by Marilyn J. Field and Christine K. Cassel. The site provides the opportunity to access the full report, which encompasses the committee's extensive effort to explore diverse issues regarding end-of-life care. Areas of interest include profiles of the dying in America, current practices in end-of-life care, legal and economic issues in end-of-life care, education of clinicians, and recommendations for improving care of the dying. Although the report was published in 1997, information contained in this important document remains current, and is frequently cited by palliative care experts because of the depth of information it contains, and the compelling arguments for the need for quality palliative care for those facing serious illness. As such, this Web site is a valuable resource for any persons hoping to gain a better understanding of the issues surrounding end-of-life care. It is an invaluable resource.

4. End-of-Life Nursing Education Consortium (ELNEC)

http://www.aacn.nche.edu/ELNEC

The End-of-Life Nursing Education Consortium (ELNEC) project is a comprehensive, national education program to improve end-of-life care by nurses. The Web site gives details regarding the ELNEC project, and links to valuable palliative resources. The ELNEC curriculum is not available online. Funded by a major grant from the Robert Wood Johnson Foundation, the ELNEC project is a partnership of the American Association of Colleges of Nursing (AACN) and City of Hope National Medical Center (COH). The goals of the project are to develop a core of expert nursing educators and to coordinate national nursing education efforts in end-of-life care. The target audience for the Web site is nursing professionals, but all health care providers will benefit from taking advantage of the easy access to comprehensive palliative resources. Information on the site is current and accurate. Some of the most useful features of the site include an extensive list of critical palliative care resource links (including a link to the Educating Physicians on End-of-Life Care [EPEC] project) and a state-specific directory of nurse educators who have completed an ELNEC course. The ELNEC trainers serve as a valuable palliative care resource in communities throughout the United States. The site contains high-level information, and is easy to navigate.

*5. Growth House

http://www.growthhouse.org

Growth House offers a wide range of resources related to life-threatening illnesses and end-of-life care issues for both professionals and the public. Many key palliative care Web sites link to Growth House. The primary mission of the organization is "to improve the quality of compassionate care for people who are dying through public education and global professional collaboration." Topics accessed at this site include care of the dying, major illnesses, and home care. A search engine of resources for end-of-life care, an online bookstore, and discussion groups are also included. This site has an enormous amount of information for both professionals and the public. Information regarding various topics in palliative care is readily accessed from the site.

6. Hospice and Palliative Care Nurses Association (HPNA)

http://www.hpna.org

The Hospice and Palliative Care Nurses Association (HPNA) Web site allows nurses to access the latest nursing innovations in both hospice and palliative care. The Web site offers opportunities to access to online discussion with peers, resources, links to important sites, and information regarding certification. Readers may also access HPNA's Journal: *Journal of Hospice and Palliative Care Nursing.* The Web site is well-organized and easy to navigate. Increased access to information is obtained through membership. Membership is free, and readers may join online. The publications and related links areas of the Web site are particularly useful.

*7. Last Acts

http://www.lastacts.org

Funded in part by the Robert Wood Johnson Foundation, Last Acts is a campaign to improve care at the end of life. The Web site gives extensive coverage of issues in palliative care. Information is targeted for health care professionals, public/families, health-care administrators, journalists, and policymakers. An electronic newsletter focuses on provider-patient communication, health system changes, ethics, and American culture and attitudes. Access to information about task forces, a database of funders interested in end-of-life projects, news releases, and resources and links to other sites is included. Information regarding the refereed journal *Innovations in End-of-Life Care* is also available on the site. Last Acts is an invaluable palliative care site. Readers are encouraged to become members, as this increases the usefulness of the site.

*8. National Hospice and Palliative Care Organization

http://www.nhpco.org

The National Hospice and Palliative Care Organization was founded in 1978. It is a nonprofit organization dedicated to "promoting and maintaining quality care for terminally ill persons and their families, and to making hospice an integral part of the U.S. health care system" for professionals and volunteers providing service to patients and their families. The Web site is an excellent source of information regarding hospice and hospice care, publications by the NHO, and opportunities for online discussion for members (apply online). Additionally, one may access information regarding conferences and educational opportunities, and related links. NHPCO's Web site offers important information regarding caring for patients and their families facing life-threatening illness.

9. Pain and Palliative Resource Center

http://prc.coh.org

The City of Hope Pain and Palliative Resource Center (COHPPRC) is one of the most important palliative care sites for nurses and other health professionals. The purpose of the site is to "serve as a clearinghouse to disseminate information and resources" that will enable other individuals and institutions to improve the quality of pain management and palliative care. COHPPRC is a central source for collecting a variety of current and accurate materials including pain assessment tools, patient education materials, quality assurance materials, research instruments and other resources. One of the most important features of this site is the provision for some materials to be accessed online. For those materials that are not available for direct download, many can be ordered by mail for a nominal fee through the City of Hope Pain Resource Center. The coordinators of the Web site invite visitors to copy materials obtained from this Web site or by mail and distribute them to whomever would benefit from this service. Many of the resources and assessment tools are available in Spanish. The appearance of the Web site is attractive, information provided is high-level, and the site is easy to use.

10.   Palliative Care: One Vision, One Voice (Palliative Care Nursing)

http://www.palliativenursing.net

This site is the result of the 'Leadership Academy in End-of-Life Care'. The Academy, which was created by the Institute for Johns Hopkins Nursing and funded by a grant from the Open Society Institute's Project on Death in America, was designed to educate, train, and organize a network of nursing leaders prepared to stimulate the nursing profession's contribution to transforming end-of-life care. The purpose of the Web site is to allow a forum where nurses may share information with other professionals about initiatives related to improving patient care at the end of life. The reader will find that information available on the site is both current and accurate. The most important features include links to organizations. An extensive report by clinicians at nine hospitals that describe how they and their colleagues established formal programs of palliative care ('Pioneer Programs') can be found under organizational links. Other features include information on educational opportunities and conferences nationwide, a media guide that links to experts in the field of palliative care, and a comprehensive resource section. The information level provided on the site is high-level, and the site is easy to navigate.

Chapter 41

Diabetes

Jenifer Lasman

D iabetes is a significant health problem that affects all communities. Diabetes is classified as gestational, nephrogenic insipidus, Type 1, or Type 2. Gestational diabetes is related to an insensitivity of maternal insulin receptors that results in high glucose levels. Nephrogenic diabetes insipidus is related to the insensitivity of nephron's collection ducts to antidiuretic hormone that results in an inability to concentrate urine. Type 1 diabetes, previously known as insulin-dependent diabetes, is characterized by the inability of the pancreas to produce insulin, resulting in high plasma glucose levels. Type 2 diabetes, previously known as noninsulin-dependent diabetes, is caused by cell receptors' inability to be affected by insulin, resulting in high plasma glucose levels. Minority groups are at increased risk for developing this form of diabetes. The World Wide Web is a useful forum for gaining information about the physical, emotional, and research dimensions of diabetes. The sites below were selected to represent the thousands of Web sites that pertain to diabetes. These sites were chosen because of their comprehensiveness and usability for nurses.

*1. American Diabetes Association (ADA)

http://www.diabetes.org

The Web site of the leading nonprofit diabetic organization, the American Diabetes Association, supplies information that is considered a gold standard for those with diabetes, their families, and their health care professionals. This excellent resource for nurses provides clinical practice recommendations including screening, medical care, nutrition, exercise, foot care, national standards for diabetic self-management education, continuous subcutaneous insulin infusion, prevention, preconception care of women, diabetic nephropathy, diabetic retinopathy, gestational diabetes, hyperglycemic crises, and insulin. Concentrating on the most significant research and information, this Web site supplies vital data but not always the most current data. All the standards are supplied on this site free of charge. A variety of other resources can be purchased from the site. In addition to standards of care, nurses may use this site to reach professional diabetic organizations, conferences, and literature. The site is sufficient for supplying basic information to clients and their families, but clients and their families must go to other sites for more detailed education. They can use this site to access information about the availability of local American Diabetic Associations. A Spanish translation is also available through this site. This is a vital site for nurses seeking clinical practice recommendations for clients' basic educational needs and local community resources. The layout of the site is deceivingly simple. Important information may be overlooked if time is not given to explore the vast amount of available data provided.

*2. Children with Diabetes

http://www.childrenwithdiabetes.com

This site is arranged to promote an online community for diabetic children, their families, and adults with diabetes. A production of the Children with Diabetes Foundation, this site has published weekly Web pages for the last 6 years. Nurses can refer parents of their young diabetic clients to this site for education and community support. This is an excellent site for parents to network with each other, but an

---

*Sites suitable for consumer use.

average site to stay informed of research and product development. Parents may enjoy the Diabetic Team section where they can ask specific questions to qualified experts about their children's conditions. Diet is emphasized through discussion and recipe sharing. The majority of information is directed toward the Type 1 diabetes community. Children will be able to find e-mailing buddies on this site but there is not much else offered for young children. The adult diabetic section is limited but helpful for networking. Although the site is only in English, Spanish-speaking e-mail buddies are available. This Internet site is published in a magazine form that lends itself to weekly explorations but may frustrate individuals looking for quick information. This is a good site for diabetic children and their families who are looking for information and support from others living with diabetes.

3. International Diabetes Federation (IDF)

http://www.idf.org

The International Diabetes Federation (IDF) Web site provides information about global diabetic advocacy with special emphasis on the developing world. IDF is the only global diabetic advocacy group. IDF works in coordination with the World Health Organization and the Pan American Health Organization. Nurses will find a unique global perspective at this Web site that is geared toward policy health care professionals. The highlights of this site are diabetic global epidemiological data, international diabetic standards, and access to ordering international publications on the subject. This site is also a forum for international networking in the diabetic community among professionals from many different part of the world. The site is repetitive and does not maximize Web pages. There is not an extensive amount of data provided, but it is relatively current. Information is available in English, French, and Spanish. This Web site is average in content but has an unrivaled international viewpoint.

4. Juvenile Diabetes Research Foundation International

http://www.jdf.org

The Juvenile Diabetes Research Foundation (JDRF) developed this site to advocate for the needs of children living with diabetes. JDRF supports fundraising for diabetic research. The site is directed toward parents of children with diabetes and those interested in supporting research. Nurses will find this to be a good source for current research direction and an excellent referral site for parents interested in research and advocacy. A unique offering on this site is the Legislative Action section. This section allows interested Internet users to become aware of policy issues involved in juvenile diabetes and how to access state and federal officials to address individual questions in regard to diabetes. The Web site also can be used to access local chapters. Although the site is only available in English, affiliations of the organization may be contacted through the site in Australia, Canada, Chile, Greece, India, Israel, Italy, Puerto Rico, and the United Kingdom. This is an excellent site for parents interested in diabetic research and research support. The site has links to many major diabetic research Internet resources in addition to an explanation of JDRF-sponsored research.

*5.   MEDLINEplus Health Information: Diabetes

http://www.nlm.nih.gov/medlineplus/diabetes.html

This site is a composite of diabetes Web site links that have been evaluated for their quality, authority, and accuracy. Developed by the National Library of Medicine and the National Institute of Health, MEDLINEplus Diabetes provides current information for health care providers and clients. The wide range of diabetic topics covered includes alternative therapy, clinical trials, diagnosis and symptoms, disease management, nutrition, prevention and screening, research, specific conditions, treatments, glossaries, directories, and organizations. MEDLINEplus Diabetes provides links that cover specific topics. Links vary from simple forms of information to higher levels of complexity. Nurses new to the field of diabetes will have fast access to the basic concepts of etiology, clinical manifestations, and treatment information. This is a good source to refer clients to who are just beginning to learn about their disease and to patients that have specific educational requirements. Many Spanish language links are included in the site. This site is well managed and kept up to date. MEDLINEplus Diabetes is an excellent source for the latest news in the diabetic community through its sampling of many sources including journals, Web sites, and newspapers. Health care professionals may feel confident referring clients to explore this site, but they will find little new information for themselves (excluding the latest news section). This is a well-organized Internet site with an outline form that is easy to investigate.

*6. National Institute of Diabetes and Digestive and Kidney Diseases (NIDDK)

http://www.niddk.nih.gov

The National Institute of Diabetes and Digestive and Kidney Diseases (NIDDK) is a subdivision of the National Institutes of Health which has developed a Web site that fosters the dissemination of diabetic research results and continued research development. This site contains superlative information for clients, families, clinicians, and researchers. The NIDDK Web site provides comprehensive current information in different forms that are appropriate for the needs of a variety of Internet users. Nurses will find many gems to help them in their clinical practices. The 50-page foot care booklet is an outstanding example of the practical information the Web site provides. This foot care booklet educates the practitioner on exams, Medicare, patient education, and tips for quality assurance. Health care practitioners may order bulk quantities of these booklets for a fee. The NIDDK site is essential for nurses interested in clinical trials for their clients offering current studies, details on inclusion criteria, and contact information. Health care researchers will be able to access information about current studies, grants, and fellowships. Diabetics will be able to download pamphlets on the etiology, clinical manifestations, and treatment of their disease. Some information for clients and families is available in Spanish. This Web site organizes information based on subject area and not on the intended user. The health professional will benefit by finding in-depth reports and patient education material at the same time, but busy nurses may be inconvenienced by the lack of separation between client and professional information. The lengthy handouts intended for professionals may overwhelm clients and families.

*7. Rick Mendosa's Diabetes Directory

http://www.mendosa.com/diabetes.htm

This Internet site is a directory of diabetic-related Web sources edited by a journalist living with diabetes. Mr. Mendosa's site bolsters the education and sense of community for those living with this illness. This is an excellent site for patient referral. Nurses may also get some valuable hints. The author has divided his site into 15 target areas: diabetic related Internet mailing lists; diabetic-related organizations and charities; universities, hospitals, physicians, and research institutions; companies dealing with diabetes; article, book, and video diabetic publications; government sites; personal Web sites; diabetes Web sites in languages other than English; Medline resources; medications; insulin; diabetes software; blood glucose meters; diabetic neuropathy; and miscellaneous. Mr. Mendosa is constantly updating his site with new Web pages and critical evaluations of these sites. This journalist's work allows those living with this disease to join the diabetic Internet community and to stay abreast of new developments. This site is unique in its concentration on the personal needs of diabetics. For example, the Internet links about glucometers and his review allow individuals to compare available products. Although well-organized, the size of this Web site may be intimidating. With 27 pages of material, Mr. Mendosa has compiled an enormous amount of information that may overwhelm the Internet user. The information is organized into usable outlines. This is an excellent site for highly motivated clients who are looking for education and support in living with their illness. Nurses will find this site a good source of practical information to pass on to their clients.

8.   Scope and Standards of Diabetes Nursing

http://www.aadenet.org/Position%20Statements/
scope_stand_nurs.html

These practice recommendations published by the American Nurses Association (ANA) in 1998 provide essential information for all nurses working in the field of diabetes. The American Association of Diabetic Educators for nurses sponsors the site. This is the most current document produced by ANA that addresses the scope and standards of diabetic nursing. The site offers the scope of diabetic clinical nursing practice, standards of care, standards of professional performance, advanced practice standards of care, and advanced practice standards of professional performance. Although the diabetic information provided on this site is not current and is minimal, the Scope and Standards of Diabetes Nursing is a fundamental bookmark for all nurses working in the field. The information on this Web site in combination with the scope and standards published by a nurse's individual state is needed for a nurse to form his or her practice. The Web site is in the form of a written document, which allows for easy downloading. Specific sections of the site are not easily accessible since the outline is not completely linked to the document.

Chapter 42

Heart Disease

Paulette Espina-Gabriel and Hussein Tahan

C ardiovascular disease affects more than 61 million Americans and is the leading cause of hospitalization in patients over 65 years of age. In 1999, about 40% of all deaths were associated with cardiovascular disease (CVD), making it the primary cause of death for both men and women and among all ethnic and racial groups. With the increasing incidence and prevalence of CVD, it is essential for health care professionals to focus on prevention and health promotion activities to reduce its occurrence. This chapter describes nine cardiovascular-related Web sites, selected for their credibility, reliability, and timeliness of information. Access to these Web sites is at no cost. All the sites include a disclaimer that advises users to always consult with a physician or health care professional for questions or concerns prior to implementation of any recommendations, as the content is presented for informational purposes only.

*1. About.com, Heart Disease/Cardiology

http://www.heartdisease.about.com

About.com, Heart Disease/Cardiology is part of the About.com Web site, which covers over 50,000 topics, 250,000 full-text articles, and

---

*Sites suitable for consumer use.

over 1 million links to well-known resources. A Guide oversees each site. The Guide is an expert on specific topics, including the latest information, important links, and discussion forums. The Guide also answers questions presented to the site. The site for Heart Disease/ Cardiology includes a listing of all relevant subjects, each with extensive link directories. Despite the complexity of the site, the information shared is current, concise, and clear, and indicates the date of posting as well as the latest date of updates. The Web pages are simply organized, making it easier to navigate and conduct multiple searches.

*2. American Heart Association

http://www.americanheart.org
http://www.strokeassociation.org

The American Heart Association (AHA) is a nonprofit multidisciplinary association of physicians, nurses, and allied health care professionals. Its goal is to reduce the incidence and prevalence of heart disease and stroke. The AHA and the American Stroke Association Web sites are primarily geared to health care professionals, but also have some consumer-related features. Some of the features of this site are "Warning Signs" which discusses the signs and symptoms of a heart attack and stroke and the importance of seeking help immediately; "Risk Assessment"—a tool that can help the consumers or health care providers to estimate their risks of having a heart attack; and "Healthy Lifestyle" which discusses health promotion and disease prevention activities. Programs include healthy diet and nutrition, exercise and fitness, lifestyle management, lowering cholesterol, "My Heart Watch" (an interactive resource program that allows consumer to discuss/chat with the experts and other consumers), and many more.

This Web site contains extensive information that health care professionals may use to educate patients, families, and caregivers regarding heart disease, treatments, and procedures. The sections of the *Heart & Stroke Encyclopedia* are arranged in an alphabetical index, and "Diseases and Conditions," includes thousands of topics. The research section discusses the "Top 10" research advances in Stroke and CVD. The AHA and Stroke Heart Association Web sites include professional and consumer features that are not clearly outlined in the main page. Although the information provided is reliable, it is not clear when it was last updated. This Web site is well-organized, making it easy for the user to navigate.

*3. Congenital Heart Information Network

http://www.tchin.org

Congenital Heart Information Network (CHIN) is a nonprofit organization created by the mother of a child with complex heart defects. The aim of the Web site is to provide information and resources to children and adults with congenital heart defects and acquired heart disease and the professionals who work with them. The educational information and resources available on this site are developed and managed by volunteers who are physicians, nurses, allied health professionals, and paraprofessionals. The CHIN Web site features the following: "Community" provides online support to children, adults, and their families through the chat rooms and e-mail lists. This site includes a family room where patients and families can share their thoughts and experiences; a memorial garden in remembrance of the patients who died of congenital heart disease; a portrait gallery and a teen lounge where children, teens, adults and their families share their stories about living with heart disease. "Resource Room" includes books and educational materials about congenital heart disease that have been previewed by the Advisory Panel for accuracy and clarity. This also includes fiction and nonfiction children's books previewed by parent volunteers to ensure that language is appropriate and understood by readers. "Internet Links" includes extensive hyperlinks to other related Web sites that are important to the families, nurses, and other health care professionals.

This Web site is simple, well-organized, and easy to navigate. The information provided is clear and concise. Although the site is patient and family focused, it offers health care professionals the opportunity to network and participate in online support groups and the development and review of education materials.

4. Heart Failure Society of America

http://www.hfsa.org
http://www.abouthf.org

The Heart Failure Society of America, Inc. (HFSA) was organized by heart failure experts to provide a forum for all health care professionals who are interested in learning more about the disease process, research, and patient care management; in playing a role in reducing health care costs; and who want to network with other providers. The Web site was created to educate physicians, nurses, and allied members of the health care profession through publications, programs, and other resources, and to enable them to enhance their practices.

The hfsa.org Web site is organized in 3 categories. These are description of the organization, its mission, corporate members, and membership information such as eligibility and benefits; a list of publications, newsletters, guidelines, and other educational materials developed or compiled by the HFSA; and announcement of annual meetings. The abouthf.org Web site includes categories such as patient education topics; frequently asked questions regarding heart failure; media center press releases; Awareness events; and free educational resources and materials for consumers and professionals.

Both Web sites are well organized and structured simply, resulting in easier navigation. The search features provide information located within the organization's publications, programs, and newsletters, as well as from their health failure link exchange sites (about 11 sites). Some information is shared in abstracts format; other is provided full-text. Information includes dates of posting and dates of recent updates. One needs the Adobe Acrobat Reader to download and print some of the full-text articles available on the site.

5. The Heart.org—Cardiology Online

http://www.theheart.org

This Web site is designed to provide information on the treatment and prevention of cardiovascular diseases. Its intended users consist of physicians and allied health care professionals. Access to the Web site is free for those who are recognized as members of professional associations or institutions. The homepage includes the following sections: "Heartwire" provides information on treatment and prevention of heart diseases, summaries of the latest developments in heart disease, clinical trial commentaries, and access to case studies; "education" offers continuing medical education (CME) and non-CME accredited case studies, seminars, and CyberSessions that are broadcast audiovisual coverage or virtual conferences that can either be live or recorded; "forum" offers the opportunity to communicate and network with expert professionals; "conference center" lists conferences, CyberSessions, courses, exams, and other events of interest to the health care professional; "collections" provides a list of archived full text articles on a specific topic that have been published on the site. This Web site is simple. Once one becomes a registered user, the site is customized to automatically provide information relevant to one's specialty. Information provided is clear and concise and posting dates are available. Printing articles or information from the site is user-friendly as unnecessary images are taken out when articles are re-formatted for printing. Participation in CyberSessions requires an up to date Java and JavaScript enabled browser.

*6.   Johns Hopkins Heart Health

http://www.jhbmc.jhu.edu/cardiology/rehab
http://www.jhbmc.jhu.edu/cardiology/rehab/profinfo.html

This Web site is developed and maintained by the Johns Hopkins Bayview Medical Center's Division of Cardiology, Cardiac Rehabilitation and Prevention, and Comprehensive Vascular Center, and is sponsored by the medical center. The site is designed to provide information and education on heart disease management and prevention, innovative treatments, clinical research studies, and resources related to cardiovascular disease for both health care professionals and consumers. The cardiology/rehab site is divided into three sections: "health conditions" provides information on the prevention and management of cardiovascular diseases; "staying healthy" provides information on nutrition, exercise, and lifestyle/behavioral changes; and "signature articles and resources" offers articles related to cardiovascular disease and provides hyperlinks to other Web sites. The professional site provides information on clinical research studies, Johns Hopkins Heart Healthy Faculty presentation on heart disease management and prevention, conferences and seminars, and links to other Web sites related to heart disease.

The site is simple and easy to navigate. Information provided is clear, concise, accurate, reliable, and includes dates of posting and dates of last updates. Adobe Acrobat Reader is required for access to some of the full-text articles. Nurses may use this site for educational purposes as well as for patient and family educational materials.

*7.   Mayo Clinic: Heart and Blood Vessels Center

http://www.mayoclinic.com

This site was developed and is now maintained by a group of physicians, nurses, health educators, researchers, and writers and is owned by the Mayo Foundation for Medical Education and Research. Although the site focuses mainly on health education of patients, families, and the general public, it offers health care professionals access to the experience and knowledge of more than 2,000 physicians and scientists of the Mayo Clinic. Mayo Clinic physicians and researchers review information available on this site. It is reliable, accurate, and timely with dates of postings explicitly stated. The homepage gives one easy access to the heart and blood center. The features of this site include: "news and features picks" which presents news briefs and alerts on the latest health information available on heart disease; "diseases and conditions, A to Z guide" which provides information about the disease process and treatments in the form of patient and family education materials; "ask the Mayo physician" which offers access to health information and education materials; and "other Web sites" which provide access to therapies, research, preventive care, and other helpful topics and resources.

Registered users can select topics of interest and have new articles in their area of interest Book marked and saved in the user's home page. The user is also notified of new articles on his/her next visit to the site. The site is well organized, free of clutter, easy to navigate, and user-friendly. Full-text articles can be downloaded and printed easily.

8. Medscape.com

*http://www.cardiology.medscape.com/Home/Topics/cardiology/
cardiology.html
http://www.medscpape.com/Home/network/nursing/nursing.html*

Medscape is one of the Web's most extensive providers of medical information and educational tools. It is organized into different sections for professionals and consumers. The professional specialty sites are divided into medical, type of profession, and other related sites. The consumer sites are subdivided into diseases and conditions and healthy lifestyles. The professional specialty sites provide reliable and up to date information for clinicians, specialists, and other health care professionals. Access to this Web site requires a one-time membership registration that automatically brings the user to the appropriate site that suits his/her profile. Customized profiles include Medscape Nurses, Medscape Cardiology, Medscape Med Student, and so on. The medical information presented on this site is relevant, constantly updated, and evaluated and approved by physicians and health care experts before it is posted.

Medscape Nurses and Medscape Cardiology are two of the specialty Web sites within Medscape that provide nurses with extensive resources on heart disease. Content comes from a wide array of peer-reviewed articles, medical and clinical journals and textbooks, medical news, late-breaking clinical updates on treatments, and next-day summaries of conferences. Each specialty Web site is organized in a consistent way, making navigation simple and less time-consuming. These Web sites contain the following features: the home page provides quick access to the sites' search features and also contains the latest news for the specialty area/field; the Continuing Medical Education Center provides a wide selection of free, continuously updated continuing education activities; conference coverage offers a brief detail of each conference session and its date(s), and geographic location; and editor's choice highlights select articles related to the site's specialty.

Medscape International Web Sites provide selections of cardiovascular-related medical information, including medical news and conference coverage, in different languages. Each of the international Web sites are formatted the same as those in the U.S. Examples of the international sites are Medscape Brazil (*http://www.medscapebrasil. com*), Medscape in Central and Eastern Europe including Czech Republic (*http://www.mediclub.cz*), Hungary (*http://www.medi centrum.hu*), Poland (*http://www.mediclub.pl*), Slovakia (*http://www. mediclub.sk*), Medscape El Mundo (*http://www.medscape.el mundo.es*), Medscape Italia (*http://www.medscapeitalia.com*), Medscape on Medipro (*http://www.so-net.ne.jp/medipro*), and Medscape Sweden, still under construction (*http://www.ronden.se*).

*9. National Heart, Lung, and Blood Institute: Information on Heart and Vascular Diseases

http://www.nhlbi.nih.gov/health/public/heart/index.htm

The National Heart, Lung, and Blood Institute (NHLBI) is one of the 17 Institutes of the National Institutes of Health (NIH) that aims to enhance people's health and well-being. The NHLBI's health information page is divided into 4 sections: patients and the general public, health care professionals, Healthy People 2010 Projects, and other health information. The health care professionals' section lists heart and vascular diseases as one of its categories and includes information about high blood pressure and provides educational materials to control and prevent high blood pressure. The National High Blood Pressure Education Program, a program for professional, patient, and public education that aims at reducing death and disability, is also available. The cholesterol section provides informational facts about cholesterol and heart disease and offers information for lowering cholesterol blood level and healthy eating. Information on the National Cholesterol Education Program aims to raise awareness about cholesterol as a risk factor in coronary heart disease. An obesity section provides information about women and heart disease, healthy weight, calculating body mass index, and physical activity. A heart attack section provides discussion and educational materials that health care professionals can use to educate the consumers on the risk factors and warning signs for heart disease and timely access to medical attention. "Other cardiovascular information" includes information on Latino cardiovascular health resources, fact sheets for heart diseases, and educational materials for healthy living. Some of these materials are provided in Spanish and English. This site has a pleasant color scheme, is well-organized, and uncluttered, making navigation easier. The information presented is clear, concise, and simple. However, it is difficult to determine whether the information shared is current because most do not include the dates when they were posted or last updated. Some information requires Acrobat Reader or Java Script capability for downloading and printing.

_____ Chapter **43**

Vascular Disease

Hussein Tahan and Paulette Espina-Gabriel

_____

L ocating information on the Internet about vascular disease presents a great challenge. Available information is most related to
cardiac rather than vascular diseases. It is mainly focused on the
needs of professional societies and associations, and most important,
those that are physician-based. However, there is one nursing society
devoted to the subject—the Society for Vascular Nursing. The characteristics of the Web sites reviewed in this chapter are similar, and in
some aspects they are the same. These are the focus on physician
practice, mainly present continuing education resources, online discussion groups and newsletters, and provision of services for members
of the professional association or society.

Use of the Web sites reviewed in this chapter is basically limited to
either enhancement of knowledge in the field of vascular diseases and
innovations in its treatment or to finding resources for patient and family
education. These sites do not have any special or unique features.
They are considered average, lack creativity or originality, and do
not require any unusual technological resources aside from Netscape
Navigator, Internet Explorer, or in a few cases Acrobat Adobe Reader.
Despite their limitations, they are still considered advantageous to

nursing and patient care. They all are easy to navigate. They also present information in a concise, clear, and simple way. They all rely on medical professionals to oversee and approve the information posted which makes their information credible, accurate, and timely. All the reviewed sites discourage any advertisement for or promotion of product sales. Additionally, they have disclaimers that release them of their responsibility toward the information posted.

*1. The American Venous Forum (AVF)

http://www.avf.org

The American Venous Forum (AVF) was founded in 1988. It provides an academic colloquium to physicians, particularly vascular surgeons, interested in research and education in the field of venous diseases. Its mission is to improve the care of patients with venous and lymphatic disorders by providing a forum for information exchange concerning basic and clinical research pertaining to venous and lymphatic systems. The site is sponsored by an unrestricted educational grant from Sanofi Sythelabo, Inc.

The Web site is organized in three parts: medical professionals, medical students, and patients. Some of the characteristics of this site that are beneficial to nurses are case presentations and discussions for society members and students, links, clinical updates on management of vascular diseases, guidelines for the diagnosis and management of vascular diseases such as deep-vein thrombosis and varicose or spider veins, and a membership directory and referral center for the treatment of vascular diseases. Information brochures can be purchased or printed from the site at no cost. The site is easy to navigate; information is clear, concise, credible, and current.

2. The Society for Cardiovascular and Interventional Radiology

http://www.SCVIR.org

The Society of Cardiovascular and Interventional Radiology (SCVIR) is a professional society for physicians who specialize in interventional

---

*Sites suitable for consumer use.

or minimally invasive procedures. SCVIR promotes education, research, health policy, and communication in this area of health care. The society's Web site includes many features related to the membership of the society and to knowledge of cardiovascular disease. However, the educational resources available are specific to interventional radiological advances and minimally invasive treatment procedures. Of particular importance to nurses are the clinical practice guidelines that define ideal practice principles to assist in providing high-quality nursing care, consumer information centers that contain separate Web pages dedicated to different diseases, online discussion boards, and links to select vascular centers of excellence.

A medical and scientific advisory board supervises the SCVIR. A membership area is only accessible to members of the society and through a protected ID and password access. Navigating the site is easy. The content of the site is concise, clear, credible, and timely.

3. Society for Vascular Medicine and Biology (SVMB)

http://www.svmb.org

The Society for Vascular Medicine and Biology (SVMB) is a community of vascular clinicians and scientists that was founded in 1989. Its goals are to improve the integration of vascular biological advances into medical practice, and to maintain high standards of clinical vascular medicine. The society believes that innovation in vascular disease results from the collaboration of all professionals involved in vascular care including nurses. Although members of the society are mostly physicians and medical scientists, nurses are encouraged to become members. The site includes several features that are helpful to nurses such as publications (journal on vascular medicine with select full-text articles and two newsletters), case study presentations, continuing medical education, and abstracts of conference proceedings. Web-based education and training are also provided on the site; this educational opportunity requires pre-registration and special ID and password access.

The SVMB recognizes vascular medicine as a medical specialty. Nurses may use the clear, concise, and timely information shared in this Web site for continuing education and professional development purposes. It is easy to access and navigate the site.

4. The Society for Vascular Nursing (SVN)

http://www.svnnet.org

The Society for Vascular Nursing (SVN) is a nursing organization dedicated to the compassionate and comprehensive care of persons with vascular diseases. The SVN Web site is specifically developed for nursing professionals, especially members of the society. Its purpose is to provide SVN members with a forum for collegial relationships and opportunities for professional growth and career development. The resources provided in this site are information about the *Online Journal on Vascular Nursing* (full access is available to subscribers and society members). Access to archived issues is available in full-text and with printing capability. Society membership applications may be completed and submitted online. A list of the national and international SVN chapters with direct e-mail access to a designated contact person for each chapter is another key feature of this site. Information is also provided on grants and research, patient education information sheets, and links.

Information posted in the SVN Web site is edited by a professional site editor and approved by the society's board of directors for accuracy, timeliness, and applicability to vascular nursing and patient care. The site is easy to navigate.

5. University of Massachusetts Medical School: An Internet Resource on Venous Thromboembolism

http://www.umassmed.edu/outcomes/dvt/
http://www.dvt.org

This Web site is sponsored by the Center for Outcomes Research at the University of Massachusetts Medical Center. It is dedicated to sharing knowledge on best practices in the area of deep-vein thrombosis and pulmonary embolism. The resource guides available on the site were developed through a partnership between the Center for Outcomes Research and the Massachusetts Peer Review Organization (MassPRO). A multidisciplinary team of professionals, including nurses, established the guides. In addition to these two guidelines, the site makes available the consensus guidelines for deep vein thrombosis and pulmonary embolism developed by the National Institutes of Health and the American College of Chest Physicians.

This Web site is helpful for nurses and can be used for continuing education. Important features of the site are availability of the guidelines in full-text with free printing, links, and teaching resources. The teaching resources include a virtual hospital, case study presentations, discussion forums, and a PowerPoint slide presentation on venous thromboembolism. Medical, nursing, and allied health professionals developed the information available on this site. It is clear, concise, credible, and easily accessible; however, it dates back mostly to 1998. The site is easy to navigate.

*6. The Vascular Disease Foundation (VDF)

http://www.vdf.org

The Vascular Disease Foundation (VDF) is a consumer-based organization that provides the public with educational resources about vascular diseases such as peripheral arterial disease, carotid disease, venous disease, and abdominal aortic aneurysm. The VDF Web site is funded by a grant from Otsuka America Pharmaceuticals, Inc. and is sponsored by several professional societies, associations, commercial entities, and pharmaceutical companies that focus on vascular disease. Although this site is not dedicated for health care professionals, it is a valuable resource for nurses that can be used for patient and family educational purposes. Some of the important resources available in this site are an online consumer newsletter about vascular diseases, educational pamphlets and fact sheets, educational videos, a section on frequently asked questions, and links. The homepage of this site appears too busy; however, it is easy to use and navigate. Available information is timely, clear, and concise. An important aspect of this site is the presentation of educational videos in a text format for those who may not have the required technology.

*7. VascularWeb: One Source for Vascular Health Information

http://www.vascularweb.org

This Web site is sponsored primarily by the American Association for Vascular Surgery (AAVS) and the Society for Vascular Surgery (SVS) in addition to several other participating organizations. It aims to further education, research, and advocacy regarding vascular diseases. The sponsors of this site are dedicated to the interests of vascular physicians and their patients, and committed to continuing medical education and the development of the scientific and technical aspects of vascular surgery. The site provides a forum for public awareness and education. Although the medical societies sponsoring this site are intended for the physicians, information available on the site is beneficial to nurses and the nursing care of patients with vascular disease.

The site contains many features such as an online newsletter for members, guidelines for membership in the society, the society's by-laws, events and conferences, contact information, online discussion forums, electronic journals, Medline Search, clinical resources, patient education resources, job opportunities, and hyperlinks to other Web sites. However, not all features are available to nurses or the public. Some require special protected access that is only available to members of the society. Resources available to nurses include clinical resources regarding diseases and techniques of care, medical and scientific articles, and radiographic images; patient and family education materials; a search feature for locating a vascular physician or surgeon; job opportunities; and online discussion forums that are open to nonphysicians as guests. However, to participate in these forums, guests must be pre-registered first.

Materials posted on the site are subject to copyright laws. The site provides limited permission for the individual user to reproduce, retransmit, and reprint for his/her own personal use. A team of several professionals specialized in vascular diseases manage the site and function as editors. Information is current, simple, credible, accurate, and concise. The site is easy to navigate.

Chapter 44

Respiratory Care

Georgia L. Narsavage

Multiple respiratory care Web sites exist and include information such as medical and nursing-focused general and disease-specific reports, specialty organization data, updated statistics—usually through government agencies, and patient education resources. The World Wide Web has progressively become a source of information that is readily accessible and easily updated, expanding capabilities to access and share knowledge. By reviewing the Web sources listed, nurses can familiarize themselves with the type of information that is available and have a quick reference list to guide searches. Web searches can be used to assist in preparing care plans and treatment protocols for respiratory patient care. Many sites link to other Web sites, facilitating deeper exploration of topics. Web sites focused on patient education and prevention of respiratory disease can also help nurses guide patients to accurate and appropriate self-care information in a user-friendly format.

*1. American Academy of Allergy, Asthma, and Immunology (AAAAI)

http://www.aaaai.org

This site provides information on the American Academy of Allergy, Asthma, and Immunology membership, mission and goals, interest sections and their professional journal. There are also sections for the media, patients and the general public, continuing education, training programs, and jobs. The section that may be of highest value to nurses is the "Physician/Clinician Reference and Patient/Public Education Materials." A drop-down menu allows easy access to these materials. The AAAAI site is well-organized, with a concise homepage and a good allergy and asthma information source. The "Just for Kids" section may be useful for pediatric nurses. The association supports another site: Allergy, Asthma and Immunology Online (*http://allergy.mcg.edu/*). This Web site is an information and news source for asthma and allergy patients, families, clinicians, and the media. Online quizzes on allergy and asthma (age-specific) let users test their knowledge of respiratory conditions while learning. Also, "Asthma Screening" is designed to alert individuals to a need for follow-up with a clinician. Finally, the information for physicians includes a Resource Manual that includes patient care guidelines, asthma checklists, treatment algorithms, therapy recommendations, and home contact worksheets. Although copyrighted, there is an online release allowing practitioners to reproduce these materials without charge for patient care. This site and the related AAAAI site are clear and focused appropriately. The intended audiences (practitioners or patients) can easily understand the text. Membership is not required for this site.

2. American Academy of Sleep Medicine (AASM)

http://www.asda.org

This professional society Web site focuses on encouraging study of and improving the practice of sleep medicine. It links through the Associated

---

*Sites suitable for consumer use.

Professional Sleep Societies (APSS) to the Sleep Research Society. This Web site should be considered in studying respiratory care due to the prevalence of sleep apnea as a major respiratory disorder and the impact of inadequate sleep on recovery from respiratory illness. A highly valuable resource linked to the ASDA Web site is "MEDSleep Educational Materials" with a comprehensive file of sleep-related case studies, problem-based learning directives and curricula, and practical guides for direct care such as "Taking a Sleep History." This site links easily from one section to another, and supplies accurate information for providers.

3. American Association for Respiratory Care (AARC)

http://www.aarc.org

The Web site of the American Association for Respiratory Care has been designed to provide respiratory therapists, nurses, managers of respiratory services, and respiratory care educators with up to date information, legislative/policy commentary along with a media kit, direct care practice resources, and career development networking. Other sections of the Web site include member services, a buyer's guide for respiratory equipment, international issues, and patient education. The "Respiratory Care Links" section provides rapid connections to many high-quality resources. A search tool, available on the homepage when the site opens, provides a quick start to the searcher. There is no password required for access, although the AARC journal and selected services are accessible only to current members. Key respiratory care information and resources such as patient education tools are particularly useful for nurses.

4. American College of Chest Physicians (ACCP)

http://www.chestnet.org

Although this is a physician-titled Web site, the information has a clinical focus appropriate for nursing. ACCP member education includes consensus statements, practice guidelines, and patient education guides. Evidence-Based Practice Guidelines include Clinician Quick Reference and Patient Education Guides on topics such as "Managing Cough." There are at least 10 Patient Education Guides that provide easy to understand information that can be used to develop discharge teaching pamphlets or to teach school-age children and parents. The presentation of guidelines in PDF format provides easily replicated and printed information. Most information is available without membership requirements for access. However, online access to the association's journal is limited to members.

*5. American Lung Association (ALA)

http://www.lungusa.org

The Web site for this "oldest voluntary health organization in the United States" provides information on programs and strategies for fighting lung disease in adults and children in community settings. Sections of the Web site include asthma care, tobacco control/prevention programs, environmental health, diseases A to Z, local ALA chapters, information for volunteers, a press center, and public education materials. The data and statistics section provides rapid information access with easily retrievable data. An ALA current initiative is reflected in the asthma care section providing detailed facts including severity, symptoms, definitions, surveys, medication information, news, and recommended publications. A focus on children with asthma describes the clinician role and the caregiver's role in home control of allergies and asthma.

6. American Thoracic Society (ATS)

http://www.thoracic.org

The American Thoracic Society Web site, originally formed in conjunction with the American Lung Association, is currently independent of the ALA and has been designed to provide physicians, nurses, and allied respiratory care professionals with expanded program information on pulmonary research, education, patient care, and advocacy. Other sections of the Web site include membership categories with costs, assembly projects, news and updates, a practitioner's page with case studies, and member-only services including a member directory and online journals. The quality-of-life resource section provides rapid connections to one of the most inclusive repositories of information on the subject. The ATS site is easily accessed and readily supports movement from one area to another. Information areas are well-developed and links are current. The search tool, available on the homepage when the site opens, is on the header and may be missed initially. There is no password required for access to most of the Web site, although the AARC journal and selected services are accessible only to current members. Practice tips and resources for research provide quality support for nurses in pulmonary specialties such as asthma education and COPD research.

*7. Asthma Information Center

http://cooke.gsf.de/asthmainfocenter

This Web site is useful for both patients and clinicians. It includes patient guidelines, bulletin boards for communications, expert comments and FAQs, surveys, and support groups that can be accessed online. Information about the Global Initiative for Asthma (GINA) is a valuable component. The informal nature of this site makes it a good first stop for clinicians needing a quick update. It provides information on a variety of areas related to asthma.

8. National Heart, Lung, and Blood Institute (NHLBI)

http://www.nhlbi.nih.gov

Federal asthma activities and smoking cessation are current initiatives that are of value to respiratory care providers. In addition to the section on asthma control and parental assessment of asthma management in school children, it includes the National Asthma Education and Prevention Program information. Epidemiology and Clinical Trials Data Sets are links on this Web site. Finally, sleep disorders research studies are coordinated and reported at this site. Although the majority of resources available on this Web site focus on cardiac conditions such as hypertension, there are topics related to respiratory disease. Clinicians with an interest in research would find this site of interest.

*9.   National Lung Health Education Program (NLHEP)

http://www.nlhep.org

The NLHEP works with government, medical, and associated professional organizations to promote lung health and prevent lung disease. With its focus on chronic obstructive pulmonary disease, the objective is to create a program for primary and secondary prevention. Resources include information for patients and physicians, as well as related Internet resources. Two useful booklets are available in PDF format to print: "Save Your Breath America" by T. Petty and D.E. Doherty with a companion one for clinicians: "Prevent Emphysema Now." Slide presentations are also available for review online by clinicians. Links to sample wellness education programs may be especially useful for community planners. The National Jewish Medical and Research Center (*www.njc.org/main*) in Colorado provides sponsorship for this site. Its organized, well-developed list of links includes descriptions of the links that are useful in directing a search for information.

10.   Respiratory Nursing Society (RNS)

http://www.respiratorynursingsociety.org

The Respiratory Nursing Society provides resources for nurses to develop respiratory knowledge and skills to promote quality care. The Web site is relatively new but provides educational resources including inexpensive patient education booklets and position statements. A core curriculum is expected to be published in 2002. The most valuable section of the current Web site is the "Related Links" section. This nursing specific list of links includes the major societies as identified in this chapter, disease-specific pages for Alpha 1 Association and the Cystic Fibrosis Foundation, Pulmonary patient support and education sites, Pharmacology, and End of Life Care sites. Although there is currently little actual information on the RNS Web site, there are indications of its potential and the linkage page alone is useful to nurses. Short descriptions of the links could add to the value of this site.

_____ Chapter 45

Genetics

Felissa R. Lashley

G enetics has become integral to health care. New diagnostic tests and therapies based on genetics continue to expand in clinical practice. Nurses often seek information on a variety of genetic-related topics including basic genetics, specific genetic disease information, information related to genetic testing, educational and teaching materials, referral sources for specialty genetic clinics, and laboratories and support groups for patients and families affected by genetic disease. Genetic sites vary widely in their focus and complexity. The sites listed below are a sampling that meets the variety of needs listed above.

1. GeneTests-GeneClinics

http://www.geneclinics.org

The purpose of this site is to serve as a medical genetic information resource developed for health care providers and researchers. It consists of *GeneReviews,* an online publication of disease reviews authored by experts, international directories of genetics clinics, prenatal diagnosis clinics, and genetic testing laboratories as well as educational materials that emphasize genetic testing and counseling concepts, a glossary, and teaching tools. It is administratively sponsored by the University of Washington School of Medicine and Children's Hospital Regional Medical Center in Seattle, Washington, with funding support from the National Institutes of Health, Health Resources and Services Administration, and the U.S. Department of Energy. It requires registration, which is free. It is up-to-date and easy to use. The disease reviews are technical. It is in English only.

*2. Genetic Alliance

http://www.geneticalliance.org

This site emphasizes support groups, resources, and public policy issues especially for individuals and families with genetic conditions. The resources page emphasizes such diverse topics as bioethics, disability resources, advocacy, policy issues, ethnocultural issues, educational resources, grief and loss, and contacting professional societies. The sponsor is the Genetic Alliance, which is an international coalition of individuals, professionals, and genetic support organizations working together to enhance the lives of everyone living with genetic conditions. The intended audience includes consumers, health care professionals, foundations, agencies, and advocates. The information is up-to-date and accurate. The site is attractive and relatively easy to use. There are links to sources in other languages such as IDEXMEDICO, a bilingual medical information service.

*3. Genetic Science Learning Center

http://gslc.genetics.utah.edu

The purpose of this site is to help people understand how genetics affects our lives and society. It is a joint project of the University of Utah Eccles Institute of Human Genetics, School of Medicine, and the Utah Museum of Natural History. It is an extremely attractive and visually appealing site. Its main divisions are basic genetics, genetic

---

*Sites suitable for consumer use.

disorders, genetics in society, and genetic thematic units. There are activities for teachers, students, parents, and families. There are engaging activities for teachers to use in teaching genetic principles to students and many interesting materials to download. The site is relatively easy to navigate, the difficulty level is low to average, and the material is up-to-date. It is in English only.

4. Genetics Education Center

http://www.kumc.edu/gec

The emphasis for this extremely comprehensive site is genetic education, the human genome project, careers in genetics, and resources. It is sponsored by the University of Kansas Medical Center. At the bottom of the page are links to the Genetic Professional Home Page (*http://www.kumc.edu/gec/geneinfo.htm*), which has more technical information and links, and the Genetic Support Group Home Page, both of which are sponsored by the same organization. The intended audience is educators interested in human genetics; however, comprehensive information is available not only about genetic education, but also about genetic conditions and support groups and ways to locate genetic experts. The resource pages for genetic education information include curricula, lesson plans, hands-on materials, computer programs, books, and videotapes. The site is easy to use and is attractive. Material varies in difficulty, but most is moderate. It is up-to-date and accurate. It is in English only.

5. Genetics Education Partnership

http://genetics-education-partnership.mbt.washington.edu

This site emphasizes genetics education from kindergarten through high school. The sponsor is the Genetics Education Partnership described as a genetics learning community including teachers, scientists, and health care professionals in the state of Washington interested in genetics. Schools, universities, and private corporations are contributors. It consists of information about why, how, and what every student should learn about genetics, detailed reviews of instructional materials, classroom activities including lesson plans and interesting tools for teaching genetics in the classroom and more. Some of these are oriented to health care such as the activities for sickle cell anemia. There are also links to additional resources. The site is attractive and easy to use. The difficulty level is easy to moderate. It is in English only.

6. Human Genome Program, Department of Energy

http://www.ornl.gov/hgmis

This site has historical and current information about the Human Genome Project. It is sponsored by the U.S. Department of Energy (DOE). Other features include News Sources, Medicine and the New Genetics, including sections on gene testing; gene therapy; specific genetic disease information and genetic counseling; publications; educational resources including videos and images; a glossary; the research programs available through DOE; aspects of the ethical, legal, and social issues section such as genetics in the courtroom and cloning; and topical fact sheets. It is an attractive site and easy to use. The level of material varies but overall is moderate. There is a guide to Web sites in Spanish.

7. National Human Genome Research Institute, National Institutes of Health

http://www.nhgri.nih.gov

This site is a major resource for information on the goals, progress, and achievements of the Human Genome Project; genetic-related policies and research initiatives; and grant and fellowship information. It has sections on genomic and genetic resources, policy and public affairs, a glossary, and an "in the news" feature. The sponsor is the National Institutes of Health (NIH). Most of the information is current but some pages are dated. It is easy to use and there are connections to the Center for Inherited Disease Research and information related to the Ethical Legal and Social Implications (ELSI) of the Human Genome Project. Many of the resources are too technical for genetic researchers. The site is moderately attractive. Information ranges from moderately to very technical. It is in English only.

8.   Office of Genetics and Disease Prevention, Centers for Disease Control and Prevention

http://www.cdc.gov/genetics/

This site specializes in the public health implications and applications of genetics. The stated goal is to provide information about human genetic discoveries and how they can be used to improve health and prevent disease. The site is sponsored by the Centers for Disease Control and Prevention (CDC). Among the information provided are reports and publications, fact sheets, glossaries, links to human genome project information, and other related CDC sites such as newborn screening, and a monthly publication on public health perspectives related to genetics. There is material in Spanish and English. The material is of easy to moderate difficulty. It is up-to-date and accurate. There is less information on specific genetic diseases and topics than other sites have.

9.   Online Mendelian Inheritance in Man (OMIM)

http://www.ncbi.nlm.nih.gov/Omim

This is a comprehensive catalog of human genes and genetic disorders as well as a database that can be searched not only by disease but also by type of inheritance, gene map, and key words. The site is authored and edited by Victor A. McKusick and colleagues at Johns Hopkins University and elsewhere, and was developed for the World Wide Web by the National Center for Biotechnology Information. There is now a link to the Entrez database of MEDLINE articles and sequence information. While fairly technical, this site has a wealth of information, pictures, references, and links to other databases, mostly of gene maps and mutations in humans and animals. The audience is for health professionals concerned with genetic disorders and genetics researchers. The site's most important feature is the current, accurate, and comprehensive information on thousands of genetic disorders. It is easy to use. It is only available in English.

_____ Chapter **46**

HIV/AIDS

Carl A. Kirton and Joseph P. Colagreco

Providers of HIV care live in a constant, dynamic world of HIV therapeutics. This area of nursing is still considered by many to be in its infancy stage—especially when compared to other well-established fields such as critical care. The progress in this field continues to grow exponentially. To remain current in HIV/AIDS care, one could spend an inordinate amount of time perusing costly academic and clinical journals. Fortunately, there are several extraordinary Web sites dedicated to various aspects of HIV/AIDS care. For most of these sites, the information is timely, accurate, and comprehensive. One merely needs to regularly consult these sites to appreciate the evolving science and care of individuals with HIV infections. A list of the ten most acclaimed sites for HIV/AIDS clinicians and researchers follows.

*1. Aegis

http://www.aegis.com/

This site professes to be the "largest HIV/AIDS web site." It also claims to be updated hourly. Of all the Web sites mentioned here, this one

---

*Sites suitable for consumer use.

has the longest tenure. It started in 1980 as a bulletin board service and has evolved into one of the most comprehensive compendiums of information for both patients and providers. To quote the site directly, "the range of information available is so vast, its quality so dependable, national and international organizations routinely log onto the system to converse or download clinical information or late-breaking news." From September 1990, to April 1995, ÆGiS operated under the auspices of the Sisters of St. Elizabeth of Hungary, a small religious community founded in 1988. In April 1995, ÆGiS was reorganized as a nonprofit charitable and educational corporation under the laws of the state of California. The site is currently sponsored by Boehringer-Ingelheim. For many, this site has become the primary source of HIV/AIDS information. Its scope covers clinical topics, newsworthy items, and legal issues. Visitors should be certain to visit the "Law Library" that in many cases includes full-text of court decisions and some law-oriented journals with content that relates to HIV/AIDS policymaking. The organization of this site is well-structured, and no topic in HIV/AIDS is excluded. One weakness of this site is the lack of links or information for persons with HIV who are Spanish speaking. This site has won more than 35 Internet awards.

*2.   AIDS Clinical Trials Information Service

http://www.actis.org/

The AIDS Clinical Trials Information Service (ACTIS) provides quick and easy access to information on federally and privately funded HIV clinical trials for adults and children. The site has several federal sponsors such as the Federal Drug Administration (FDA), The Centers for Disease Control (CDC), and the National Library of Medicine (NLM). This site is designed for use by both health care professionals and laypersons. For example, the site can be personalized to provide information in layman's terms or professional clinical information can be provided in a research-oriented format. For the clinician, there is a feature that displays brief descriptions of clinical trials in the database that are currently recruiting participants and those that are closed to enrollment. When results from a trial have been published or presented at a conference, a reference to the article or paper is provided. As additional trial data are published, the bibliographic references are updated. This site is also dedicated to providing education to those who are considering, or actively participating in, clinical trials; it provides the ability to speak with ACTIS health information specialists and several of the documents intended for patients are in both English and Spanish. The content of this site is accurate and current. Clinical trials are covered in enough breadth so that the clinician can use this site as a day-to-day resource. The site is well-constructed and very user-friendly.

3. Association of Nurses in AIDS Care

http://www.anacnet.org/

ANAC, The Association of Nurses in AIDS Care, is a "non-profit professional nursing organization committed to fostering the individual and collective professional development of nurses involved in the delivery of health care to persons infected or affected by the Human Immunodeficiency Virus (HIV) and to promoting the health, welfare, and rights of all HIV infected persons." This site is sponsored by Ortho-Biotech, but the content is managed by ANAC. This site provides information primarily about the nursing organization, i.e., membership, conferences, certification, and as such its original offerings are few. It mainly provides links to other Web sites such as links to nursing programs with AIDS specialization courses and a variety of links to other sites of interest to nurses who work in the field of HIV and AIDS. There are two nursing continuing education programs available online and a link to other learning opportunities which are mainly links to other conferences or continuing education programs. The site meets its intended outcome by providing information to and for its members. Someone wanting information about HIV/AIDS or HIV/AIDS nursing might not find this site particularly useful. Thus, for its membership, it is well-organized and a useful resource.

*4. Center for AIDS Prevention Studies at the University of California San Francisco

http://www.caps.ucsf.edu/

CAPS is an acronym for the Center for AIDS Prevention Studies, and is the premier authority of information related to prevention of HIV infection. This center, located at the University of California, San Francisco (UCSF), sponsors a voluminous number of projects—too many to mention here. It has links to some of its model prevention programs. Program planners and designers can access instruments and surveys that have been designed and tested by CAPS scientists. In most cases, they provide the full curriculum for their model programs online. The many monographs and reports produced by the center are also available for download. Bibliographies and abstracts are provided for contributors to this site, which includes more than 30 content areas in HIV/AIDS. The site contains a page with HIV Prevention Fact Sheets that are referenced summaries of specific topics important to HIV prevention. These sheets are mailed to over 6,000 service providers, researchers, policymakers, media, and members of the public. Topics for the Fact Sheets are chosen on the basis of timeliness, what the community needs to know, and what scientific matters are of particular importance. The HIV Prevention Fact Sheets address the question of "what works"—programs that have been found to be effective in reducing HIV infection or modifying HIV-risk-related behavior. Each Fact Sheet emphasizes programs that have been scientifically evaluated and found effective, as well as aspects of programs that are lacking, and directions for future prevention efforts. Fact Sheets are available in English, Spanish, and Kiswahili in both hypertext markup language (HTML) and portable document format (PDF). The site content is an excellent compendium of information on this topic and is useful to nurses. It provides evidence for practice in all areas of prevention. For example, do you want to know if sex education works in prevention? This fact sheet give you simple, nontechnical facts based on current evidence. The site is well-organized and comprehensive, yet simplistic in its design and style.

5. Centers for Disease Control Divisions of HIV/AIDS Prevention

http://www.cdc.gov/nchstp/hiv_aids/dhap.htm

The Centers for Disease Control and Prevention, Division of HIV/AIDS Prevention, sponsors this site. It is a clearinghouse for HIV/AIDS information. The site features links to *Morbidity and Mortality Weekly Reports* that contain information related to HIV/AIDS. Most of the material is available in both HTML and PDF format. Most notable, this site offers slide sets of the latest HIV/AIDS surveillance data that can be downloaded into PowerPoint. By supplying an e-mail address, the CDC will notify you when new slide sets are posted to the Web site. Another unique offering of this site is the ability to download software that is free of charge from the CDC. For example, "CDC EZ-Text" is a qualitative software program developed to assist researchers to create, manage, and analyze semistructured qualitative databases. Equally appealing to researchers is the public use database and analysis software for AIDS cases reported through 1999. The content of the site is accurate, relevant, and essential to those in the field of HIV. Its scope of coverage is broad so that any individual wanting information in the field of HIV/AIDS can find it located on this site. Because it is so comprehensive, a novice to the Internet can be easily intimidated by all that this site offers.

*6. The HIV Drug Interactions Web Site

http://www.hiv-druginteractions.org/index.htm

Based in the Department of Pharmacology and Therapeutics at the University of Liverpool, this Web site was designed for use both by clinicians and patients as a straightforward, up to date reference on anti-HIV drugs. The Liverpool HIV Pharmacology Research group (LHPG) is led by Professor David Back and comprises clinical and nursing staff, research personnel, and PhD students. The LHPG has an extensive track record in the investigation of major pharmacological issues in HIV therapy and has research projects that are both laboratory-based and patient-led. This Web site is supported by educational grants from Roche and Glaxo Wellcome. This Web site should be bookmarked on every clinician's desktop for easy access to valuable and comprehensive information about HIV drug-drug interactions. The site design is attractive, eye-catching, and very easy to use. There is a FAQ section about drug-drug interactions and other related drug topics on issues that clinicians face daily. There are some full-text links to papers published as a result of the work of this research group.

7. HIV InSite

http://www.hivinsite.ucsf.edu/InSite

For one-stop shopping, every HIV clinician, researcher, educator, and policy analyst should be sure to visit this site sponsored by the University of California, San Francisco (UCSF). The site has many sponsors including private, government, and pharmaceutical support. The homepage has been recently revised, is attractive, and easy to navigate. The site is organized into categorical information on HIV/AIDS treatment, policy, and prevention. There is an excellent international section. New to the site is a link to its companion, youth-oriented site, *http://www.whatudo.org/*. Its design makes it somewhat difficult to determine how the authors defined "youth" and some of the links make it more confusing, e.g., a link to the national parent and teacher organization, *http://www.pta.org/* and a link to the National Association of State Boards of Education, *http://www.nasbe.org/HealthySchools/index.mgi*.

Nonetheless, it includes citations from various clinical and governmental agencies and in some cases full-text articles from some journals. As an added feature, *The HIV InSite Knowledge Base* (HKB), is available free online. The HKB is a "hypertextbook," has over 100 chapters, and not only continues to make its chapters widely available free of charge, but also organizes and provides access to related materials, both within HIV InSite and wherever else they may be available on the World Wide Web. In the HKB's completed form, each chapter links to a page of "Related Resources," organized into categories including guidelines, fact sheets, and journal articles. Previously the site contained a feature to ask an expert clinician advice and consultation online. This feature no longer seems to be available. There is an *Ask HIV Insite* page that contains the answers to submitted questions, but currently there is no mechanism to submit questions. Visit the site regularly for slides and audio lectures from experts in the field. The content of the site is extremely accurate and useful to both clinicians and researchers. The site is well-maintained with an extremely user-friendly interface.

8. International Association of Physicians in AIDS Care

http://www.iapac.org/

The Web site of the International Association of Physicians in AIDS Care (IAPAC), which claims to be *"the only global organization exclusively representing HIV care providers,"* falls short of representing providers other than physicians, but can be a resource to nurses who are particularly interested in international initiatives in HIV/AIDS. The site has a strong focus on issues of poverty and dehumanization—with equally strong sections on public policy and human rights. IAPAC has several initiatives that are worth examining, such as *International Drug Access Monitoring*. In collaboration with the United Nations, IAPAC serves as an official monitor of prototype programs designed to improve access to drugs and related technologies in less industrialized nations. IAPAC's *God Bless the Child* initiative coordinates a global network of sponsors to underwrite the cost of antiretroviral drugs and diagnostic technologies for HIV-infected children in less industrialized nations where such drugs and technologies may not be available. Visit the Web site to learn about IAPAC's transmission reduction, vaccine, and sexual counseling initiatives. Surprisingly, some of the posted information in the professional section is old. For example, the most recent article in the antiretroviral drug resistance section is from 1997. Moreover, a quick perusal of the authors on many of the clinical articles are United States physicians. There seems to be a lack of international authors. The content of the site is accurate and meets its intended outcome of providing an international perspective on HIV and AIDS. The design of the site is simplistic, making it easy to navigate. However, it falls short of being a clinical resource for health care professionals.

*9. Johns Hopkins AIDS Service

http://www.hopkins-aids.edu/

Equal to the UCSF site (HIV InSite) in its breadth and quality of HIV information is the John Hopkins AIDS Service Web site. It too provides late breaking, accurate, scientific and clinical information. An added feature is a literary corner that provides excerpts from recently published books dealing with HIV/AIDS issues. Another fun feature is the animation of the life cycle of HIV that one can view with the appropriate browser plug-in. One of the features that distinguishes this site from the aforementioned site is its coverage of managed care issues related to HIV. It is well worth a regular visit. Three HIV/AIDS publications are available free online. They are the Medical Management of HIV Infection, a clinical handbook of HIV/AIDS care written by Drs. John G. Bartlett and Joel E. Gallant of the Johns Hopkins University Division of Infectious Diseases. This book, which is fully updated every year, represents the standard of care of both the Johns Hopkins University AIDS Service and quality assurance for Maryland Medicaid. This handbook often represents the standard of care for many clinical professionals and is widely cited. The Hopkins HIV Report, a bimonthly HIV/AIDS care newsletter for health care professionals, written by faculty of The Johns Hopkins University, is also available online. This newsletter is mailed to thousands of health care professionals and remains an invaluable resource to busy clinicians. Online, the newsletter is available in both HTML and PDF formats. The Moore News Quarterly is a quarterly newsletter for patients that is written and published by the faculty, staff, and patients of the Johns Hopkins AIDS Service. The Moore News Quarterly is also available online. The content of the site is extremely accurate and useful to both professionals and consumers.

10. The National AIDS Treatment Advocacy Project

http://www.natap.org/

The National AIDS Treatment Advocacy Project (NATAP) mission is to educate individuals about HIV and hepatitis treatments and to advocate on the behalf of all people living with HIV/AIDS and Hepatitis C Virus (HCV). Primarily intended as a site for the HIV- or HCV-infected patient, it provides the reader with the very latest in HIV drug development, research, and treatment information on its Web site. The writing sophistication and coverage makes this an excellent resource for nurses. The strength of this site lies in its coverage of important AIDS science conferences from all over the world. After the conferences, follow-up reports are frequently posted to this site. *NATAP Reports,* the project's newsletter, is available online. The site has been revamped since we last wrote about it. Previously, the Web frames were so large that it made reading an article online a burdensome task. This has been corrected. The site has a fresh new look, is easy to navigate, and now includes PDF files for many important articles on HIV.

Chapter 47

Cancer

Trudy Johnson and Françoise Juste

Web sites related to clinical oncology and cancer care are designed to attract several different users. The users are broadly defined as consumers and health care professionals. The Web sites originate from organizations that service cancer patients and families of patients with cancer, related professional organizations, and government agencies with services for cancer care or research. There are numerous sites available to choose from. Many sites are dedicated specifically to subspecialties of cancer care and links for these sites are found within the sites described herein. Cancer sites targeted to consumers usually provide educational material regarding prevention, treatment, clinical trials; how and where to obtain support services; and how to advocate for public policy related to cancer care and research. Some of these sites provide recommendations for professionals to refer to consumers.

*1. American Cancer Society (ACS)

http://www.cancer.org

The American Cancer Society is a community focused nonprofit health care organization with divisions throughout the country. The organiza-

---

*Sites suitable for consumer use.

tion's mission is the commitment to eliminate cancer as a major health problem through prevention, research, education, advocacy, community, and services. A national board of directors, mostly volunteers, is responsible for the overall planning, coordination, education, and administration of various programs of research. The intended audience is mainly health care professionals and persons interesting in learning about preventing cancer and diminishing suffering from cancer through research and education. The Web site is consistent with this mission and is comprehensive in its approach for consumers and health care professionals. The index is simple and easy to navigate for any user. The *Patient Services* section includes the common type of information available on cancer Web sites. The free brochures and pamphlets are a valuable resource for consumers and clinicians. The topics can readily be searched for by key words. The documents are available in English or Spanish and include guidelines for clinicians as well.

Research is an important focus for this organization. It is the largest U.S. not-for-profit source of funds for scientific study of cancer that focuses on investigator-initiated, peer-reviewed research proposals. The *Research* section includes a newsletter that gives updates on treatment recommendations, cancer activities in the news, and reports from around the country to meet the varying interests of consumers and professionals. The *Media Services* section complements this nicely with archives of article abstracts, news releases, and statistics about cancer displayed graphically. The site is kept current with news updates posted within one week of the review. In general, this resource is valuable for consumers and professionals and could be referred to consumers for their use in order to obtain comprehensive information covering cancer education and research.

*2. American Society of Clinical Oncology (ASCO)

http://www.asco.org

This nonprofit organization has over 10,000 members involved in clinical oncology. Members are from the disciplines of medicine, nursing, and other health care professions who work in the many subspecialties of clinical oncology. The society fosters the exchange of information about cancer through scientific programs, educational programs, and other initiatives. ASCO was founded by a small group of physicians, members of the American Association of Cancer research (AACR), in

1964. The mission of the organization is to facilitate the delivery of quality care, to optimize the communication among various specialties concerned about cancer care, and to promote different ideas related to patient-oriented clinical research. The site design allows the user to easily scan the index by using dropdown menus from the four major index links at the top of the homepage. The site is subdivided for members, oncology professionals, consumers, "people living with cancer," and a media center. The site is easy to use and navigate. This design ensures that when someone only looks at one section of the index the person will see all the related links whether they are a consumer or professional, thereby optimizing the use of all pages on the site. Readers may also subscribe or renew their subscriptions to *The Journal on Clinical Oncology.*

The *Policy and Practice* section for professionals includes links to other credible sources of cancer information, public policy statements related to oncology concerns, and clinical practice guidelines. The evidence-based guidelines published by ASCO cover general and specialty topics, for example *Recommendations for use of anti-emetics* or *Recommended breast cancer surveillance guidelines.* Complimentary patient guides are also available such as *Follow-up care for breast cancer.* These guides are available via PDF format and print an attractive, easy-to-read format that could be copied for patients. Overall, this site is extremely useful to professionals and to consumers. It offers an array of information related to Cancer information, research, and treatment.

*3. Cancer Care, Inc.

http://www.cancercare.org

Cancer Care, Inc. is a national organization whose mission is to provide emotional support, and information to assist patients and families coping with cancer. Services are available to people of all ages, with all types of cancer. This is an excellent source for professionals to keep abreast of legislation related to cancer, current research, patient/family education guides, and other available resources. Cancer Care Inc. has a list of all the organizations and companies that helped sponsor and bring information to this site including numerous pharmaceutical companies such as Pfizer, Glaxo-Wellcome, and Ortho Biotech Oncology. The intended audience is directed toward health care professionals, people with cancer, family members of persons with cancer, and caregivers. The design is efficient and includes a text-only option from the homepage index. Unique to this site is the local support services section, which offers a search function to find the nearest support group in the user's region. Teleconferences are also a vital service of the organization and these are posted on the Web site. Patient/family education material is also included, some of which is available in Spanish. Overall the site is efficient, easy to use and to follow. The site is a comprehensive tool for professionals and consumers.

*4. Cancernet

http://www.cancernet.nci.nih.gov

Cancernet is a service of the National Cancer Institute (NCI) that provides current information on cancer. The material on the site has recent information published within one month of the author's review. The information is revised and updated by experts in oncology and related cancer specialties. The purpose of this site is to make information accessible regarding types of cancer, usual topics of diagnosis, treatment, clinical trials, fact sheets for patient/family education, support services and cancer literature. The intended audience is anyone interested in cancer, professionals, patients, researchers, and caregivers. The clinical trials section allows a search by disease stage and open-versus-closed trials to narrow the search findings. Unique to this site is an additional search directory to find genetic counselors specializing in genetic risk for cancer. Also available from this site is the NCI's Comprehensive Cancer Database to search for other information. This information is also useful for clinical nurses who are not expert in oncology nursing. An additional feature of this site is that the information is available in Spanish. The design is very easy to read and to follow. For first-time visitors, the site offers a user-friendly map, which helps one navigate and search for various topics of interests.

5. City of Hope Pain and Palliative Care Resource Center for Nursing Research and Education

http://www.cityofhope.org/mayday

The purpose of City of Hope Pain and Palliative Resource Center is to serve as a clearinghouse for information to facilitate individuals and organizations to improve pain management for persons with cancer. This is a repository of a variety of materials for pain management including pain assessment tools, patient/family education materials, research tools and numerous other resources. Articles are available for a $3.00 copyright fee. The index covers nursing knowledge, home care, pain in the elderly, pain and family, nonmalignant pain, ethics, pain in pediatrics, and costs related to pain. Clinical pathways or standards of care from other hospitals, educational program modules and professional competency guidelines from major medical centers, video series and quality-of-life instruments to measure pain are also available from this site. The information is very simple.

*6. National Alliance of Breast Cancer Organizations (NABCO)

http://www.nabco.org

The National Alliance of Breast Cancer Organizations (NABCO) is a network of breast cancer organizations that provides information and assistance to persons interested in cancer. This organization advocates for the concerns of breast cancer survivors and women at risk. The major sections are similar to other sites including news, resources, clinical trials, and support groups. This site is targeted primarily for consumers. The news is understandable for consumers, but this section does not include recently dated materials. In addition to the links and publications the resource section also includes educational information. This factual information regarding cancer care and special programs may also be valuable to professionals depending on their level of expertise in oncology. The information regarding prevention and treatment would be beneficial to provide patient teaching in the ambulatory setting. The best section of the site is related to clinical trials. It helps patients and families understand the implications of participating in a clinical trial. Additionally, it provides a breast cancer trial directory available in any language and was developed in collaboration with the National Cancer Institute. The level of information of this site is average, but does not contain valuable information for the health care professional. In addition, NABCO works closely with state and federal levels for regulatory changes related to women at risk.

*7. National Coalition for Cancer Survivorship

http://www.cansearch.org

National Coalition for Cancer Survivorship (NCCS) is a patient-led organization working for people with cancer and those caring for them. It is a leading national advocacy organization and frequently provides testimony before Congress and other government agencies. The mission of this site is to ensure quality care for all Americans. This site is also available in Spanish. NCCS strives to positively unite everyone who has been affected by cancer. NCCS, based in Maryland, is recognized as a leader in cancer survivorship and is recognized as a founding member of cancer organizations such as National Breast Cancer Coalition, and U.S. TOO International Prostate Cancer organization. This site is most valuable for keeping abreast of what is important to consumers to ensure that their needs are met and that clinicians consider what the lay public values as important for their treatment and support services. The *Conference and Events* listing was not extensive at the time of review, but it does provide a link to the National Cancer Institute meeting calendar. The level of information of this site is average and the content is beneficial to health care professionals and consumers. The design of this site is easy to use and to navigate.

*8. Oncolink

http://www.oncolink.com

Cancer specialists at the University of Pennsylvania Cancer Center (UPCC) founded this site to provide free information related to cancer. The site is appropriate for patients, families and health care professionals. The site has several sponsors including Amgen, AstraZeneca, Aventis, Elsevier Science, Pfizer, Ortho Biotech, and Varian, Inc. Comprehensive resources are available for both consumers and professionals. Topics include updates on specific types of cancer treatment and news about advances in research. Menus are user-friendly and easy to navigate. The disease-oriented menus for *Types of Cases* and *Treatment Options* are quite comprehensive. The most valuable feature of the site is the "Ask the Experts" page where questions can be submitted and are later published on the site; an archive of these questions is also maintained. The *Featured Sections* provides highlights of various topics related to coping with cancer that are useful for consumers and professionals. *Cancer News* links to recently published articles from *Reuters Health Information.* The *Hot Spot* section includes information from conferences, including abstracts of scientific publications. Additionally, the *Oncolink Library* has extensive resources for consumers and professionals. It includes book/video reviews, journal reviews, and peer-reviewed journals. The best section in the library is "Coping with

Cancer" which includes excerpts from online books. The only limitation of the online books is that plug-ins are needed for display. The level of information is average and is updated daily to provide accurate, precise, and credible information.

*9. Oncology Nursing Society (ONS)

http://www.ons.org

Oncology Nursing Society (ONS) online is a cancer information service developed for ONS members, other health care providers, oncology nurses, people with cancer, and their families and friends. The mission of ONS is to lead the transformation of cancer care by initiating and actively supporting educational, legislative, and public awareness to positively improve the care of people with cancer. ONS is a national organization of oncology nurses who are committed to excellence and advancing education in oncology. Corporate sponsors include Aventis Oncology, Brystol Myers Squibb Oncology, Purdue, Glaxo, Smith Kline, and Amgen. The "Research" link offers the reader information about ONS and nursing research funding. This link provides nurses with current information on trends and guidelines regarding cancer diagnosis, treatment, and care management.

Chapter 48

Maternity

Kristen S. Montgomery

This section presents current clinical information resources on the Web appropriate for Certified Nurse Midwives (CNMs) and clinical nurses caring for childbearing families. A variety of sites have been selected, including clinical information, legislative issues and statistics, professional organizations, and some sites that address the technological aspects of pregnancy care. A plethora of information on pregnancy and pregnancy care for expectant and new parents is available. However, professional information and resources were minimal in comparison.

1. American College of Nurse-Midwives (ACNM)

http://www.acnm.org

The American College of Nurse-Midwives Web page provides information related to midwifery. The ACNM is the governing body for nurse-midwifery in the U.S. and provides a wealth of information on the site. The site includes information on finding a nurse-midwife, professional information, midwifery education, products, events, and services. The professional information section includes information about the credentialing process, certificate maintenance, resources and bibliographic information, policy and political action documents, and information on *The Journal of Midwifery and Women's Health.* One of the highlights of this site is the Department of Global Outreach Information. This department provides information on programs in place to help midwives across the globe, including a Lifesaving Skills Training Program, Community Partnerships for Safe Motherhood, midwifery associations, Family Centered Maternity Care, a meta-analysis on traditional birth attendant care, and distance learning and in-service education. Overall, this is an excellent site. The information is current, it is well-organized, and easy to navigate. Text is clear and concise and is provided at an average level in English.

2. Association for Reproductive Health Professionals (ARHP)

http://www.arhp.org

The Association for Reproductive Health Professionals is an interdisciplinary association of professionals in health care, research, and policy dedicated to promoting reproductive health care through education, research, and advocacy. The association was founded in 1963. The Web site includes news, online CME (continuing medical education), member login, and feedback. The purpose of the Web site is to provide information regarding the organization. Information on advocacy, programs, publications, and resources is included. The advocacy section includes legislative news and the option to sign up for free updates regarding legislation. The programs section provides information on various programs relating to reproductive health and includes past, current, and future events. This is an excellent site that provides a wealth of current and accurate information to the user. The sections are quite detailed and comprehensive. The text is clear and concise and provided at an average level.

3. Association for Women's Health, Obstetrics, and Neonatal Nurses (AWHONN)

http://www.awhonn.org

AWHONN is a nonprofit organization of 22,000 nurses dedicated to the health of women and newborns. The AWHONN homepage features new items of interest with a corresponding posted date, and the following main categories of information: continuing education, annual convention, health policy, AWHONN store, fetal monitoring and others. Also included are a fax-on-demand service, products, position statements, press releases, career opportunities, membership information, and chapters/sections. A staff directory is also provided. A table of contents section is available for *JOGNN: Journal of Obstetric, Gynecologic, and Neonatal Nursing,* the official journal of the organization. Overall, this is an excellent site. The site is well-organized, comprehensive, and easy to navigate.

*4. Helping After Neonatal Death

http://www.h-a-n-d.org

HAND is a California nonprofit 501(c)3 corporation founded in 1981 to help parents, their families, and health care providers cope with the loss of a baby before, during, or after birth. HAND is a resource network of parents, professionals, and supportive volunteers. The site includes separate sections for professionals and consumers. The professionals section includes details about what to do at the hospital and for follow-up, special considerations, and care for the caregiver. There is an excellent section for parents on dealing with family and friends after the loss. The site also includes parent stories and a section on cultural considerations. The entire site can be printed via PDF files. A resources list includes information on local support groups, publications, links, and a book list. The site is presented at a simple level in English.

*5. Lamaze International

http://www.lamaze-childbirth.com

Lamaze international is dedicated to promoting natural childbirth through education, advocacy, and reform. The homepage is divided into several sections that address different audiences who are interested in the Lamaze method of childbirth preparation. There is information

---

*Sites suitable for consumer use.

provided on being a Lamaze-approved provider, a Lamaze-certified childbirth educator locator service for expectant parents, reading materials for both professionals and parents, certification options, and accredited programs. There is also a section on continuing education available through Lamaze International, The Mother-Friendly Childbirth Initiative, *The Journal of Perinatal Education* (selected articles), and information on Lamaze International, including membership. Overall, this is a good site. It is very comprehensive and provides detailed, up to date information presented at a simple to average level. The homepage is, however, a bit cluttered.

*6. March of Dimes

http://www.modimes.org

The March of Dimes is a nonprofit organization devoted to ensuring healthy lives and futures for babies. Their main focus is on the prevention of birth defects through healthy behaviors during pregnancy. They function to support research and education for both the public and health care providers. The homepage for the March of Dimes includes the following main categories of information: health library, research, support, programs, and public affairs. The health library contains information on national perinatal statistics, including live births, incidence of low birth weight, prematurity, and infant mortality. The public policies studies section provides results from March of Dimes-initiated research projects. Birth defects information is also included in the health library. Discussion of the Children's Health Act of 2000, which created the National Center on Birth Defects and Developmental Disabilities, is also included, as this initiative was led by the March of Dimes. A very comprehensive listing of "fact sheets" is also provided; these are ideal for distribution to patients, families, or staff new to the obstetrical and pediatric areas. Opportunities to obtain nursing continuing education requirements are also provided. The public affairs section includes information on issues and priorities, advocacy, policy research RFPs (request for proposals), and links to state and congressional Web sites. Finally, a mechanism is also provided to search for one's local chapter via zip code. This can be particularly useful for nurses who care for pregnant patients or patients who need the support and education provided by the March of Dimes. Overall this is a very good site.

Information is current, accurate, and easy to access. The text is easy to understand.

7. OB Ultrasounds

http://www.ob-ultrasound.net

This is a comprehensive site on ultrasounds, developed by Dr. Joseph Woo. It includes a brief introduction to and background information on ultrasound use and technology, and discusses why and when ultrasound is used in pregnancy. Health care providers are the intended audience. Types of fetal ultrasound measurements are reviewed with real ultrasound pictures showing the measurements. Schedules for ultrasound use during the nine gestational months are provided. Additionally, there are sections addressing the controversies of ultrasound use during pregnancy (i.e., whether it is really necessary), safety of ultrasound during pregnancy, a picture gallery, and a section where fetal heartbeat can be heard. In addition, there is a discussion of the history of ultrasound use in obstetrics and gynecology and a compilation of Web pages that address certain fetal anomalies that are diagnosable via ultrasound. This is an excellent site. The site is very comprehensive and provides a vast amount of knowledge on ultrasound use during pregnancy. The content provided on the site is accurate and up to date. The organization is clear and easy to follow.

*8. ObGyn.net

http://www.obgyn.net

An international resource for obstetrics and gynecology professionals and patients, this site provides current reference information, search tools, forums, practice guidelines, Cochrane reviews, chat rooms, directories, education resources, publications, and clinical reference collections. It is sponsored by MediSpeciality.com, a commercial Web site producer based in Austin, Texas. The obstetrics and gynecology section includes a variety of topics on labor, delivery, and postpartum care. In addition, there are resources directed toward nurse-midwifery practice. This site also features articles on women's health. The center section of the homepage features news events, upcoming conferences and meetings, and new information added to the feature sections. An association spotlight is also provided. Interactive career tools include a Medline knowledge finder, event calendar, career search, glossary of acronyms, search, and health headlines. Interested persons may sign up to receive an e-mail newsletter and Pap smear and mammogram e-mail reminders. An extensive collection of PowerPoint slide presentations is made available on this site. Information is also provided on The Center for the Study of Multiple Birth. More than 50 women's health and general health associations are linked to this site. Blinking ads on this Web site were multiple. The sections are extensive, however, the appearance of the site is a bit cluttered, though this has improved since the original review in the first edition of this text. There is much good information on the site; it just takes some sorting to find it.

*9. Office of Population Affairs

http://www.dhhs.gov/progorg/opa

The OPA is part of the Office of Public Health and Science of the Department of Health and Human Services. It provides information on population, family planning, reproductive health, and adolescent pregnancy. The Web site contains the Offices of Family Planning and Adolescent Pregnancy Programs. The intended audience is both researchers and clinicians and the general public. Included in the site are sections that address grant availability, current legislation, and an information clearinghouse. The Office of Population Affairs administers two grant programs: The Title X Family Planning Program and The Title XX Adolescent Family Life Program. Descriptions of both sections include extensive statistical information regarding their topic areas. The section on grant availability includes information on currently available grants, grants that are in progress, and past awards. The OPA clearinghouse collects, develops, and distributes information on family planning, adolescent pregnancy, abstinence, adoption, reproductive health care, and sexually transmitted diseases. The Office of Population Affairs Web site is very comprehensive and offers valuable information to the user. The site is well organized, up to date, and easy to search. Text is clear and concise.

Chapter 49

Breastfeeding

Kristen S. Montgomery

Breastfeeding is recommended by the American Academy of Pediatrics (AAP). It offers substantial benefits to both the infant and mother, including immunological protection for the infant, particularly for respiratory, gastrointestinal, and ear infection and reduced risk for certain types of reproductive cancers for the mother. This chapter includes Web resources on general breastfeeding information, professional organizations, and information related to lactation consultant certification.

1. Academy of Breastfeeding Medicine (ABM)

http://www.bfmed.org

The Academy of Breastfeeding Medicine is a worldwide organization of physicians dedicated to the promotion, protection, and support of breastfeeding and human lactation. The goals of the organization are physician education, increased knowledge in both breastfeeding science and human lactation, and facilitation of optimal breastfeeding practices. The organization was founded in 1994 and is located in San Diego, California. The organization is international and multi-specialty, with over 500 members in 25 countries. A toll-free contact number is provided. The site is intended for physicians, but is useful to all health care providers. Content is current and accurate. A detailed protocol is available online regarding glucose monitoring and treatment of hypoglycemia in term breastfed neonates. The protocol features a recent "approved date." Information is also provided on the annual meeting (all can attend), newsletter subscription, and a very comprehensive list of links. The site is easy to navigate and is presented in an average level of English.

*2. Australian Department of Health and Ageing: Breastfeeding

http://www.health.gov.au/pubhlth/strateg/brfeed/

This is the breastfeeding section of the Australian Department of Health and Aging. The purpose of the site is to provide breastfeeding information to a wide audience, including both consumers and health care providers. Information provided on the site is current and accurate. The Web site includes the following main sections: family education, national accreditation standards for maternal and infant services, health professional education, antenatal education, and the *National Breastfeeding Strategy Summary Report.* The Web site addresses each of the focus areas identified in the report. Each of these categories has detailed information that can be downloaded via PDF files. Some of the patient education materials in the family education section are available in Arabic, Turkish, Chinese, Spanish, and Vietnamese. These include *Balancing Breastfeeding and Work, 7 Helpful Hints for Learning to Breastfeed, and 7 Helpful Hints for Breastfeeding Problems.* The text is available in a simple to average level. The site is very well organized and easy to use.

*3. Breastfeeding.com

http://www.breastfeeding.com

The Breastfeeding.com Web site is the-everything-you-ever-wanted-to-know-about-breastfeeding-site. The information ranges from news,

---

*Sites suitable for consumer use.

fun, and shopping, to information on the benefits of breastfeeding, what to do prior to delivery and at delivery, and problem solving. It features photographs and video clips for things like positioning techniques, a lactation consultant directory, videotapes, articles, message boards, and mother-to-mother support. A newer feature to the Web site is the availability of leading breastfeeding physician Dr. Ruth Lawrence to answer questions about breastfeeding. Dr. Lawrence is author of *Breastfeeding: A Guide for the Medical Profession*, a comprehensive, well-respected lactation resource. Breastfeeding.com is a private company owned and published by Victor and Joan Babbitt, who are based in Colorado. This is a very comprehensive site that provides good information for both professionals and consumers. While there is some overlap in information that is appropriate for health care providers and consumers, it is often difficult to locate the more professionally oriented information. Additionally, the pages within the site are a bit cluttered.

4. International Board of Lactation Consultant Examiners (IBLCE)

http://www.iblce.org

IBLCE is a nonprofit corporation established in 1985 to develop and administer a voluntary certification program for lactation consultants (LCs) to become International Board Certified Lactation Consultants (IBCLCs). The exam is offered annually and thus far has been written in 8 languages at numerous sites around the globe. The Web site is intended for individuals, who may or may not be health care providers, who are interested in sitting for the IBLCE exam. The information provided on the site is current, accurate, and up to date. Highlights of the site include the benefits of board certification, exam information, the IBLCE Code of Ethics, exam blueprint, an international registry of certified lactation consultants (IBCLCs), contact information, and a suggested reading list to prepare for the exam. The exam is held the last Monday in July each year. Applications are accepted August 1 through May 15. Detailed educational and practical criteria to qualify to sit for the exam are provided on the Web site. The text is only available in English and is presented at a simple level.

5. International Lactation Consultant Association (ILCA)

http://www.ilca.org

The International Lactation Consultant Association (ILCA) promotes the professional development, advancement, and recognition of lactation consultants worldwide for the benefit of breastfeeding women, infants, and children. Information is provided on contacting ILCA, a bulletin board, annual conference, and publications. A link is provided to the *Journal of Human Lactation*, the official journal of the society. Position papers and reports are also available online. Information provided on this site is current, accurate, and available at a simple level in English.

*6.   La Leche League International (LLLI)

http://www.lalecheleague.com

La Leche League International is a breastfeeding information and support network for mothers. There is also information available for health care providers who work with breastfeeding women. Information is available on the organization, becoming a La Leche League leader, and special events and conferences. The information on the site is current and accurate and available in English. A link is provided to other Web sites that feature additional languages including Chinese, Czech, Dutch, Flemish, German, Hebrew, Italian, Japanese, Lithuanian, Portuguese, Slovenian, and Spanish. Some articles are available in Spanish and Italian. Another link is provided to assist with access to printed materials in other languages. One of the best features of this site is the index of local LLLI groups with a listing of over 600 groups. Contact information is provided. The site is easy to use and features a wide range of culturally diverse photos of mothers and infants.

*7.   Medela

http://www.medela.com

Medela, Inc. is a supplier and manufacturer of breast pumps and other breastfeeding supplies. The company was founded in 1979. The company Web site provides information on the company, its products, and establishing corporate lactation programs. The site is geared toward business professionals, consumers, and health care providers who work with breastfeeding women. The section on establishing corporate lactation programs is one of the key features of this site. Information is provided on how supporting breastfeeding can lower absenteeism and decrease employee turnover. There is also information available on how breastfeeding can reduce health care costs, balancing family life, and tips for a successful program. Separate sections are provided for consumers and health care providers. Extensive information is available on the features of different Medela products and searching capabilities area also provided. Information is provided in English at a simple level. The site is easy to use and is not cluttered with excessive advertisements. Information is current and accurate.

*8. ProMOM

http://www.promom.org

This site was developed by Promotion of Mother's Milk, Inc., a nonprofit organization dedicated to increasing public awareness and public acceptance of breastfeeding. The homepage features several main categories of information including breastfeeding information, 101 reasons to breastfeed, discussion forums, 3-minute activist, photo gallery, shopping, and join ProMOM. A site index is also included. The site is geared toward health care providers, consumers, and others interested in breastfeeding. The site is accurate and up to date and very well referenced. The "101 Reasons to Breastfeed" section includes references to support the reasons and in some cases provides a direct link to the information source. The "3-Minute Activist" section includes an updated list of current legislative activities with highlights and successes of previous efforts. Information is presented at an average level in English. The site is easy to navigate.

*9. United States Breastfeeding Committee

http://www.usbreastfeeding.org

This is the public Web site for the U.S. Breastfeeding Committee whose mission is "to improve the nation's health by working collaboratively to protect, promote, and support breastfeeding." This site is geared toward a wide audience that includes health care providers and is sponsored by the U.S. Department of Health and Human Services (DHHS). The site is current and accurate. Some of the highlights of the site are "About USBC," "Events," "Resources," and the new "Strategic Plan." The site is a bit brief at present, but additional information is anticipated as the Committee continues its work. The site is available in English and is presented at an average level. The site is easy to use and free of clutter.

10. World Alliance for Breastfeeding Action (WABA)

http://www.waba.org.br/

WABA is "a global network of organizations and individuals who believe breastfeeding is the right of all children and mothers and who dedicate themselves to protect, promote, and support this right." WABA is geared toward health care providers and works in liaison with UNICEF. The Web site is accurate and current. Features of the site include information on the organization's goals and structure, activities, action sheets, action folders, international seminars, and global participatory action research. The site also features extensive links, including *Nurturing the Future,* a breastfeeding site appropriate for children, and a photo gallery and virtual tour. The Web site is available in Chinese, Dutch, Spanish, French, Italian, Japanese, Portuguese, Swedish, and English. The content is presented at a simple level. The Web site is easy to use and free from distracting information.

_____ Chapter **50**

Complementary and Alternative Therapies

Kristen A. Guadalupe

W eb sites for complementary and alternative therapies are especially difficult to assess. There is a vast multitude of alternative health Web sites, but on closer inspection, many are commercial in focus. Although folk practices have been used throughout time in many different cultures, only recently has the scientific community begun a rigorous scientific evaluation of complementary and alternative medicine (CAM) therapies. In 1998, the National Institutes of Health (NIH), in response to a congressional mandate, established the National Center for Complementary and Alternative Medicine (NCCAM). This center serves as a structure to coordinate CAM research at the NIH and to provide information for professionals and the general public. NCCAM has established 13 research centers to evaluate alternative treatments for diverse health concerns.

*1.   Alternative Health News Online

http://www.altmedicine.com

The Web site cited above presents a number of alternative medicine techniques and approaches that consumers can discuss with their

_____
*Sites suitable for consumer use.

physician or health care provider. The site offers scientifically based interventions, as well as what the site labels as "hogwash interventions" in alternative medicine. The purpose of this site is to report on wellness and approaches to staying healthy and living longer. The site is produced by Frank Grazian, publisher of Alternative Health News Online, Inc. The intended audience of this site are health care consumers, however, nurses may benefit from using this site because some of the information (e.g., research funding opportunities) comes directly from the Office of Alternative and Complementary Medicine at the National Institutes of Health (NIH). The information is updated daily and weekly and is taken from scientific studies at major universities. The best feature of this site is that most of the information provided is scientifically based and referenced. A weak point is a disclaimer of understanding on the homepage that appears to be irrelevant to the site's purpose. The site is only available in English, but there is a section for questions where readers could ask if the information is available in other languages. Overall, I would rate the level of information in this site as average to high depending on which content areas are accessed. Only general information of research studies is presented in the site. The site's overall appearance is organized and easy to follow, with the exception of the disclaimer on the homepage. The site can be recommended to nurses for general information on research funding opportunities and for information on studies of alternative medicine.

*2. Complementary/Alternative Therapies Center

http://www.colaradohealthnet.org/

The Web site cited above provides comprehensive information on holistic therapies, and other health care topics such as chronic illnesses. The purpose of the site is to present information on alternative and complementary therapies to health care consumers and providers. The site is produced by The Colorado Healthsite. The site is beneficial for nurses because it provides definitions and facts about alternative and complementary therapies. In addition, the site offers a section of patient questions with physician answers that may assist nurses in answering questions that patients may have. The information appears current, however, the site does not say how often it is updated. The best feature of this site is a link to NIH and the patient question and answer section.

Another strong point of this site is the section that lists commonly used herbs, their potential side effects, and their intended medicinal purposes. A weak point of this site is the amount of information that is somewhat limited with regard to depth of topics. The information is provided in English and additional languages were not noted. Overall, the level of information is average but easy to read. The site is well-organized; most of the information presented is referenced. The site can be recommended to nurses and to health care consumers because it answers many pertinent questions and presents the basics of alternative and complementary therapies.

3. Dr. Bower's Complementary Medicine Home Page

http://www.peterbower.com

The Web site cited above claims to be the first and longest running Web site on complementary medicine. The purpose of the site is to stimulate curiosity, to engage the intellectual, and to foster a broader understanding of the underpinnings of many complementary medicine traditions and techniques. The site was developed by Peter Bower, M.D. The intended audience of this site is intellectuals interested in complementary medicine who will use the information provided as a basis for serious scientific inquiry. The site is useful for nursing scholars who are skeptical by nature and are interested in learning the foundations of complementary medicine. This site offers many ideas for future research focused in the area of complementary medicine. The most important feature is a list of various complementary medicine techniques, which allows the reader to choose a specific area of interest without wasting time in other areas. For example, nurses researching the effects of tai chi can directly access information that is pertinent to their study. A weak point is that the site is not well-organized and easy for a layperson to use. The information is available in English, Spanish, and Chinese. Overall, the level of information on this site is high because of the format of the site and the depth of information that is provided. The site can be recommended to all nursing scholars interested in exploring the effects of complementary medicine on health. The site is very thought-provoking and informative.

*4. Holistic Healing Web Page

http://www.holisticmed.com

The Web site cited above provides information on alternative and complementary therapies for health care consumers to discuss with their physician or health care providers. The purpose of the site is to present ideas, not advice, which patients can discuss with health care professionals. The site is produced by The Holistic Medicine Resource Center. The intended audience for this site is health care consumers, however, nurses may benefit from this information as it provides general information on alternative and complementary therapies that can be easily accessed. It is difficult to determine how current the information is because it does not state how often the information is updated. However, research studies conducted in 2001 are presented. The most important feature of this site is the link that provides a list of associations and organizations specializing in different aspects of holistic medicine. The list serves as an excellent reference for nurses and patients interested in learning more about this topic. A weak point is the lack of references on the information that is presented. However, the site clearly points out that its purpose is not to provide medical advice to its readers. The information is presented in English with no mention of availability in other languages. Overall, the level of information on this site is average because the terms and definitions are presented in a manner that is easily understood. The site's overall appearance is slightly overwhelming at first glance because of the broad area of topics that are presented on the homepage. However, the site can be recommended because once the reader is able to decipher where his/her topic of interest is, the organizational format of the site is not difficult.

*5. Holistic-Online.com

http://www.holisticonline.com

The Web site cited above offers comprehensive information about health featuring alternative, integrative, and mind-body medicine. The purpose of this site is to offer its readers choices about health, other than those offered by conventional medicine. Holisticonline is sponsored by International Cyber Business Services, Inc. (ICBS). The site's intended audience appears to be the general public, however, nurses may greatly benefit from the information provided. For example, the site describes alternative therapies for various diagnoses, and describes potential drug interactions with common household items such as grapefruits and antihistamines. The information on this site would be very useful for nurses to share with patients and families. The information is current and accurate, revised in December 2001, and offers a section on bioterrorism and anthrax. The best feature of this site is the information on the effects of stress at various stages and interventions to prevent the short- and long-term effects of untreated stress. A weak point is that the information is not referenced. The site does have a section where readers can find health care practitioners in and outside of the United States who specialize in alternative and complementary medicine. The information is presented in English and there is an e-mail address where questions about the site may be asked. Overall, the level of the information presented on this site is average because there is not a lot of medical jargon used. The overall appearance of the site is very organized and easy to use. For example, each section is systematically organized to present the information in sequence. As a result, the reader is able to clearly follow along. The site can be recommended to nurses as a reference and for patient education information.

6.   National Center for Complementary and Alternative Medicine (NCCAM)

http://www.nccam.nih.gov

The Web site cited above explores complementary and alternative healing practices in the context of rigorous science. The purpose of the site is to disseminate information about alternative and complementary therapies to health care professionals, particularly those interested in research. The site is sponsored by the National Institutes of Health (NIH) and is especially useful for nursing scholars interested in studying nonconventional therapies and their effect on health. The most important feature of this site is the scientific foundation from which it is built. A weak point of this site is the lack of general information that is user-friendly to a general audience. Information is presented in English with no mention of information being available in other languages. Overall, the level of information is high, because of the site's research focus. The site is organized and gives educational, research, and employment opportunities for nurses at all levels. The site can be recommended to all nurses because it provides information that is useful to the nursing discipline.

Chapter 51

Disaster Preparedness

Tener Goodwin Veenema

The wealth of Internet resources continues to grow at an astonishing pace. Following the devastating attacks of September 11, 2001 in New York, Washington, and Pennsylvania, the number of sites focused on Disaster Preparedness has grown. Sorting through these Web sites in order to find specific information can be cumbersome and time-intensive. Many Web sites are either difficult to navigate, not designed for use by health providers, or have commercial purposes as their goal, thus providing little value to nurses. Web sites were selected based on their sponsorship by well-known and highly regarded organizations or agencies, depth and scope of the content presented, and relevance to nursing practice.

*1. American Hospital Association Hospital Preparedness For Mass Casualties

http://www/ahapolicyforum.org/policyresources/Modisaster.asp

This Web site contains a 32-page report of the March 2000 proceedings of the invitational forum convened by the American Hospital Association

---

*Sites suitable for consumer use.

with the support of the Office of Emergency Preparedness, U.S. Department of Health and Human Services. Recognizing that most hospital disaster plans do not address disasters and incidents with hundreds or thousands of casualties, the forum addressed the issues of community-wide preparedness, staffing, communications, and public policy. The report provides recommendations for hospitals and communities with regard to each of the four topic areas, to guide them in disaster preparation.

2. Chemical and Biological Terrorism: Research and Development to Improve Civilian Medical Response

http://www.nap.edu/terror

This site connects to the book *Chemical and Biological Terrorism: Research and Development to Improve Civilian Medical Response* (1999), produced by the Institute of Medicine and published by National Academy Press. The book is available full text online and represents one of the best resources available for information on this topic. The book contains the results of 2 years of work by a committee of national experts convened by the Institute of Medicine to analyze national preparedness and present recommendations for improvement in that area. The level of information is very high, with emphasis on clinical detail. An executive summary is included that concisely presents the conclusions and recommendations of the committee. This book is most valuable for nurses involved in strategic emergency response planning in their organization or health department.

3. International Nursing Coalition for Mass Casualty Education

http://www.vanderbilt.edu/nursing

Sponsored by the Vanderbilt School of Nursing, the International Nursing Coalition for Mass Casualty Education was formed in March, 2001 to address the educational needs of nurses across the nation regarding disaster preparedness and bioterrorism. The organizational members of this coalition represent leading schools of nursing, nursing accrediting bodies, governmental nursing/health and military agencies, and professional nursing societies. The coalition is currently identifying educational content for nurses and core competencies in disaster preparedness, and provides access to experts in the field. The Web site is undergoing redesign to enhance public access and serves as a valuable resource for nurses and nursing faculty.

4. Johns Hopkins Center for Civilian Defense

http://www.hopkins-biodefense.org/

Johns Hopkins University's Web site provides news, resources, coordination guidelines, and case studies on biological threats. This is a well-designed and easy to use Web site for anyone seeking information on bioterrorism. The site is sponsored by the Alfred P. Sloan Foundation and the Robert Wood Johnson Foundation. The information is accurate and timely and includes news, events, biological agent background information, and access to library resources and staff at the Center. The site includes the JAMA consensus statements and proceeds of congressional hearings on national preparedness for a bioterrorist attack. This site contains moderate to high level information and is a great resource for nurses.

5. Joint Commission Resources

http://www.jcrinc.com/subscribers/perspectives.asp?durki=187

Joint Commission Resources, Inc. (JCR) is a global, knowledge-based organization that disseminates information regarding accreditation, standards development and compliance, good practices, and health care quality improvement. JCR, a subsidiary of the Joint Commission on Accreditation of Healthcare Organizations, offers a wide variety of resources to organizations including consulting and custom educational programs. Its board of directors includes national and international health systems experts. The Web site includes a link to the current edition of the online journal, *Perspectives,* which is focused entirely on preparation for a national bioterrorism response. While the journal articles are based on using JCAHO standards as a starting point to prepare for an emergency, the site presents several of the most current and user-friendly guidelines for disaster planning and emergency management. Topics addressed include analysis of organizations' vulnerability to hazards, developing practical emergency management education programs, and preparing for a mass casualty event.

6. National Domestic Preparedness Office (NDPO)

http://www.ndpo.gov

The National Domestic Preparedness Office is the clearinghouse for state, local, and federal weapons of mass destruction information and assistance. Its mission is to coordinate all federal efforts, including those of the Department of Defense, Federal Bureau of Investigation, Federal Emergency Management Agency, Department of Health and Human Services, Department of Energy, and the Environmental Protection Agency, to assist state and local emergency responders with planning, training, equipment, and exercise needs necessary to respond to a weapon of mass destruction incident. This Web site is designed primarily for emergency providers and agencies. It includes a vast communication network and information resource standard, the NDPO's Common Communication Link, to assist state and local communities in preparedness. The CCL includes a common e-mail system, computer conferencing, news groups, community planning, and links to other weapons of mass destruction Web sites.

7. National Safety Council (NSC)

http://www.crossroads.nsc.org/cbion.cfm

The National Safety Council's Web site is a safety, health, and environmental search engine and news network created to provide safety, health, and environmental (SHE) managers with information and links to topics related to chemical safety. The "Nerve and Biological Agents" Web page provides news updates with links to many other organizations and agencies dealing with chemical and biological agents. For the most part, the news releases are timely and the site is regularly updated.

8.   U.S. Public Health Service Office of Emergency Preparedness

http://www.ndms.dhhs.gov

This is the official Web site of the U.S. Department of Health and Human Services, Office of Emergency Preparedness (OEP). The site is geared to professionals (disaster responders, public health officials, and some providers) and is updated once a month. OEP works in partnership with the Federal Emergency Management Agency (FEMA) to serve as the lead agency for health and medical services within the Federal Response Plan. The site provides information specific to health, medical and social services, and recovery, to major emergencies and federally declared disasters including natural disasters, technological disasters, major transportation accidents, and terrorism. OEP also directs and manages the National Disaster Medical System (NDMS) and the site includes access to information regarding the system. There is a comprehensive online training program for response team training and a library.

9.   What We Know about Terrorism, Disaster and Health

http://www.stti.iupui.edu/library/ojksn/homepage.html

The *Online Journal of Knowledge Synthesis for Nursing* (OJKSN) is the peer-reviewed online journal of Sigma Theta Tau International, the honor society of nursing. Authors can search, review, and extract the clinical meaning from research articles on a number of topics. The *OJKSN* is expediting publications reflecting what is known about health interventions and disaster response and has compiled a bibliography of references to essential literature on disaster care. This site is particularly valuable because of its ability to offer evidence to guide quality health care and to offer it in a highly accessible, online form, rapid-turnaround fashion. Click on the flag icon on the homepage, and the reader is taken to "What We Know About Terrorism, Disaster and Health," a comprehensive set of bibliographies that reflects resources in disaster care. The bibliographies incorporate a broad array of evidence, classified into categories that reflect the strength of the evidence. The bibliographies provided include Systematic Reviews, Clinical Practice Guidelines, Research and other Resources for General Disasters, Post Disaster Care (both physical and psychological), Post-Traumatic Stress Disorder & Crisis Intervention, Terrorism/Bioterrorism, and Disaster Management.

_____ Chapter **52**

Bioterrorism

Tener Goodwin Veenema

_____

his chapter provides a selection of the most valid and reliable
Web sites addressing topics related to disaster preparedness
and bioterrorism. Web sites were selected based on their sponsorship by well-known and highly regarded organizations or agencies,
depth and scope of the content presented, and relevance to nursing
practice. Web sites chosen are known to be current and updated on
a regular basis; include an easy-to-use site map, and provide the user
with valuable, time-saving links to other resources of interest. Whether
searching for sites for application to clinical practice, research or educational content, these were selected as the best Web sites on bioterrorism available for nurses at this time.

1. American College of Emergency Physicians

http://www.acep.org

Sponsored by the American College of Emergency Physicians, this
easy-to-use Web site is a valuable resource for nurses as well. Go

to the homepage and click on the icon "Bioterrorism Resources for Emergency Physicians" and a site map appears containing current news, policy statements, articles, self-study exercises, and links to other bioterrorism-related Web sites. The site contains valuable clinical guidelines for practitioners regarding distinguishing anthrax from influenza and the treatment of pregnant women with anthrax. The news section includes the current issue of the CDC's *Morbidity and Mortality Weekly Report*. Full-text articles in the journal *Annals of Emergency Medicine* are password-protected and limited to ACEP members, however, abstracts are available. ACEP has granted access to lessons in "Critical Decisions in Emergency Medicine," their online self-study program—"Emergency Department Preparedness in the Event of Bioterrorism," and "Chemical Weapons: History, Identification, and Management."

2. Armed Forces Institute of Pathology

http://anthrax.radpath.orh/index.html

This Armed Forces Institute of Pathology (AFIP) site provides information about the pathogenesis and imaging of inhalational anthrax. The content is the result of collaboration between the AFIP and the American Registry of Pathology and INOVA Fairfax Hospital, Fairfax, Virginia.

3. Centers for Disease Control Bioterrorism Preparedness and Response

http://www.bt.cdc.gov

The CDC serves as the national center for developing and applying disease prevention and control, environmental health, and health promotion and education activities designed to improve the health of the people of the United States. This vast Web site provides information on Diseases, Injuries, Disabilities, Health Risks, Specific Populations, and Prevention Guidelines and Strategies. The site provides disease surveillance and as such, it is the clearinghouse for up to date public health emergency response and preparedness information. The CDC site contains Databases and Health Statistics, publications, software and products, and funding information for health care researchers. The Centers for Disease Control and Prevention has developed a special Web site to deal specifically with bioterrorism threats, and can be reached directly through the following link: *http://www.bt.cdc.gov*. The CDC Web site contains a wealth of information on bioterrorism and is currently the best Web site available to locate timely and accurate information. This site offers information on emergency contacts, maintains an index of restricted agents, and protocols for bioterrorism management. The CDC operates a large number of infectious disease surveillance systems, most, of which are based on voluntary collaboration with state and local health departments. The most well-recognized of these, the National Notifiable Disease Surveillance System, currently includes many, but not all, of the diseases considered likely to be used in warfare.

The Centers for Disease Control and Prevention (CDC) and the National Immunization Program (NIP) have created a homepage specific to anthrax, that can be reached directly with the following link: CDC Anthrax Homepage and NIP Vaccine Recommendations *http://www.cdc.gov/diseases/anthrax/*. This site is valuable as a valid and reliable quick reference on all aspects of the confirmation and management of an anthrax emergency. The site contains an "information for everyone" section, current news releases, specific information for health care providers, data and statistics, and an update on international efforts. Users can conduct a NIP site search on any question related to vaccines and immunization. All of the CDC sponsored Web sites are provided in Spanish as well as English.

The CDC Web site also includes Bioterrorism-Related Inhalational Anthrax: The First 10 Cases Reported in the U.S. at *http://www.cdc.gov/ncidod/eid/vol7no6/jerigan.htm*. The November-December 2001 issue of *Emerging Infectious Diseases* published by CDC presents this research article describing the clinical presentation and course of the first 10 cases of bioterrorism-related inhalational anthrax.

The CDC has released "Interim Smallpox Response Plan and Guidelines," located at *http://www.cdc.gov/nip/diseases/smallpox/*, which outlines CDC's strategies for responding to a smallpox emergency. The plan, which recommends the ring vaccination concept, has been sent to all state bioterrorism coordinators, state health officers, state epidemiologists, and state immunization program managers for review and comment. An executive summary is provided detailing the plan. Nurses should visit this Web site for updates as the smallpox guidelines will soon be revised.

4. National Library of Medicine's MEDLINEplus Biological and Chemical Weapons (Includes AMA consensus statements)

http://www.nlm.gov/medlineplus/biologicalandchemicalweapons.html

One of the best sites on the Web, MEDLINEplus is a goldmine of health information from the world's largest library, the National Library of Medicine. The quality, authority, and accuracy of its contents are of the very highest level. The site is continually maintained and provides unique information regarding biological and chemical weapons with a minimum of redundancy and overlap between resources. MED-LINEplus has developed a very large detailed Web site focusing on a number of topics related to bioterrorism. The site map allows users to jump quickly between traditional and alternative therapies, coping, prevention & screening, research, and information specific to children and teenagers. The Web site is in both English and Spanish. Users can hyperlink to other MEDLINEplus related pages such as anthrax, disasters and emergency preparedness, immunization/vaccination, general infectious disease, smallpox, and poisoning/toxicology and environmental health.

5. Organization for the Prohibition of Chemical Weapons

http://www.opcw.nl/chemhaz/cwagents.htm

Prepared and maintained by the Organization for the Prohibition of Chemical Weapons, this site details the chemistry and pharmacology of chemical weapons and their countermeasures. The Chemical Weapons Convention (CWC) or, as the complete title reads, the "Convention on the Prohibition of the Production, Stockpiling and Use of Chemical Weapons and on their Destruction," was opened for signature in 1993. It is one of the most complex international conventions ever negotiated and presently 174 nations have signed or acceded to it. The full-text of the convention is accessible on the Web site. While intended for the authorities who are implementing the treaty, it is an interesting site with detailed information on chemicals/toxicology and may be of some interest to nurses.

6. U.S. Army Treatment of Biological Warfare Casualties

http://www.vnh.org/FM8284/index.html

This Web site contains the field manual written by the Headquarters Departments of the Army, the Navy and The Air Force and Commandant of the Marine Corps and published in July 2000. While developed for use by the military, this highly detailed and well-organized manual provides a concise resource for all aspects of the management of a biological terrorist event. Chapters address classification and handling of biological agents, therapy, prevention, protective equipment, as well as detailed information on specific bacterial agents, viral agents, toxins, and the medical management and treatment of each.

7. U.S. Army Medical Research Institute of Infectious Diseases. Medical Management of Biological Casualties

http://www.nbc-med.org/SiteContent/Homepage/WhatsNew/
MedManual/Feb01/handbook.htm

This site contains the fourth edition of *Medical Management of Biological Casualties Handbook* published in February 2001 by the U.S. Army Medical Research Institute of Infectious Disease. The handbook details characteristics of biological agents, patient isolation precautions, management and laboratory diagnosis of samples, and some guidelines for differential diagnosis. It provides an appendix containing a comprehensive collection of references (journal articles, books, Web resources) and a list of emergency response contacts, including a telephone directory of each State and Territorial Public Health Director and the field offices of the Federal Bureau of Investigation.

8. World Health Organization: Global Outbreak Alert & Response Network

http://www.who.int/emc/deliberate_epi.html

Internationally, the World Health Organization (WHO) monitors disease outbreaks through The Global Outbreak Alert and Response Network. This Network was formally launched in April 2000 and links together 72 existing networks from around the world, several of which were uniquely designed to diagnose unusual agents and to handle dangerous pathogens. It electronically links the expertise and the skills needed to keep the international community constantly alert to the threat of outbreaks and ready to respond (World Health Organization, *http://www.who.int/emc/deliberate_epi.html*).

The Network has four primary tasks:

1. Systematic disease intelligence and detection. The first responsibility of the WHO is to systematically gather global disease intelligence drawing from a wide net of resources, both formal and informal. Ministries of Health, WHO country offices, government and military centers, and academic institutions all file regular formal reports with the Global Outbreak Alert and Response Network. An informal network scours world communications for rumors of unusual health events.

2. Outbreak verification. Preliminary intelligence reports from all sources, both formal and informal, are then reviewed and converted into meaningful intelligence by the WHO Outbreak Alert and Response Team, which makes the final determination whether a reported event warrants cause for international concern.

3. Immediate alert. A large network of electronically connected WHO member nations, disease experts, health institutions, agencies, and laboratories is kept continually informed of rumored and confirmed outbreaks. The WHO also maintains and regularly updates an Outbreak Verification List, which provides a detailed status report on all currently verified outbreaks.

4. Rapid response. When the Outbreak Alert and Response Team determines that an international response is needed to contain an outbreak, it enlists the help of its partners in the global network. Specific assistance available includes targeted investiga-

tions, confirmation of diagnoses, handling of dangerous biohazards (biosafety level IV pathogens), patient care and management, containment, and logistical support in terms of staff and supplies (World Health Organization, *http://www.who.int/emc/deliberate_epi.html*).

_____ Part **III**

Evaluation Information

Chapter 53

Web Sites with Evaluation Guidelines

Gail L. Ingersoll

S everal online resources are available to assist with the evaluation of Web sites and the information contained within them. The depth of these sources varies widely, however, as does their usefulness to nurses and others interested in the quality of online information. Some of the assessment strategies described on these Web sites are targeted at primary and secondary school educators and students, while others are geared to a more diverse audience. Materials included on the Web sites pertain to the evaluation of Web sites for purposes of data collection or targeted research and to evaluation strategies for measuring the effect of online learning on participant outcome. The sites identified in this review contain content relevant to nurses interested in evaluating Web sites for usefulness in clinical practice, for potential for educating others, and for contribution to the investigation of health-related phenomena.

1. American Medical Association

http://jama.ama-assn.org/issues/v283n12/ffull/jsc00054.html

An excellent resource available through the American Medical Association's (AMA) Web site, or directly through the *Journal of the American*

Medical Association, is a publication of proposed guidelines for medical and health information sites on the Internet (Winker et al., 2000). Although developed primarily for oversight of AMA Web sites, the authors of the report note the relevance of the content to health care providers as a whole and to individuals involved in creating and monitoring Web sites that provide health information to professionals and consumers. Several important dimensions of health-related Web site evaluation are covered in this document. Among the evaluation concerns of particular relevance to health-related sites are the mechanisms used to protect visitor privacy. This aspect of Web site evaluation is not covered in other reviews of evaluation procedures and warrants particular attention for nurses developing and evaluating Web sites for use by consumers and participants in online research protocols. The second important issue highlighted in this review is the need for an ongoing evaluation of Web sites. Because of the constantly evolving nature of Web sites, information validated by a single assessment will not be sufficient for assuring the continued quality of the site.

   Included is a discussion of the need for peer review prior to the Web site's inclusion of health-related content. This aspect of professional responsibility also is not covered in most of the other reviews of Web site evaluation and is particularly important for nurses and other health care professionals. Other assessment areas covered in this document include the credibility of the authors, the attribution of content to sources, the disclosure of funding and competing interests, and the timeliness of information presented. Factors relevant to the inclusion of e-commerce also are described. This Web site is relevant to nurse clinicians, researchers, and others seeking confirmation on the quality and accuracy of information, including online research reports, published articles, and statements of best practice. Although targeted for medical Web sites, the information is relevant to all health-related sources of online information.

2.   Johns Hopkins Center for Communication Programs

http://www.med.jhu.edu/ccp/ppt/casey/eval.htm

The Johns Hopkins Center for Communication Programs' (JHCCP) Web page includes a conceptual model for the evaluation of Web sites and several linkages to papers developed by authors at Cornell University (Becker, 1996; Bowen, 1996; Cirillo, 1996; Fitzelle & Trochim, 1996). The model used at JHCCP incorporates four phases in which Web site evaluation occurs—conceptualization of the Web site content domain, development of the Web site content, implementation of the Web site and outcome evaluation of the Web site, and its effects. A general depiction of the model's application to Web site development is incorporated, although no clear indication of the ways in which the model is used to assess each of the four phases of Web site development is included.

The links contained in this Web site connect to articles describing methods for gathering data about a Web site (Becker, 1996), issues associated with experimental and quasi-experimental Web site evaluation designs (Bowen, 1996), strategies for measuring Web site access (Cirillo, 1996) and the impact of Web site instruction on learning outcomes (Fitzelle & Trochim, 1996). The second and third papers cited are most useful for nurse researchers interested in developing methods for collecting data related to Web site usage and user self-reports (of any type of information). The first and fourth describe the findings of an investigation of undergraduate students' learning outcomes using Web-based instructional interventions.

The Becker (1996) and Cirillo (1996) articles provide useful information for nurse researchers with limited experience in the development of Web site data collection strategies. Each paper contains introductory information about the mechanics of the electronic data collection process and examples to clarify their content. In addition, the Becker discussion includes a step-by-step process for developing a data collection instrument and for testing it prior to its widespread use. Access to these articles, in combination with the conceptual model identified on the primary Web site, makes this Web site a beneficial one for nurses newly involved in collecting data through the use of the Web.

3. Oregon Public Education Network (OPEN)

http://www.open.k12.or.us/jitt/charact.html
http://www.open.k12.or.us/jitt/evalform.html

This Web site, developed by the Oregon Public Education Network, contains a useful Web site evaluation checklist and helpful criteria for determining an acceptability rating for Web sites. The overall rating is computed by summing the individual ratings of each of 10 desired characteristics. These characteristics pertain to the Web site's format, content, and potential for learning. Format characteristics relate to user-friendliness, courtesy, and aesthetics. Content characteristics address credibility, usefulness, richness of information, and interdisciplinary nature of material. Learner aspects cover higher-order thinking, engagement of learner process, and use of multiple learning strategies.

Included with the evaluation checklist are assessment criteria to guide the assignment of desired characteristic rating. These assessment criteria are easy to interpret and representative of the items commonly considered as important to Web site evaluation. A link is provided at the end of each list of attributes to bring the reader back to the evaluation checklist for purposes of assigning a rating score. The checklist and supporting documents are covered by copyright and use of the format and materials require copyright release from the owner. The information contained in the checklist and supporting assessment criteria provide a useful framework for individuals interested in developing a reasonably rapid, comprehensive evaluation tool for Web site review.

Although designed for educators of elementary and secondary schools, the content contained within the Web site is relevant to nurses and others interested in developing and evaluating Web sites as learning instruments. The limitation evident with this assessment tool is its absence of any reliability and validity information. Consequently, nurses wishing to use the evaluation elements should plan for and complete reliability and validity assessments, including a consideration of the tool's utility for assessing health-related sites.

4. VirtualSalt

http://www.virtualsalt.com/evalu8it.htm

The VirtualSalt Web site contains a step-by-step process for evaluating Internet research sources. Although targeted for researchers wishing to evaluate scientific information contained on the Web, the document is valuable to anyone undertaking a comprehensive review of Web site material. The author of this Web-based document (Harris, 1997) begins his discussion with a statement of the need to define what is being sought in the review prior to evaluating any specific Web site. He notes the importance of determining whether the review will serve to provide new ideas or information, offer factual or reasoned support for a position, clarify general understanding about a phenomenon, or disprove an idea. This process facilitates the screening of potential sources, thereby increasing the efficiency of the Web-based search. Included in this pre-assessment step is the deliberation over which sources are most credible for the information desired and which are likely to be fair, objective, and designed in keeping with the expectations for quality control. Once this pre-assessment work is done, the author recommends using the CARS (credibility, accuracy, reasonableness, support) checklist for evaluating information quality. These criteria are consistent with several other recommended strategies for Web site review.

5. World Wide Web Virtual Library

http://www.vuw.ac.nz/~agsmith/evaln/evaln.htm

This site is designed for librarians and individuals interested in assessing the quality of Internet information. It is an excellent first-stop resource for nurses seeking information about how to evaluate Web sites. The Web site is housed in the Information Quality section of the World-Wide Virtual Library and contains multiple linkages to other on-line and print sources, many of which provide connections to other sources as well. Each of the listings is linked to the original source and is grouped according to category—general selection criteria, selection criteria for specific sources, and commentary. The site also contains a notation of the date on which the information was modified, assuring the reader of the timeliness of listings.

Included with each listing is a brief (one sentence) description of the content. The listings include a broad range of topics, with an equally broad range of content depth. As a result, the reviewer needs to critically examine each source for its relevance. Although some indication of the listing's usefulness is included, the reviews are much too brief to allow for sole reliance on their assessment. Among the listings included is a link to a policy paper and information quality tool developed by the Health Summit Working Group, convened by the Health Information Technology Institute of Mitretek Systems and supported by the Agency for Healthcare Research and Quality (Mitretek Systems, 1999). The criteria for evaluating Internet health information are similar to those identified at other sites, although the availability of an instrument, with a clear rationale for each criterion, is a useful addition. Caution should be used with the adoption of this instrument, however, as no reliability or validity information is provided. Moreover, the weighting system is not clearly defined. This Web site identifies many more relevant listings than appear with general search engine outputs. As a result, it is a highly useful resource for nurses beginning a review of Web site evaluation discussions and those seeking updates as new information is published.

REFERENCES

Becker, R. M. (1996). *Gathering evaluation data on a website using the Web.* Available at *http://trochim.human.cornell.edu/webeval/webforms/webforms.htm.* Accessed 12/28/01.

Bowen, D. A. (1996). *Website evaluation: experimental and quasi-experimental design issues.* Available at *http://trochim.human.cornell.edu/webeval/webexper/webexpr.htm.* Accessed 12/24/01.

Cirillio, D. (1996). *Evaluating Web site access.* Available at *http://trochim.human.cornell.edu/webeval/weblog/weblog.htm.* Accessed 12/28/01.

Fitzelle, G. T., & Trochim, W. M. K. (1996). *Survey evaluation of Web site instructional technology: Does it increase student learning?* Available at *http://trochim.human.cornell.edu/webeval/webques.htm.* Accessed 12/28/01.

Harris, R. (1997). *Evaluating Internet research resources.* Available at *http://www.virtualsalt.com/evalu8it.htm.* Accessed 12/24/01.

Mitretek Systems. (1999). *Criteria for assessing the quality of health information on the Internet—Policy paper.* Available at *http://hitiweb.mitretek.org/hswg/.* Accessed 12/28/01.

Winker, M. A., Flanagin, A., Chi-Lum, B., White, J., Andrews, K., Kennett, R. L., DeAngelis, C. D., & Musacchio, R. A. (2000). Guidelines for medical and health information sites on the Internet. Principles governing ANA Web sites. *Journal of the American Medical Association, 283,* 1600–1606.

Alphabetical Index of Web Sites

Site Name	Section	Language	Appropriate for Consumers
About.com Heart Disease/Cardiology *http://www.heart disease.about.com*	Heart Disease	English	•
Academy of Breastfeeding Medicine (ABM) *http://www.bfmed.org*	Breastfeeding	English	
Acid-Base Tutorial *http://www.acid-base.com/*	Critical Care	English	
Advanced Physical Assessment: Breast *http:// nsweb.nursingspectrum.com/ ce/ce85.htm*	Physical Assessment	English	

Site Name	Section	Language	Appropriate for Consumers
Agency for Healthcare Research and Quality (AHRQ) *http://www.ahrq.gov/ clinic/epcix.htm*	Administration, Clinical Decision Making, Economics, Evidence-Based Practice, General Health Care, Government, Outcomes, Primary Care	English, Some Spanish	•
AIDS Clinical Trials Information Service *http://www.actis.org*	HIV/AIDS	English, Patient Education Materials are Available in English and Spanish	•
All Nurses: International *http://allnurses.com/ Boards_of_Nursing/ International*	International	English	
Alternative Health News Online *http:// www.altmedicine.com*	Complementary and Alternative Medicine	English	•
Alternative Link *http://www. alternativelink.com*	Nursing Classification Systems	English	
Alzheimer's Association *http://www.alz.org*	Mental Health	English, Some Spanish	•
American Academy of Allergy, Asthma, and Immunology (AAAAI) *http://www.aaaai.org*	Respiratory	English	•
American Academy of Hospice and Palliative Medicine (AAHPM) *http://www.aahpm.org*	Palliative Care	English	

Site Name	Section	Language	Appropriate for Consumers
American Academy of Nurse Practitioners *http://www.aanp.org*	Jobs, Professional Organizations	English	
American Academy of Pain Management *http://www.aapain manage.org/*	Pain	English	•
American Academy of Pediatrics (AAP) *http://www.aap.org*	Community Health; Infants, Children, and Adolescents	English	•
American Academy of Sleep Medicine *http://www.asda.org*	Respiratory	English	
American Association of Colleges of Nursing *http:// www.aacn.nche.edu*	Education	English	
American Association of Critical Care Nurses (AACN) *http://www.aacn.org*	Critical Care, Emergency, Professional Organizations	English	
American Association of Managed Care Nurses (AAMCN) *http://www.aamcn.org*	Managed Care	English	
American Association for Respiratory Care *http://www.aarc.org*	Respiratory	English	
American Cancer Society *http://www.cancer.org*	Cancer	English, Spanish	•
American Case Management Association (ACMA) *http:// www.acmaweb.org*	Case Management	English	

Site Name	Section	Language	Appropriate for Consumers
American College of Chest Physicians (ACCP) *http://www.chestnet.org*	Respiratory	English	
American College of Emergency Physicians *http://www.acep.org*	Bioterrorism	English	
American College of Nurse-Midwives (ACNM) *http://www.acnm.org*	Maternity	English	
American Diabetes Association (ADA) *http://www.diabetes.org*	Diabetes	English, Spanish	•
American Dietetic Association *http://www.eatright.org*	Nutrition	English, Some Spanish	•
American Heart Association *http:// www.americanheart.org http://www.stroke association.org*	Heart Disease	English	
American Hospital Association (AHA) *http://www. ahacentraloffice.org/*	Economics	English	
American Hospital Association Hospital Preparedness for Mass Casualties *http://www. ahapolicyforum.org/ policyresources/ Modisaster.asp*	Disaster Preparedness	English	•

Site Name	Section	Language	Appropriate for Consumers
American International Health Alliance *http://www.aiha.com/ english/programs/phc/ index.cfm#overview*	Primary Care	English and Russian Translations of the Multilingual Library	
American Lung Association *http://www.lungusa.org*	Respiratory	English	
American Medical Association *http://jama.ama-assn.org/issues/ v283n12/ffull/ jsc00054.html*	Evaluation	English	
American Medical Informatics Association (AMIA) *http://www.amia.org/*	Nursing Informatics	English	
American Medical Women's Association *http:// www.amwa.doc.org*	Women's Health	English	
American Nephrology Nurses Association (ANNA) *http:// www.annanurse.org*	Professional Organizations	English	
American Nurses Association (ANA) *http://www.ana.org*	Careers, Education, Health Policy, Jobs, Professional Organizations	English	
American Nurses Association *http:// www.nursingworld.org*	Education	English with French and Spanish Web sites available	

Site Name	Section	Language	Appropriate for Consumers
American Nurses Foundation (ANF) *http://www.ana.org/anf/inc/index.htm*	International, Research and Grants	English	
American Nursing Informatics Association (ANIA) *http://www.ania.org*	Nursing Informatics	English	
American Organization of Nurse Executives (AONE) *http://www.aone.org*	Administration	English	
American Psychiatric Nurses Association *http://www.apna.org*	Mental Health	English	
American Public Health Association (APHA) *http://www.apha.org*	Community Health	English	
American Society of Clinical Oncology *http://www.asco.org*	Cancer	English	●
American Thoracic Society *http://www.thoracic.org*	Respiratory	English	
American Trauma Society *http://www.amtrauma.org*	Emergency	English	
American Venous Forum *http://www.avf.org*	Vascular Disease	English	●
Americans for Better Care of the Dying (ABCD) *http://www.abcd-caring.org*	Palliative Care	English	●

Site Name	Section	Language	Appropriate for Consumers
Anthony and Associates *http://anthony.case management.com*	Case Management	English	
Anthony J. Jannetti, Inc. *http://www.ajj.com*	Publishing Companies	English	
Approaching Death: Improving Care at the End of Life *http://www.nap.edu/ readingrooms/books/ approaching*	Palliative Care	English	•
Arbor Nutrition Guide *http:// www.arborcom.com*	Nutrition	English, French, German, Portuguese, and Spanish and French Links	•
Armed Forces Institute of Pathology *http:// anthrax.radpath.orh/ index.html*	Dister Preparedness	English	
Army Leadership Development *http://www.army.mil*	Leadership	English	
Aspen Publishers, Inc. *http://www.aspen publishers.com*	Heart Disease	English	
Assessment of Abnormal Growth Curves *http://www.aafp.org/afp/ 980700ap/legler.html*	Physical Assessment	English	

Site Name	Section	Language	Appropriate for Consumers
Assessment Tips and Techniques *http:// www.nursing.about. com/cs/assessment skills/index.htm*	Physical Assessment	English	
Association of Fundraising Professionals *http://www.afpnet.org*	Fundraising	English	
Association of Healthcare Philanthropy (AHP) *http://www.go-ahp.org*	Fundraising	English	
Association of Nurses in AIDS Care *http://www.anacnet.org/*	HIV/AIDS	English	
Association of PeriOperative Registered Nurses (AORN) *http://www.aorn.org*	Professional Organizations	English	
Association for Reproductive Health Professionals (ARHP) *http://www.arhp.org*	Maternity	English	
Association of Women's Health, Obstetrics, and Neonatal Nurses (AWHONN) *http://www.awhonn.org*	Maternity	English	
Asthma Information Center *http://cooke.gsf.de/ asthmainfocenter*	Respiratory	English	

Site Name	Section	Language	Appropriate for Consumers
The Auscultation Assistant *http://www.wilkes. med.ucla.edu/ index.htm*	Physical Assessment	English	
Australian Department of Health and Ageing: Breastfeeding *http:// www.health.gov.au/ pubhlth/strateg/brfeed/*	Breastfeeding	English Some Patient Education Materials are Available in Arabic, Chinese, Spanish, Turkish, and Vietnamese	
Australian Electronic Journal of Nursing Education *http://www.scu.edu.au/ schools/nhcp/aejne/*	Online Journals	English	
Bandido Books *http://www. bandidobooks.com*	Education	English	
Bandolier *http://www.jr2.ox.ac.uk/ bandolier/index.html*	Evidence-Based Practice	English, Spanish	
Bioterrorism-Related Inhalational Anthrax: The First 10 Cases Reported in the U.S. *http://www.cdc.gov/ ncidod/eid/vol7no6/ jerigan.htm*	Disaster Preparedness	English	
Bioterrorism Overview *http://www.omaha medical.com/ biobittner.asp*	Disaster Preparedness	English	

Site Name	Section	Language	Appropriate for Consumers
Bioterrorism Resources for Emergency Physicians *http://acep.org*	Disaster Preparedness	English	
Blackboard *http:// www.blackboard.com*	Education	English, Some Other Languages Available for Discussion Groups	
Breastfeeding.com *http://www. breastfeeding.com*	Breastfeeding	English	•
Bright Futures *http:// www.brightfutures.org*	Infants, Children, and Adolescents	English, Spanish	•
Bureau of Labor Statistics (BLS) *http://www.bls.gov/*	Economics	English	
Canadian-International Nurse Researcher Database *http://www.nurse researcher.com*	Research and Grants	English, French	
Cancer Care, Inc. *http:// www.cancercare.org*	Cancer	English, Some Spanish	•
Cancernet *http://www.cancernet. nci.nih.gov*	Cancer	English, Spanish	•
Cardiac Trace Tutorials *http://www.healthsci. utas.edu.au/physiol/ tute1/Intro.html*	Critical Care	English	
Cardiovascular Exam *http:// www.medinfo.ufl.edu/ year1/bcs/clist/ index.html*	Physical Assessment	English	

Site Name	Section	Language	Appropriate for Consumers
Case Management Resource Guide *http://www.cmrg.com/*	Case Management	English	
Case Management Society of America (CMSA) *http://www.cmsa.org/*	Case Management	English	
Center for AIDS Prevention Studies at the University of California San Francisco *http:// www.caps.ucsf.edu/*	HIV/AIDS	Fact Sheets are Available in English, Kiswahili, and Spanish	•
Center for Case Management (CCM) *http://www.cfcm.com/*	Case Management	English, Some Japanese	
Center for Clinical Informatics *http://www.clinical-informatics.com/jlarc*	Outcomes	English	
Center for Creative Leadership, *http:// www.ccl.org/capabilities*	Leadership	English	
Center for Leadership and Change Management *http://leadership. wharton.upenn.edu*	Leadership	English	
Centers for Disease Control Adolescent and School Health *http://www.cdc.gov/ nccdphp/dash*	Infants, Children, and Adolescents	English	

Site Name	Section	Language	Appropriate for Consumers
Centers for Disease Control Bioterrorism Preparedness and Response *http://www.bt.cdc.gov*	Disaster Preparedness	English	
Centers for Medicare and Medicaid Services *http://www.cms.hhs.gov*	Government, Managed Care, Outcomes	English	•
Center for Nursing Classification *http://www.nursing. uiowa.edu/cnc*	Nursing Classification Systems	English	
Center Watch *http:// www.centerwatch.com*	Pharmaceuticals	English	
Centers for Disease Control and Prevention (CDC) *http://www.cdc.gov*	Community Health, Consumer Health, Disaster Preparedness, General Health Care	Some Spanish	•
Centers for Disease Control Anthrax Homepage and National Immunization Program Vaccine Recommendations *http://www.cdc.gov/ diseases/anthrax/*	Disaster Preparedness	English, Spanish	
Centers for Disease Control Bioterrorism Preparedness and Response *http://www.bt.cdc.gov*	Disaster Preparedness	English	
Centers for Disease Control Divisions of HIV/AIDS Prevention *http://www.cdc.gov/ nchstp/hiv_aids/ dhap.htm*	HIV/AIDS	English	

Site Name	Section	Language	Appropriate for Consumers
Centers for Disease Control Interim Smallpox Response Plan and Guidelines *http://www.cdc.gov/nip/ diseases/smallpox*	Disaster Preparedness	English	
Centers for Medicare and Medicaid Services (CMS) *http://cms.hhs.gov/*	Economics	English	
CenterWatch *http:// www.centerwatch.com*	Clinical Decision-Making	English	•
Centre for Evidence-Based Medicine *http://cebm.jr2.ox.ac.uk*	Clinical Decision-Making	English	
Chemical and Biological Terrorism: Research and Development to Improve Civilian Medical Response *http://www.nap.edu/ terror*	Disaster Preparedness	English	
Chemical/Biological Agents Treatment Chart *http://www.hcms.org/ biochem1005.doc*	Disaster Preparedness	English	
Children with diabetes *http://www.children withdiabetes.com*	Diabetes	English, Some Spanish Emailing Buddies Are Available	•

Site Name	Section	Language	Appropriate for Consumers
Children's Intensive Caring *http://www.intensive caring.com*	Infants, Children, and Adolescents	English	•
Children's Safety Network National Injury and Violence Prevention Resource Center *http://www.edc.org/ HHD/csn*	Emergency	English	
The Chronicle of Higher Education Career Network *http:// www.chronicle.com*	Careers, Jobs	English	
Chronicle of Philanthropy *http:// www.philanthropy.com*	Fundraising	English	
City of Hope Pain and Palliative Care Resource Center for Nursing Research and Education *http:// www.cityofhope.org/ mayday*	Cancer	English	
Cochrane Clinical Reviews *http:// www.cochrane.org/ cochrane/revabstr/ mainindex.htm*	Clinical Decision-Making	English	

Site Name	Section	Language	Appropriate for Consumers
Cochrane Collaboration http:// www.cochrane.org	APN, Evidence-Based Practice; Clinical Decision-Making, Outcomes	Abstracts are available in Italian Centers in Various Countries have Web sites in the Native Language including: Spain, Germany, France, Netherlands, Brazil, Italy, China, and South Africa	
Cochrane Collaboration Abstracts http://www.update-software.com/ccweb/ cochrane/revabstr/ mainindex.htm	APN	English Italian	
The Comfort Line http://www.uakron.edu/ comfort	Nursing Theory	English	
Complementary/ Alternative Therapies Center http://www.colorado healthnet.org	Complimentary and Alternative Health	English	•
Computers in Nursing http:// www.nursingcenter.com/ journals	Nursing Informatics	English	

Site Name	Section	Language	Appropriate for Consumers
Congenital Heart Information Network *http://www.tchin.org*	Heart Disease	English	•
The Cost Utility Analysis (CUA) Data Base *http:// www.hsph.harvard.edu/ organizations/hcra/ cuadatabase.intro.html*	Economics	English	
Council for Aid to Education (CAE) *http://www.cae.org*	Fundraising	English	
Council for the Advancement and Support of Education (CASE) *http://www.case.org*	Fundraising	English	
The Council on Foundations *http://www.cof.org*	Fundraising	English	
Council on Graduate Education for Administration in Nursing (CGEAN) *http://www.unc.edu/ ~sengleba/CGEAN/*	Administration	English	
The Cross Cultural Health Care Program *http://www.Xculture.org*	Culturally Competent Care	English	•
Delmar Nursing *http://www.delmar nursing.com*	Publishing Companies	English	
Dick Chapman's Pain Research Home Page *http:// painresearch.utah.edu/ crchome/*	Pain	English	

Site Name	Section	Language	Appropriate for Consumers
Diversity Rx *http:// www.DiversityRx.org*	Culturally Competent Care	English	•
Division of Nursing, Health Resources and Services Administration (HRSA) *http:// www.bhpr.hrsa.gov/dn*	Outcomes	English	
Dr. Bower's Complementary Medicine Home Page *http:// www.peterbower.com*	Complimentary and Alternative Medicine	Chinese, English, and Spanish	
Duke Health Policy CyberExchange *http:// www.hpolicy.duke.edu/ cyberexchange/*	Health Policy	English	
EBN On-line *http:// ebn.bmjjournals.com/*	Evidence-Based Practice	English	
The ECG Library *http:// www.ecglibrary.com/ ecghome.html*	Critical Care	English	
Education World *http://www.education- world.com*	Education	English	
Electronic Policy Network (EPN) *http://www.epn.org/*	Health Policy	English	
11 Rules of Writing *http://www.junket studies.com/rulesofw/*	Writing	English	
Emergency Medical Services for Children *http://www.ems-c.org*	Emergency	English	

Site Name	Section	Language	Appropriate for Consumers
The Emergency Medicine and Primary Care Home Page *http://www.embbs.com/*	Primary Care	English	
Emergency Nurses Association *http://www.ena.org*	Emergency	English	
Emergency Nursing (UK) *http://www.emergency-nurse.com/resource/turtorials.htm*	Emergency	English	
End of Life Nursing Education Consortium (ELNEC) *http:// www.aacn.nche.edu/ ELNEC*	Palliative Care	English	
Erickson and Associates, Inc. *http:// www.nursesearch.com*	Careers	English	
EthnoMed *http:// www.ethnomed.org*	Culturally Competent Care	English, Patient Information Available in a Variety of Languages, Some Videos in Chinese	
Federal Drug Administration (FDA) *http://www.fda.gov*	Government	English	•
Federal Reserve Bank of St. Louis *http://www.stls.frb.org/ index.html*	Economics	English	

Site Name	Section	Language	Appropriate for Consumers
Financial Aid http://www.finaid.org	Returning to School	English	
Food and Agriculture Organization of the United Nations http://www.fao.org	Nutrition	Arabic, Chinese, French, and Spanish	
Food and Nutrition Information Center http:// www.nal.usda.gov/fnic/	Nutrition	English	•
Food Safety and Nutrition Info: International Food Information Council http:// www.ificinfo.health.org/	Nutrition	English	
Food Service and Nutrition Journals http:// www.sciencekomm.at/ journals/food.html	Nutrition	English	
The Foundation Center http:// www.fdncenter.org	Fundraising	English	
GeneTests- GeneClinics http:// www.geneclinics.org	Genetics	English	
Genetic Alliance http://www.genetic alliance.org	Genetics	English with Links to Other Languages	•

Site Name	Section	Language	Appropriate for Consumers
Genetic Science Learning Center *http:// gslc.genetics.utah.edu*	Genetics	English	•
Genetics Education Center *http://www.kumc.edu/ gec*	Genetics	English	
Genetics Education Partnership *http://genetics- education-partnership. mbt.Washington.edu*	Genetics	English	
Geriatric Assessment *http://www.vhct.org/ case1199/index.shtml*	Physical Assessment	English	
Geriatric Care Managers (GCM) *http:// www.caremanager.org/*	Case Management	English	•
Global Health Council *http:// www.globalhealth.org*	International	English	
Global Initiative for Chronic Obstructive Lung Disease *http:// www.goldcopd.com*	Respiratory	English	
Gloria's Critical Care and Nursing Pages *http://w3.one.net/ ~gloriamc/index.html*	Critical Care	English	
Go60.com *http://www.go60.com*	Older Adults	English	•
Graduate Research in Nursing and Research for Nursing Practice *http://www.graduate research.com/ index.shtml*	Online Journals	English	

Site Name	Section	Language	Appropriate for Consumers
Graduate Schools http:// www.gradschools.com	Returning to School	English	
GRE Web Site http://www.gre.org	Returning to School	English	•
Growth House http:// www.growthhouse.org	Palliative Care	English	•
Harborview Injury Prevention and Research Center http:// depts.washington.edu/ hiprc/	Emergency	English	
Harcourt Health Sciences http://www.harcourt health.com/	Publishing Companies	English	
HCPro http://www.hcpro.com	Administration	English	
Health and Age http://www.health andage.com/	Older Adults	English	•
Health Information Management Systems Society (HIMSS) http://www.himss.org	Nursing Informatics	English	
Health Level 7 (HL7) http:// www.students.tut.fi/ ~viigipuu/HL7/ about.html	Nursing Classification Systems	English, Finnish	
Health on the Net Foundation http://www.hon.ch/ Global/HON	Administration	English	

Site Name	Section	Language	Appropriate for Consumers
Health Resources and Services Administration (HRSA) *http://www.hrsa.gov/*	Infants, Children, and Adolescents; Health Policy	English	•
Health Resources and Services Administration (HRSA) Focus on Child Health *http:// www.hrsa.dhhs.gov/ childhealth*	Infants, Children and Adolescents	English	•
Healthcare Financial Management Association *http://www.hfma.org/ index.html*	Economics	English	
Healthcare Informatics *http://www.healthcare-informatics.com/*	Nursing Informatics	English	
Healthfinder® *http:// www.healthfinder.gov*	Consumer Health	English, Some Spanish	•
HealthWeb *http:// www.healthweb.org*	Consumer Health	English	•
Heart Failure Society of America *http://www.hfsa.org http://www.aboutf.org*	Heart Disease	English	
The Heart.org-Cardiology Online *http://www.theheart.org*	Heart Disease	English	
Helping After Neonatal Death *http://www.h-a-n-d.org*	Maternity	English	•
The HIV Daily Briefing *http://www.aegis.com/*	HIV/AIDS	English	•

Site Name	Section	Language	Appropriate for Consumers
The HIV Drug Interactions Web Site *http://www.hiv-druginteractions.org/index.htm*	HIV/AIDS	English	•
HIV InSite *http:// www.hivinsite.ucsf.edu/ InSite*	Consumer, HIV/AIDS	English, Patient Fact Sheets are Available in English, French, and Spanish	•
Holistic Healing Web Page *http:// www.holisticmed.com*	Complementary and Alternative Medicine	English	•
Holistic-Online.com *http:// www.holisticonline.com*	Complementary and Alternative Therapies	English	•
Home Health Care Classification System (HHCC) *http:// www.sabacare.com*	Nursing Classification Systems	Dutch, English, German, Portuguese, and Spanish	
Hospice and Palliative Care Nurses Association (HPNA) *http://www.hpna.org*	Palliative Care	English	
Hot Nurse Jobs *http:// www.hotnursejobs.com*	Jobs	English	
HSLS Health Resources *http://www.hsls.pitt.edu/ intre/health/pharm.html*	Pharmaceuticals	English	•

Site Name	Section	Language	Appropriate for Consumers
Human Genome Program, Department of Energy *http://www.ornl.gov/ hgmis*	Genetics	English with a Guide to Web Sites in Spanish	
Identifying Structural Hip and Knee Problems *http:// www.postgradmed.com/ issues/1999/12_99/ skinner.htm http:// www.postgradmed.com/ pearls.htm*	Physical Assessment	English	
Indiana University-Purdue University Indianapolis (IUPUI) Center on Philanthropy *http:// www.philanthropy. iupui.edu*	Fundraising	English	
Indispensable Writing Resources *http:// www.quintcareers.com/ writing*	Writing	English	
InfoMIN: Medical Information Network for Chronic Pain, CFS, FMS, and Other Medical Resources *http://www2.rpa.net/ ~lrandall/index.html*	Pain	English	•
Institute for Child Health Policy *http://www.ichp.edu*	Infants, Children, and Adolescents	English	
Institute for Nursing Healthcare Leadership *http://www.care group.org/inhl*	Leadership	English	

Site Name	Section	Language	Appropriate for Consumers
Institute for Nursing Leadership (INL) *http:// www.nursingworld.org/ tan/98julaaug/ enhance.htm*	Leadership	English	
International Association of Physicians in AIDS Care *http://www.iapac.org/*	HIV/AIDS	English	
International Board of Lactation Consultant Examiners (IBLCE) *http://www.iblce.org*	Breastfeeding	English	
International Classification of Nursing Practice (ICNP) *http://www.icn.ch/ icnp.htm*	Nursing Classification Systems	English, French, and Spanish	
International Council of Nurses (ICN) *http://www.icn.ch/*	Health Policy	English, Links to Spanish and French Translations	
International Diabetes Federation (IDF) *http://www.idf.org*	Diabetes	English, French, Spanish	
International Lactation Consultant Association (ILCA) *http://www.ilca.org*	Breastfeeding	English	
International Network for Doctoral Education in Nursing (INDEN) *http://www.umich.edu/ ~inden/*	International	English	

Site Name	Section	Language	Appropriate for Consumers
International Nursing Center, American Nurses Foundation (ANF) *http://www.ana.org/anf/inc/index.htm*	International	English	
International Nursing Coalition for Mass Casualty Education *http://www.vanderbilt.edu/nursing*	Disaster Preparedness	English	
International Society for Quality in Health Care (ISQHC) *http://www.isqua.org.au*	International	English	
The Internet Journal of Advanced Nursing Practice *http://www.ispub.com/journals/ijanp.htm*	Online Journals	English	
Internet Mental Health *http://www.mentalhealth.com*	Mental Health	English, French, German, Italian, Portuguese, and Spanish	•
Internet Resources for Nurse Practitioner Students *http://nurseweb.ucsf.edu/www.arwwebpg.htm*	APN, Education	English	
Institute for Child Health Policy *http://www.ichp.edu*	Infants, Children, and Adolescents		•
Jacobs Institute of Women's Health *http://www.jiwh.org*	Women's Health	English	

Site Name	Section	Language	Appropriate for Consumers
The Joanna Briggs Institute *http://www.joanna briggs.edu.au/*	Evidence-Based Practice	English	
Johns Hopkins AIDS Service *http://www.hopkins-aids.edu/*	HIV/AIDS	English	
Johns Hopkins Center for Civilian Defense *http://www.hopkins-biodefense.org/*	Disaster Preparedness	English	
Johns Hopkins Center for Communication Programs *http:// www.med.jhu.edu/ccp/ ppt/casey/eval.htm*	Evaluation	English	
Johns Hopkins Heart Health *http:// www.jhbmc.jhu.edu/ cardiology/rehab http:// www.jhbmc.jhu.edu/ cardiology/rehab/ proinfo.html*	Heart Disease	English	•
Johnson & Johnson's Discover Nursing *http://www.discover nursing.com*	Careers	English	•
Joint Commission on Accreditation of Healthcare Organizations (JACHO) *http://www.jcaho.org*	Administration	English	

Site Name	Section	Language	Appropriate for Consumers
Joint Commission Resources *http://www.jcrinc.com/ subscribers/ perspectives. asp?durki=187*	Disaster Preparedness	English	
Journal of the American Medical Association Women's Health Information Center *http://www.ama-assn.org/special/womh/ womh.htm*	Women's Health	English	
Journal of Undergraduate Nursing Scholarship http://juns.nursing. arizona.edu/Default.htm	Online Journals	English	
Juvenile Diabetes Research Foundation International *http://www.jdf.org*	Diabetes	English, Links Available to Sites in Australia, Canada, Chile, Greece, India, Israel, Italy, Puerto Rico, and the United Kingdom	
Kaisernetwork.org Health Policy As It Happens *http:// www.kaisernetwork.org*	Health Policy	English	•

Site Name	Section	Language	Appropriate for Consumers
Kaplan Educational Centers *http://www.kaplan.com*	Careers, Returning to School	English	
KinderStart *http:// www.kinderstart.com*	Community Health	English, Some Spanish	•
La Leche League International (LLLI) *http://www.laleche league.com*	Breastfeeding	English with links to other sites in Chinese, Czech, Dutch, Flemish, German, Hebrew, Italian, Japanese, Lithuanian, Portuguese, Slovenian, and Spanish	•
Lamaze International *http://www.lamaze-childbirth.com*	Maternity	English	•
Last Acts *http://www.lastacts.org*	Palliative Care	English	•
LEAP Program *http:// www.bphs.hrsa.gov/ leap/default.htm*	Physical Assessment	English Spanish	
Library of Congress *http://www.loc.gov*	Government	English	
Lippincott, Williams, and Wilkins *http:// www.lippincott.com http:// www.wwilkins.com*	Publishing Companies	English	

Site Name	Section	Language	Appropriate for Consumers
March of Dimes *http:// www.modimes.org*	Maternity	English	•
Martindale's "Virtual" Nursing Center *http://sun2.lib.uci.edu/ ~martindale/ Nursing.html*	General Health Care	English	
Mature Connections *http://www.mature connections.com/*	Older Adults	English	•
Mayo Clinic *http:// www.mayoclinic.com*	Consumer Health, Heart Disease, Pharmaceuticals	English	•
Mayo Clinic.com Food and Nutrition Center *http:// www.mayohealth.org* Click "Healthy Living Centers" Click "Food and Nutrition"	Nutrition	English	•
McGill University Virtual Stethoscope *http:// sprojects.mmi.mcgill.ca/ mvs/mvsteth.htm*	Physical Assessment	English	
McMaster University Evidence-Based Health Care Resources *http://www.cochrane. mcmaster.ca/ evidence-based.htm*	Evidence-Based Practice	English	
MD Consult *http:// www.mdconsult.com/*	APN	English	

Site Name	Section	Language	Appropriate for Consumers
Med Bulletin *http:// www.medbulletin.com*	Jobs	English	
Medela *http://www.medela.com*	Breastfeeding	English	•
Medem™ *http://www.medem.com*	Consumer Health	English, Some Spanish	•
MedExplorer *http:// www.medexplorer.com*	Pharmaceuticals	English	•
MedHunters *http:// www.medhunters.com*	Jobs	English	
Medical Matrix: Decision Making and Tools *http://www.medmatrix. org/_spages/Decision_ Making_and_Tools.asp*	Clinical Decision-Making	English	
Medical Outcomes Trust *http://www.outcomes-trust.org/ instruments.htm*	Outcomes	Web site is in English Some Instruments are Available in Additional Languages	
Medical World Search (MWS) *http:// www.mwsearch.com*	Pharmaceuticals	English	
MEDLINEplus *http:// www.medlineplus.gov/*	Consumer Health, Diabetes	Some Spanish	•

Site Name	Section	Language	Appropriate for Consumers
MEDLINEplus Health Information: Diabetes *http://www.nlm.nih.gov/ medlineplus/ diabetes.html*	Diabetes	English	•
Medscape Cardiology *http:// www.medscpape.com/ Home/network/nursing/ nursing.html*	Heart Disease	English	
Medscape for Nurses *http:// www.medscape.com/ Home/network/nursing/ nursing.html*	General Health Care	English	
Medscape Primary Care *http:// PrimaryCare.medscape.com/ Home/Topics/ PrimaryCare/ PrimaryCare.html*	Primary Care	English	
Medscape Psychiatry and Mental Health *http:// www.medscape.com/ Home/Topics/ psychiatry/ psychiatry.html*	Mental Health	English	
Medscape.com *http://www.cardiology. medscape.com/Home/ Topics/cardiology/ cardiology.html*	General Health Care, Heart Disease, Mental Health, Primary Care	English	

Site Name	Section	Language	Appropriate for Consumers
Mental Disorders in Primary Care *http://www.who.int/msa/ mnh/ems/primacare/ edukit/*	Primary Care	English	
Mental Health InfoSource *http:// www.mhsource.com/*	Mental Health	English	•
Mental Help Net *http://mentalhelp.net*	Mental Health	English	•
The Merck Manual *http://www.merck.com/ pubs/mmanual/*	APN, Pharmaceuticals	English	•
Midwest Nursing Research Society *http://www.mnrs.org*	Research and Grants	English	
Midwifejobs.com *http:// www.midwifejobs.com*	Jobs	English	
Monster.com *http:// www.monster.com*	Jobs	English	
Mosby *http://www.mosby.com/ ijtn* *http://www.mosby.com/ jen*	Emergency	English	
Motherwear *http:// www.motherwear.com*	Breastfeeding	English	

Site Name	Section	Language	Appropriate for Consumers
MSNBC Children's Health Headlines *http://www.msnbc.com/ news/ CHILDRENSHEALTH_ front.asp*	Infants, Children, and Adolescents	English	•
Narelle's NetNurse Pages *http://www-personal.usyd.edu.au/ ~nacolema/ njc_nursing.html*	Critical Care	English	
National Academy for State Health Policy *http://www.nashp.org*	Health Policy	English	
The National AIDS Treatment Advocacy Project *http://www.natap.org/*	HIV/AIDS	English	
National Alliance of Breast Cancer Organizations (NABCO) *http://www.nabco.org*	Cancer	English	•
National Alliance for the Mentally Ill *http://www.nami.org*	Mental Health	English, Some Spanish	•
National Archives and Records Administration *http://www.nara.gov*	Government	English	
National Center for Complementary and Alternative Medicine (NCCAM) *http:// www.nccam.nih.gov*	Complimentary and Alternative Medicine	English	

Site Name	Section	Language	Appropriate for Consumers
National Center for Injury Prevention and Control *http://www.cdc.gov/ ncipc*	Emergency	English	
National Center for Youth Law *http://www.youthlaw.org*	Infants, Children, and Adolescents	English	•
National Center on Elder Abuse (NCEA) *http://www.elder abusecenter.org*	Community Health	English	•
National Coalition for Cancer Survivorship *http:// www.cansearch.org*	Cancer	English	•
National Council of State Boards of Nursing (NCSBN) *http://www.ncsbn.org*	Education	English	
National Depressive and Manic-Depressive Association *http://www.ndmda.org*	Mental Health	English	•
National Domestic Preparedness Office (NDPO) *http://www.ndpo.gov*	Disaster Preparedness	English	
National Guideline Clearinghouse *http:// www.guidelines.gov*	APN, Evidence-Based Practice, Clinical Decision Making, Government	English	
National Healthy Start Association *http://www.healthy startassoc.org*	Infants, Children, and Adolescents	English	
National Heart, Lung, and Blood Institute (NHLBI) *http://www.nhlbi.nih.gov*	Heart Disease, Respiratory	English	•

Site Name	Section	Language	Appropriate for Consumers
National Highway Traffic Safety Administration *http:// www.nhtsa.dot.gov/ people/injury/ems/*	Emergency	English	
National Hospice and Palliative Care Organization (NHPCO) *http://www.nhpco.org*	Palliative Care	English	•
National Human Genome Research Institute *http:// www.nhgri.nih.gov*	Genetics	English	
National Institute of Child Health and Human Development *http://156.40.88.3/ default.htm*	Infants, Children, and Adolescents	English	•
National Institute of Diabetes and Digestive and Kidney Diseases (NIDDK) *http:// www.niddk.nih.gov*	Diabetes	Some Spanish	•
National Institute of Mental Health *http://www.nimh.nih.gov*	Mental Health	English, Some Spanish	•
National Institute of Nursing Research (NINR) *http://www.nih.gov/ninr*	Outcomes, Research and Grants	English	
National Institutes of Health (NIH) *http://www.nih.gov*	Community Health, General Health Care, Government, Health Policy	English, Some Spanish	•

Site Name	Section	Language	Appropriate for Consumers
National League for Nursing (NLN) *http://www.nln.org*	Education	English	
National Library of Medicine (NLM) *http://www.nlm.nih.gov*	Clinical Decision Making	English and Spanish	•
National Library of Medicine's MEDLINEplus Biological and Chemical Weapons *http://www.nlm.gov/ medlineplus/ biologicalandchemical weapons.html*	Disaster Preparedness	English and Spanish	
National Lung Health Education Program (NLHEP) *http://www.nlhep.org*	Respiratory	English	•
National Mental Health Association *http://www.nmha.org*	Mental Health	English	•
National Patient Safety Foundation *http://www.npsf.org*	Administration	English	
National Safekids Campaign *http://www.safekids.org*	Emergency	English	•
National Safety Council (NSC) *http://www.crossroads. nsc.org/cbion.cfm*	Disaster Preparedness	English	
National Student Nurses Association Leadership University Facilities *http://www.NSNA. leadershipu.org/ library.htm*	Education, Leadership	English	

Site Name	Section	Language	Appropriate for Consumers
The National Women's Health Information Center (NWHIC) *http://www.4woman.org*	Consumer Health, Women's Health	Some Spanish	•
NOAH: New York Online Access to Health *http://www.noah-health.org/*	Consumer Health, Pain	English, Spanish	•
North American Chronic Pain Association of Canada *http://www.chronic paincanada.org*	Pain	English	•
North American Nursing Diagnosis Association (NANDA) *http://www.nanda.org*	Nursing Classification Systems	English	
NP Central *http://www.nurse.net/*	APN	English	
NurseScribe *http:// www.enursescribe.com/ link.htm*	Nursing Theory	English	
Nurseweek *http:// www.nurseweek.com*	Careers	English	
Nursing Around the World *http://world-nurse.com http://world-nurse.com/ Nursing_Resources/ Nursing_Theory*	Nursing Theory	English	

Site Name	Section	Language	Appropriate for Consumers
Nursing Center *http://www.nursing* *center.com*	Careers, Publishing Companies	English	
Nursing- Informatics.com *http://www.nursing-* *informatics.com/*	Nursing Informatics	English	
Nursing Informatics.net *http://* *www.lemmus.demon.co.uk/* *inf_main.htm*	Nursing Informatics	English	
Nursing Information and Data Set Evaluation Center (NIDSEC) *http://* *www.nursingworld.org/* *nidsec*	Nursing Classification Systems	English	
Nursing Leadership *Forum* *http://www.springer* *journals.com/nlf/* *home.htm*	Leadership	English	
Nursing Network Forum *http://* *www.nursingnet.org*	Careers	English, Spanish	
Nursing Spectrum: Career Fitness On Line *http://www.nursing* *spectrum.com*	Careers	English	
Nursing Theory Link Page *http://* *healthsci.clayton.edu/* *eichelberger/* *nursing.htm*	Nursing Theory	English	

Site Name	Section	Language	Appropriate for Consumers
The Nursing Theory Page http://www.ualberta.ca/~jrnorris/nt/theory.html	Nursing Theory	English and Some French	
Nutrition and the Pregnant Adolescent http:// www.epi.umn.edu/let/ nmpabook.html	Nutrition	English	
Ob Gyn.net http://www.obgyn.net	Maternity	English	•
OB Ultrasounds http://www.ob-ultrasound.net	Maternity	English	
Office of Disease Prevention and Health Promotion http://odphp. osophs.dhhs.gov/ odphpfact.htm	Primary Care	English, Some Consumer Information in Spanish	•
Office of Genetics and Disease Prevention, Centers for Disease Control and Prevention http://www.cdc.gov/ genetics/	Genetics	English and Spanish	
Office of Minority Health, Department of Health and Human Services http://www.omh.gov	Culturally Competent Care	English	•
Office of Population Affairs http://www.dhhs.gov/ progorg/opa	Maternity	English	•

Site Name	Section	Language	Appropriate for Consumers
Omaha System *http://omahasystem.org*	Nursing Classification System	English	
Oncolink *http:// www.oncolink.com*	Cancer, Consumer Health	English	•
Oncology Nursing Society (ONS) *http://www.ons.org*	Cancer, Professional Organizations	English	•
Online Journal of Clinical Innovations *http://www.cinahl.com/ cexpress/ojcionline3/ index.html*	Online Journals	English	
Online Journal of Issues in Nursing *http:// www.nursingworld.org/ ojin*	Online Journals	English	
Online Journal of Knowledge Synthesis for Nursing *http:// www.stti.iupui.edu/ library/ojksn/*	Online Journals	English	
Online Journal of Nursing Informatics *http:// www.hhdev.psu.edu/ nurs/ojni/index.htm*	Online Journals	English	
Online Mendelian Inheritance in Man (OMIM) *http:// www.ncbi.nlm.nih.gov/ Omim*	Genetics	English	

Site Name	Section	Language	Appropriate for Consumers
ONLINE Nursing Editors™ http:// members.aol.com/ suzannehj.naed.htm	Publishing Companies	English	
Opening Doors http://www.opening-doors.org	Culturally Competent Care	English	
Oregon Public Education Network (OPEN) http:// www.open.k12.or.us/jitt/ charact.html http:// www.open.k12.or.us/jitt/ evalform.html	Evaluation	English	
Organization for the Prohibition of Chemical Weapons http://www.opcw.nl/ chemhaz/cwagents.htm	Bioterrorism	English	
Ottawa Health Decision Center http://www.ohri.ca/ programs/ clinical_epidemiology/ OHDEC/decision.asp	Clinical Decision Making	English	
Pain and Palliative Resource Center http://prc.coh.org	Palliative Care	Many resources and assessment tools are available in Spanish	

Site Name	Section	Language	Appropriate for Consumers
Pain.com *http://www.pain.com*	Pain	English	•
PainLink *http://www.edc.org/ PainLink/*	Pain	English	
PainNet, Inc. *http://www.painnet.com/*	Pain	English	
Palliative Care: One Vision, One Voice (Palliative Care Nursing) *http://www.palliative nursing.net*	Palliative Care	English	
Pan American Health Organization (PAHO) *http://www.paho.org*	International	English, Spanish	
Pathogenesis and Imaging of Inhalational Anthrax *http:// anthrax.radpath.orh/ index.html*	Disaster Preparedness	English	
Pediatric Assessment in the Home *http:// nursing.about.com/gi/ dynamic/offsite.htm*	Physical Assessment	English	
Pediatric Critical Care Medicine (PedsCCM) *http:// PedsCCM.wustl.edu*	Critical Care	English with Some Areas Available in French, Russian, and Spanish	

Site Name	Section	Language	Appropriate for Consumers
Pediatric Pain *http://is.dal.ca/ %7Epedpain/ pedpain.html*	Pain	English	
Peterson's *http:// www.petersons.com*	Returning to School	English	
PharmInfoNet *http://pharminfo.com*	Clinical Decision Making	English	•
Physical Assessment of the Well Woman *http:// www.umanitoba.ca/ womens_health/ nephys.htm*	Physical Assessment	English	
Physical Exam Study Guides *http:// www.medinfo.ufl.edu/ year1/bcs/clist/ index.html*	Physical Assessment	English	
Portfolio of British Nursing Web Sites *http://www.british-nursing.com*	International	English	
Prenatal Screening and Assessment Tool *http:// nursing.about.com/gi/ dynamic/offsite.htm*	Physical Assessment	English	
Primary Care Clinical Practice Guidelines *http:// medicine.ucsf.edu/ resources/guidelines/*	APN, Primary Care	English	

Site Name	Section	Language	Appropriate for Consumers
ProMOM *http://www.promom.org*	Breastfeeding	English	•
PubMed *http:// www.ncbi.nlm.nih.gov/ PubMed/*	General Health Care Resources	English	
The Quality Center of the Bureau of Primary Health Care *http://bphc.hrsa.gov/ quality*	Primary Care	English, Some Spanish	
RALE (Respiration Acoustic Laboratory Equipment) Repository *http://www.RALE.ca/ Recordings.htm*	Physical Assessment	English	
Rehobth McKinley Christian Emergency Department *http://www.rmcg.org/ erlinks.htm*	Emergency	English	
Research! America *http://www.research america.org*	Research and Grants	English	
Respiratory Nursing Society (RNS) *http://www.respiratory nursingsociety.org*	Respiratory	English	
Responding to Chemical Terrorism *http://www.opcw.nl/ chemhaz/cwagents.htm*	Disaster Preparedness	English	
Rick Mendosa's Diabetes Directory *http:// www.mendosa.com/ diabetes.htm*	Diabetes	Links to Other Languages	•

Site Name	Section	Language	Appropriate for Consumers
RNWanted.com http:// www.rnwanted.com	Jobs	English	
Robert Wood Johnson Executive Nurse Leadership Program http://www.future health.ucsf.edu/rwj.html	Leadership	English	
Royal College of Nursing's Research and Development Co-ordinating Centre http://www.man.ac.uk/ rcn	Research and Grants	English	
The Royal Windsor Society for Nursing Research http:// www.windsor.igs.net/ ~nhodgins	Research and Grants	English	
RxList http://www.rxlist.com	Pharmaceuticals	English, Spanish	•
RxMed http://www.rxmed.com	Pharmaceuticals	English	•
Sarah Cole Hirsh Institute http:// www.hirshinstitute.com/ default.htm	Evidence-Based Practice	English	
Scope and Standards of Diabetes Nursing http://www.aadenet.org/ Position% 20Statements/scope_ stand_nurs.html	Diabetes	English	
Senior Net http:// www.seniornet.org	Older Adults	English	•

Site Name	Section	Language	Appropriate for Consumers
Sigma Theta Tau International *http:// www.nursingsociety.org http://www.nursing society.org/programs/ chiron.html*	Careers, Leadership, Professional Organizations	English	
Slack, Inc. *http:// www.slackinc.com/*	Publishing Companies	English	
The SmartStudent™ Guide to Financial Aid *http://www.finaid.org*	Returning to School	English	
SNOMED *http://www.snomed.org*	Nursing Classification Systems	English	
The Society for Cardiovascular and Interventional Radiology *http://www.SCVIR.org*	Vascular Disease	English	
Society for Medical Decision-Making *http://www.smdm.org*	Clinical Decision Making	English	
Society for Vascular Medicine and Biology (SVMB) *http://www.svmb.org*	Vascular Disease	English	
The Society for Vascular Nursing *http://www.svnnet.org*	Vascular Disease	English	
Society for Women's Health Research *http://www.womens-health.org*	Women's Health	English	

Site Name	Section	Language	Appropriate for Consumers
Southern Nursing Research Society (SNRS) http://www.snrs.org	Research and Grants	English	
Springer Publishing Company http:// www.springerpub.com	Publishing Companies	English	
Springhouse Corporation http:// www.springnet.com	Publishing Companies	English	
SpringNet http:// www.springnet.com	Administration, Careers, Critical Care	English	
Systematized Nomenclature of Medicine (SNOMED) http:// www.snomed.org/	Nursing Informatics	English Some Spanish	
TCP Web.com http://www.tcpweb.com	Returning to School	English	
10 Lessons on Writing for Publications http:// www.springnet.com/ jrdescr/wlesson.htm	Writing	English	
Topics in Advanced Practice Nursing http:// nursing.medscape.com/ Medscape/nurses/ journal/public/ nursing.journal.html	Online Journals	English	

Site Name	Section	Language	Appropriate for Consumers
Tufts Nutrition Navigator *http:// navigator.tufts.edu/*	Nutrition	English	
United Anesthesia Associates, Inc. *http://www.united anesthesia.com*	Jobs	English	
United Nations (UN) *http://www.un.org*	International	Arabic, Chinese, English, French, Russian, Spanish	
United States Breastfeeding Committee *http://www.usbreast feeding.org*			
United States Food and Drug Administration Center for Drug Evaluation and Research *http://www.fda.gov/cder*	Pharmaceuticals	English	
University of Massachusetts Medical School: An Internet Resource on Venous Thromobembolism *http:// www.umassmed.edu/ outcomes/dvt* *http://www.dvt.org*	Vascular Disease	English	
University of Michigan Health System Primary and Preventative Health *http:// www.med.umich.edu/ 1libr/primry/prim00.htm*	Primary Care	English	•

Site Name	Section	Language	Appropriate for Consumers
University of Rochester Center for Nursing *http://www.urmc. rochester.edu/son/ research/crebp.html*	Evidence-Based Practice	English	
University of Washington Writer Toolkit *http://www.healthlinks. washington.edu/ toolkits/writer.html*	Writing	English	
University of York Centre for Evidence-Based Nursing (EBN) *http://www.york.ac.uk/ depts/hstd/centres/ evidence/ev-intro.htm*	Evidence-Based Practice	English	
U.S. Army Medical Research Institute of Infectious Diseases Medical Management of Biological Casualties *http://www.nbc-med.org/SiteContent/ Homepage/WhatsNew/ MedManual/Feb01/ handbook.htm*	Disaster Preparedness	English	
U.S. Army Treatment of Biological Warfare Casualties *http://www.vnh.org/ FM8284/index.html*	Disaster Preparedness	English	
U.S. Breastfeeding Committee *http://www.usbreast feeding.org*	Breastfeeding	English	

Site Name	Section	Language	Appropriate for Consumers
U.S. Department of Health and Human Services (DHHS) *http://www.dhhs.gov*	Community Health, Government	English	
U.S. News and World Reports *http://www.usnews.com*	Returning to School	English	
U.S. Public Health Service Office of Emergency Preparedness *http:// www.ndms.dhhs.gov*	Disaster Preparedness	English	
Vanderbilt Shock Trauma Information Center *http:// www.mc.vanderbilt.edu/ surgery/trauma/ MDvsticfp.htm*	Emergency	English	
The Vascular Disease Foundation *http://www.vdf.org*	Vascular Disease	English	
VascularWeb: One Source for Vascular Health Information *http:// www.vascularweb.org*	Vascular Disease	English	•
Virtual Hospital *http://www.vh.org/*	Primary Care	English	
VirtualSalt *http:// www.virtualsalt.com/ evalu8it.htm*	Evaluation	English	

Site Name	Section	Language	Appropriate for Consumers
Voices for Health http://www. voicesforhealth. org	Culturally Competent Care	English Spanish Courses Online Many Languages for Interpretation Services	
Watson's Theory of Human Caring http://www.uchsc.edu/ ctrsinst/chc/index.htm	Nursing Theory	English	
What We Know About Terrorism, Disaster, and Health http:// www.stti.iupui.edu/ library/ojksn/ homepage.html	Disaster Preparedness	English	
Women's Health Interactive http://www.womens-health.com	Women's Health	English	•
World Alliance for Breastfeeding Action (WABA) http://www.waba.org.br/	Breastfeeding	Chinese, Dutch, English, French, Italian, Japanese, Portuguese, Spanish, Swedish	
World Health Organization (WHO) http://www.who.org	Disaster Preparedness; Infants, Children, and Adolescents; International	English, French, Spanish	

Site Name	Section	Language	Appropriate for Consumers
World Health Organization (WHO) Child and Adolescent Health and Development *http://www.who.int/ child-adolescent-health*	Infants, Children/ Adolescents	English	
World Health Organization Global Outbreak Alert and Response Network *http://www.who.int/emc/ deliberate_epi.html*	Bioterrorism	English	•
World Wide Nurse: Nursing Research Funding *http:// www.wwnurse.com/ nursing/research-funding.shtml*	Research and Grants	English	
World Wide Web Virtual Library *http://www.vuw.ac.nz/ ~agsmith/evaln/ evaln.htm*	Evaluation	English	
Yahoo Seniors *http://www.seniors. yahoo.com/*	Older Adults	English	•

Index

Springer Publishing Company

Telecommunications for Health Professionals

Providing Successful Distance Education and TeleHealth

Myrna L. Armstrong, EdD, RN, FAAN, Editor

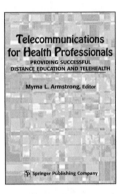

"It is a book that describes how creative people, often taking a fresh approach, can get the best out of what modern distance communications technology has to offer." —from the Foreword by **Susan M. Sparks, RN, PhD, FAAN** and Michael J. Ackerman, PhD

This book is a guide to creating and managing programs in distance education and patient care, written by thirty two health care professionals with direct and extensive experience with these programs. The technical and human aspects of providing distance education and health care are addressed, along with practical information on how modern telecommunications technology can extend the skills of both the clinician and the educator.

Partial Contents:

Part I. The Exploding Field of Distance Education
• Working With Audiographics, *S. Frazier, B.A. Gessner and M. Monson*
• Faculty Development, *D. Scott and M.L. Armstrong*
• The Culture of Distance Learning, *M.L. Bond and M.E. Jones*
• Multidisiplinary Continuing Education for Distant Sites, *S.A. Ramirez*

Part II. The Impact of TeleHealth on Direct Patient Care
• TeleHealth and Direct Health Care Delivery: An Introduction, *J.D. Long*
• Improving Telemedicine Consultation with TeleDoc, *C.S. Hickman and W.M. Dyer*

Part III. Telecommunications Issues for Health Care Professionals
• Ethics and Legal Perspectives for Distance Education and TeleHealth, *K.D. Menix*
• Public Policy Issues: Achieving Public Access to Technology at Reasonable Cost, *S. Cotton*
• Resources: Organizations, Conferences, Publications, and Internet Sites, *G.P. Connick*

1998   352pp   0-8261-9840-6   hard

536 Broadway, New York, NY 10012-3955 • (212) 431-4370 • Fax (212) 941-7842
Order Toll-Free: (877) 687-7476 • www.springerpub.com

Springer Publishing Company

Annual Review of Nursing Education: *Volume I*

Marilyn H. Oermann, PhD, RN, FAAN, Editor
Kathleen T. Heinrich, PhD, RN, Associate Editor

Interested in the latest trends in nursing education written by the nurse educators pioneering these innovations? Then welcome to the first volume of the Annual Review of Nursing Education. This Review focuses on the practice of teaching. It describes educational strategies you can adapt to your own settings and is written for educators in associate, baccalaureate, and graduate nursing programs, staff development, and continuing education. The goal of the Review is to keep educators updated on this year's innovations in nursing education across all settings.

Partial Contents:
Part I: Nursing Education and the Community
- Community-Based Curricula at BSN and Graduate Levels, *D. M. Wink*
  - Community-Based Curricula at ADN Level: A Service-Learning Model, *M. E. Tagliareni and E. Speakman*

Part II: Mentoring and Preceptorship
- Strategies for Promoting Nontraditional Student Retention and Success, *M. R. Jeffreys*
  - Preceptorship: A Quintessential Component of Nursing Education, *F. Myrick and O. Yonge*

Part III: Distance Education
- Community-Based Model of Distance Education for Nurse-Midwives and Nurse Practitioners, *S. E. Stone*
- Issues in Rural Health: Model for a Web-Based Course, *A. Bushy*
- International Distance Learning Collaboration to Prepare Nurse Educators in Malaysia, *D. M. Billings and contributors*

Part IV: Innovative Strategies
- Interdisciplinary Education: Breaking Out of the Silos, *Denise G. Link*
- Using Clinical Scenarios in Nursing Education, *Catherine Nored Dearman*

Feb. 2003   352pp (est.)   0-8261-2444-5   hard

536 Broadway, New York, NY 10012-3955 • (212) 431-4370 • Fax (212) 941-7842
Order Toll-Free: (877) 687-7476 • www.springerpub.com